Drug Abuse Prevention

A School and Community Partnership

Second Edition

Drug Abuse Prevention

A School and Community Partnership

Second Edition

Richard Wilson
Cheryl Kolander

JONES AND BARTLETT PUBLISHERS

Sudbury, Massachusetts

BOSTON   TORONTO   LONDON   SINGAPORE

World Headquarters

Jones and Bartlett Publishers
40 Tall Pine Drive
Sudbury, MA 01776
978-443-5000
info@jbpub.com
www.jbpub.com

Jones and Bartlett Publishers
 Canada
6339 Ormindale Way
Mississauga, ON L5V 1J2
CANADA

Jones and Bartlett Publishers
 International
Barb House, Barb Mews
London W6 7PA
UK

Jones and Bartlett's books and products are available through most bookstores and online booksellers. To contact Jones and Bartlett Publishers directly, call 800-832-0034, fax 978-443-8000, or visit our website at www.jbpub.com.

Substantial discounts on bulk quantities of Jones and Bartlett's publications are available to corporations, professional associations, and other qualified organizations. For details and specific discount information, contact the special sales department at Jones and Bartlett via the above contact information or send an email to specialsales@jbpub.com.

ISBN-13: 978-0-7637-5380-1

PRODUCTION CREDITS

Acquisitions Editor: Kristin L. Ellis
Production Editor: Julie C. Bolduc
Editorial Assistant: Nicole Quinn
Associate Marketing Manager: Ed McKenna
Director of Interactive Technology: Adam Alboyadjian
Web Site Designer: Kristin E. Ohlin

Manufacturing Buyer: Therese Braüer
Composition: International Typesetting and Composition
Text and Cover Design: Anne Spencer
Printing and Binding: Odyssey Press
Cover Printing: Odyssey Press

LIBRARY OF CONGRESS CATALOGING-IN-PUBLICATION DATA
Wilson, Richard W., Dr.
  Drug abuse prevention : a school and community partnership / Richard
Wilson, Cheryl Kolander.-- 2nd ed.
     p. ; cm.
Includes bibliographical references and index.
  ISBN 0-7637-1461-5 (alk. paper)
  1. Drug abuse--United States--Prevention. 2. Drug abuse--Study and
teaching--United States.
  [DNLM: 1. Substance-Related Disorders--prevention &
control--Adolescence. 2. Health Education--methods. 3. Health
Promotion--methods.] I. Kolander, Cheryl A. II. Title.
  HV5825.W536 2003
  362.29'17'0973--dc21
6048   2002156046

Printed in the United States of America
11 10 09 08 07   10 9 8 7 6 5 4 3 2

To Tristan, a promising new edition.
R.W.

To my students who are seeking growth and fulfillment through positive life choices, and are currently living free or working toward freedom from the influence of tobacco, alcohol, or other drugs.
C.K.

Contents

Chapter 4   Other Drugs, Mostly Legal   59

Chapter 5   Other Drugs, Mostly Illegal   75

| Chapter 6 | **School and Community Violence Prevention** | **99** |

| Chapter 7 | **Single-Focus Approaches to Prevention** | **121** |

| Chapter 8 | **Current Prevention Approaches** | **141** |

Chapter 11 — Early Intervention with Drug Abuse and Related Problems   221

Chapter 12 — Treatment of Alcohol, Tobacco, and Drug Addiction   245

| Chapter 13 | **Needs Assessment and Program Evaluation** | **265** |

Features

FYI

Hints & Tips

Viewpoints

Preface

From an author's perspective, there is something to be said for writing a novel or a short story. Once it is finished, it is finished forever, to be judged on its merits from its first day forward. Charles Dickens didn't have to eventually update to *A Tale of Three Cities*. Nathaniel Hawthorne didn't have to revise for *House of the Eight Gables*.

Unlike nonfiction works, most academic disciplines are constantly changing because of inquisitive and creative researchers and changing social circumstances. The field of drug abuse prevention is no exception. When *Drug Abuse Prevention: A School and Community Partnership* was first written, new developments had occurred even before the first copies arrived in bookstores.

The fact that content for the book needed to be updated to keep up with new knowledge and trends in drug abuse prevention was not surprising to us. The authors have each taught prevention courses for years and are accustomed to updating class material every semester. However, we did not anticipate changes that have occurred from the first to second edition in the writing process or the rapid evolution in higher education with respect to how text and reference material is used in higher education.

When we were writing the first edition, much time was spent in the library, researching education, public health, and behavioral science literature and poring over vast collections of government documents. The work for the second edition was mostly done electronically, via the Internet and electronic databases maintained by libraries. Rarely was it necessary to leave the computer because the wealth of data on which the revisions are based could be found electronically with a few keystrokes.

Even more striking has been the way that the idea of a textbook has changed. In our earlier years as scholars and instructors, a textbook contained the bulk of the material students needed to know, with the exception of material needed for research paper development. That is becoming less true as instructors rely more and more on Internet-based materials and electronic formats. It wouldn't be shocking if the next edition of this text were no longer recognizable as a book printed on paper, but rather took the form of some new technology.

In any case, we are excited about the opportunity to update and improve on the first edition of *Drug Abuse Prevention: A School and Community Partnership*. Every chapter in the book has been modified. In the drug information chapters, statistics have been brought up to date. Many changes have occurred regarding local and national efforts to minimize tobacco use and alcohol abuse, and several illegal drugs have taken on greater prominence, such as the so-called club drugs, a term new since the first edition was written, describing old drugs used in a new context.

An even more important change in the content is found in the chapters on school and community prevention. The multibillion dollar annual investments in local, state, and national drug abuse prevention activities have created huge pressures for accountability. It has become apparent that much of what's been done in the past did not work. Right now there are tighter, more stringent regulations that force the application of science-based best practices in prevention. Students need to know about those concepts, and will find this important new material in Chapters 7 to 9.

Since the first edition, schools and communities have been continuing to struggle with drug abuse and, more recently, with youth violence. The violence problem is not new, but over the last few years there has been a significant increase in the proportion of schools that have organized programs and policies dealing with violence. The drug problem and youth violence are intertwined in many ways, which is recognized by a new chapter on violence prevention.

Finally, while the earlier edition of *Drug Abuse Prevention* had extensive appendices on many different issues, this edition has moved most of that material to an electronic format, accessible on the Internet. The importance of this change to students is that fewer printed pages holds down the cost of producing and purchasing the book. More important, it creates the opportunity of regularly updating this material without having to wait for the next edition to be published.

We are excited about this second edition, and anxiously anticipate feedback from students and instructors as it is incorporated into drug education courses and continuing education workshops and seminars. We believe in prevention, and are excited about teaching concepts and skills to help people be more effective in the ATOD programs in their schools and communities. We hope students will sense and absorb our energy and enthusiasm as they read the lines of our work.

Drug Abuse Prevention

web resources

The Web site for this book offers many useful resources for educators, students, and professional counselors and is a great source for additional information. Visit the site at **http://healtheducation.jbpub.com/drugabuse/.**

Chapter Learning Objectives

Upon completion of this chapter, students will be able to:

1. Define and correctly use the terms *drug, drug abuse, addiction, prevention, intervention,* and *treatment.*

2. Differentiate between "no-use" prevention and harm reduction prevention.

3. Briefly summarize the concept of science-based prevention.

4. Discuss the concepts of high risk and resiliency and propose some implications for drug abuse prevention.

5. Describe the public health model and explain its importance as an approach to comprehensive drug abuse prevention.

6. Compare and contrast several sources of national drug use data.

Scenario

Michelyn Guthrie has recently been hired by the executive board of a regional drug abuse prevention coalition. She will serve as the program coordinator and administrator for all day-to-day activities. Prior to taking this position she completed a master's degree in public health education, with an emphasis on issues regarding alcohol, tobacco, and other drugs (ATOD). In addition, she has worked in drug abuse prevention positions in government and the private sector for a number of years.

Prior to Michelyn's arrival, the coalition had been in operation for about 10 years. During that time, it has become very well known in the community. It enjoys a lot of support from prominent politicians, business leaders, clergy, and officials with the school system because the executive board has always taken pains to curry the favor of important community leaders, and has conducted programs with wide community support.

One month after her start date, Ms. Guthrie presented her program plans to the executive board. She proposed significant changes from activities that the coalition had sponsored in the past. For all of the last 10 years, the coalition had been a sponsor of the Drug Abuse Resistance Education (DARE) program, implemented in the local middle and high schools. However, Michelyn has been persuaded by evaluation research that the DARE program is ineffective, and so she is recommending that the coalition provide seed money for schools to invest in other curricula that have evidence of effectiveness or at least have a strong evaluation component. She is also proposing that the coalition

Chapter

An Introduction to Drug Education

Introduction

Throughout history there are instances in which drug use and abuse have been ignored or even encouraged by social institutions. On the other hand, many people and institutions have made efforts to limit the use and abuse of various drugs, mostly through legal sanctions and restrictions enforced by governments. However, as democracy has proliferated, there has also been reliance on voluntary limits promoted by education. This is not to say that government controls are not still widely implemented—a look at U.S. government spending patterns shows otherwise—but it is to say that drug education has developed into a movement and an industry over the last 40 years.

sponsor training workshops for teachers to learn new curricula and principles of effective prevention.

Michelyn also believes the coalition needs to put much more emphasis on tobacco prevention, for two reasons. First, because in the long run, tobacco does more damage in disease and death than all other drugs. Second, because she believes that if children and youth can be discouraged from smoking, they are much less likely to become users of other drugs.

Upon hearing these plans, the executive board is alarmed and apprehensive. Some members are angry. After all, the DARE program has been around for a long time. It is well liked by teachers. Law enforcement agencies see it as a good opportunity for enhancing their relations with the community. Finally, they are skeptical of anything coming from those "radi-cal" universities with liberal professors who don't really understand the drug problem and "our values." They are not convinced that whatever replaces DARE will be better.

In addition, the board members are very concerned that making tobacco a focus will hurt the coalition's support from the agricultural interests in the state and the local business community. Some think tobacco programming is a waste of time and that the coalition should be addressing the "real" drug problems.

After this lukewarm and even antagonistic response from the board, Michelyn is reconsidering how to proceed. Should she stick to her principles, or should she make compromises in the short run until she has more credibility with the board, at which time she can safely be more assertive with her ideas?

This proliferation of drug education raises many questions for educators and policymakers in schools and other government agencies. What is drug education? What is the goal of drug education? Why is the subject taught? Can drug education be taught effectively and, if so, how? These issues will be discussed at length in this text. At this point, it may be helpful to comment briefly on some of these questions.

Drug education is teaching and communicating to help people avoid harm caused by the abuse of various drugs. Drug education is done most intensively with young people in schools, but it is also taught in diverse community settings to both the young and old. Although it is usually thought of as a classroom activity for individuals or groups, it may also be done through mass media or as part of events that are not primarily educational but in which education may be incorporated, such as sporting events or art festivals. (See **Figure 1.1.**) A drug education program may be a distinct event or experience that is carefully designed; however, an individual may also receive drug education in many forms and from uncoordinated sources that may have differing theoretical and philosophical bases. All of this presents a substantial challenge for program evaluation.

Drugs have received such bad publicity over the years that many people respond, almost as a reflex,

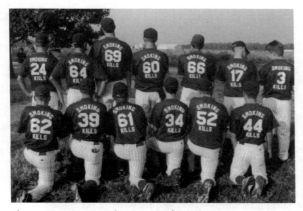

Figure 1.1 **Community Drug Education** Drug education is usually done in schools, but may occur in many community sites. An example is the Smoking Kills baseball team in Kentucky. (Photo courtesy Coach Mike Sawyer)

that we should get rid of all drugs forever. This is a pretty tall order. Even if it were possible, is it really what we want? Often people support prohibiting or restricting drugs that other people use or value, but not their own drugs of choice. Although there is no doubt that many people suffer harm from drug abuse, there is no consensus about which drugs should be the focus of drug education or whether we should strive for total abstinence or something less ambitious.

Mainstream U.S. culture seems to agree that restrictions should be placed on drug use by young people. However, many distinctions are made among drugs and about the earliest age at which use is deemed acceptable. For example, some cultures and social groups have permissive attitudes toward children's use of alcohol. Evidence does not clearly show that those cultures' drug problems are any greater than in less permissive cultures and social groups.

This issue will not be solved here, but it must be resolved in local communities. Outcome evaluation studies can help by clarifying when abstinence-oriented education is effective and when moderation-oriented or responsible-use-oriented education is effective. However, the uncertainty created by this lack of consensus makes drug education planning difficult. Drug education is challenging in many other ways as well.

Federal, state, and local governments spend billions of dollars for drug education interventions.[1] Although many people feel that such programs are underfunded, this spending still amounts to a great deal of money. Surveys may show declines in youth drug use,[2] but it is a fair question to ask whether, and how, drug education contributed to that progress. Unfortunately, much of what has been done in the name of drug education has not been well evaluated, and information about what does and does not work has not been disseminated effectively.[3] Consequently, drug education planners at the local level are faced with a barrage of materials, strategies, and program ideas but have little capacity for making sound decisions in this regard. Often the most immediate source of information to guide them is one with a commercial conflict of interest.

Another difficulty faced by those committed to drug education is the lack of consensus regarding the value of drug education in the first place. Policymakers and other administrators may have different priorities, question the need for drug education at all, or have differing opinions on the size of the investment that should be made. In states where tobacco is grown there has been great reluctance, until recently, to include tobacco in school drug education and prevention programs because of the political ramifications. This ambivalence may result in a reluctance to address the drug problem at all or in a greater concern with other approaches to the problem, such as treatment. Consequently, drug educators often fight battles on two fronts: on the side of applying effective education strategies and, on the institutional side, of trying to maintain and build program support.

As our experience with drug education has developed and been charted, it has become apparent that effective efforts need to be comprehensive.[4] A classroom teacher's efforts must be reinforced by schoolwide drug abuse prevention activities, and these must in turn be supported by interventions in all aspects of community life. Furthermore, it is not enough merely to address the surface issue of drug use behavior; we must also address the environmental circumstances that contribute to such problems. This complex issue presents a great challenge to drug educators, but it also calls for a restructuring, sometimes called a **paradigm shift**, of many of our social institutions and the way they interact.[5] For example, faith-based organizations are generally uninvolved in drug abuse prevention, except to condemn drug abuse. For them to have an organized and planned role in prevention will require a shift in their thinking about their goals and what type of programs they should sponsor. Establishing referral networks, service linkages, and collaborative relationships among community agencies and individuals is a difficult hurdle.

Whether or not this is done, drug education professionals often do not know the long-term results of their work because the outcome occurs in the future, when educators no longer have contact with the objects of their efforts. Satisfaction may come from reviewing data trends as the years unfold, but this is not as gratifying as the immediate results that may come from participating in drug treatment or other kinds of human service work in which success is more immediately apparent. Of course, the flip side is that failure also is not recognized. Prevention efforts are repeated because they are well received or because of the inherent satisfaction of doing them. The fact that they have no impact may not be realized without careful evaluation.

There has been a new push by the U.S. government to demand that state and local prevention programs, when funded by state and federal dollars, be "science based." The expectation is that programs should show some evidence, prior to implementation, that they will actually affect youth drug use. The background to this effort is that enthusiasm and genuine concern for preventing adolescent drug abuse have often been translated into activities that are enjoyable but not carefully examined and tested. Schools have used funds to purchase t-shirts and ribbons, hire expensive motivational speakers, and to acquire videotapes and untested curriculum material without any assurance that such expenditures have led in the past, or will lead in the future, to decreases in youth drug use. However, there remains a large chasm of uncertainty regarding the criteria of science-based evaluation and how much flexibility can be used in applying the criteria. This effort to promote accountability and quality control is commendable and will be discussed further in later chapters.

In spite of all of these hurdles, drug education is an exciting challenge. It offers the opportunity to relieve a significant source of human suffering. In its most complete form, it contributes to a better life in a holistic way, not just by addressing drug-abuse-mediated problems. It is intellectually stimulating for an educator to come to grips with the complexity of having an impact on individuals in the social and institutional context. And as drug educators gain greater understanding of the causes and circumstances of drug use behavior, they develop a fuller understanding of self and the human family.

Drug Education Terminology

To understand the rest of this book and be an effective drug educator requires that you recognize some common terms. It must be appreciated, though, that heterogeneous, pluralistic societies don't work entirely in sync. The meanings of terms that are provided here are those with the most universal acceptance. Be alert to alternate understandings and uses!

Drug

It is possible to define the term **drug** in a number of ways. Drugs include a wide range of substances that alter the structure and function of the body. Drugs that are commonly abused specifically alter the function of the nervous system: They are "mind altering." More important than the definition is the recognition that this term may include over-the-counter and prescription medicines, caffeinated beverages, alcohol, tobacco, illegal substances, herbs, and volatile chemicals such as airplane glue, correction fluid, and paint.

Drug Abuse

Drug abuse generally refers to chronic, excessive use of a drug, such that physical or other personal harm is very likely to occur. Drug abuse and addiction usually occur together, but they are not the same thing. Theoretically, all drugs may be abused; however, some drugs are more commonly abused than others. A subset of drug abuse is **drug misuse,** which is potentially harmful consumption that is not chronic but only an isolated episode. Examples include taking more than the recommended dosage of an over-the-counter drug, drinking alcohol to excess only on New Year's Eve, and mistakenly taking the wrong medication.

Addiction

Addiction is uncontrolled compulsion to use a drug in spite of the physical, emotional, or social problems that result. Addiction is characterized by physical dependence, which is tolerance to a drug and the avoidance of the withdrawal symptoms that occur when consumption is ended and intoxication wanes. **Tolerance** is characterized by failure of the drug to cause the usual effect or the need for a higher dose to bring about the desired effect.

Withdrawal consists of a variety of physical and emotional symptoms that occur when an accustomed dose level of a drug is abruptly cut off. The nature and magnitude of withdrawal vary with the drug and the user.

Another characteristic of addiction is psychological dependence, which occurs when a drug's properties reinforce certain behaviors and emotions of the user. Psychological dependence leads a user to maintain a state of mind and perception more pleasurable than a normal state or to relieve the pain and discontent of living in reality.

Some drugs have little potential to cause addiction. Some drugs may cause psychological but not physical dependence, whereas other drugs will cause both. Addiction occurs more readily if the mind-altering properties of a drug are pronounced and if the effects occur and cease rapidly. There is major debate over what causes addiction and whether the term can be applied appropriately to other forms of compulsive behavior such as overeating, gambling, and shopping. These issues are discussed more fully in Chapter 12.

Prevention

In the broadest sense, **prevention** is organized activity designed to avoid or decrease health problems. In the context of this book, *prevention* refers to steps that might be taken to avoid alcohol and other drug problems. The focus of prevention might be on drugs, individuals, or community environments, and prevention activities may be done in homes, schools, churches, and a variety of other community agencies and settings. Education is the most commonly used prevention strategy; its impact will be much greater if it is reinforced by other prevention activities.

The word *prevention* as used in this book is synonymous with the public health term *primary prevention*. The public health terms *secondary* and *tertiary prevention* refer to remediating or repairing a problem that has already occurred. However, this book avoids using those designations; when the word *prevention* is used it will always refer to activities designed to hinder the development of drug abuse problems. Activities designed to respond to drug abuse problems that already exist will be called *intervention* or *treatment*.

Intervention

Steps taken for early identification and treatment of an alcohol or other drug problem that has already begun constitute **intervention**. The concept is that intervention will facilitate and hasten the drug abuser's entrance into treatment, thereby minimizing the harm that may occur. Intervention may take place in homes, schools, worksites, and other settings. The process usually includes recognition of a problem, referral, and follow-up.

There is a second, but also important, definition of intervention. Health educators, prevention specialists, and public health workers commonly use the word *intervention* to refer to any strategy to prevent, treat, or otherwise control a health or social problem. For example, distribution of clean needles in an urban neighborhood is an intervention to break the transmission of the human immunodeficiency virus (HIV). Within this text, *intervention* will be used in the first way cited earlier. However, in the world of drug abuse prevention, the other definition sometimes will be intended.

Treatment

Activities done with the objective of eliminating an individual's drug abuse and repairing some of the damage and disability that have occurred are called **treatment**. Such activities may be applied by trained professionals or by nonprofessionals in self-help groups. To be successful, treatment requires the individual's active participation and commitment. Addicts' significant others often have an important role in treatment.

Attitudes About Prevention

Drug issues are emotionally charged and very controversial. In American society there is a great difference of opinion regarding the use of alcohol and other drugs. The view of many people is that using illegal drugs and (to a lesser extent) alcohol is immoral and unacceptable. Others with different roots and values believe that drug use is an acceptable way to smooth the rough edges of life and bring pleasure to daily existence. This latter group does not think of drugs in terms of right or wrong. Perhaps most Americans are found in the middle

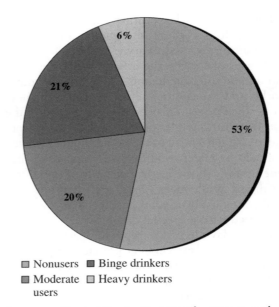

Nonusers   Binge drinkers
Moderate   Heavy drinkers
users

Figure 1.2 Alcohol Use in Past Month, Ages 12 and Older, 2000

Source: National Household Survey on Drug Abuse.

of these extreme poles. It is a striking paradox that among developed nations, the United States has a large proportion of adults who are alcohol abstainers, yet it has one of the highest rates of alcoholism and alcohol problems. (See **Figure 1.2.**)

Added to this is the fact that the majority's disapproval of drugs has in the past been linked with suspicions and fears associated with immigrants and other minorities whose values and customs may differ from those of the dominant culture.[6] At times society's abhorrence of certain drugs has been a proxy for racial and ethnic bias, class struggles, and competition for favored status in communities.[7,8]

Because alcohol and tobacco have long been associated with mainstream society, including major commercial interests, these drugs are much more accepted. Consumption of alcohol and tobacco is legal and socially acceptable, and abuse of them is not viewed with the revulsion and disgust reserved for other drugs. Crack babies make headlines; babies malformed due to their mothers' tobacco or alcohol use are almost totally ignored by the media.

For much of the last century, the so-called illicit drugs, such as cocaine, marijuana, and heroin, were not openly used, but were mostly found on the fringes of society: the urban ghetto, the criminal underworld, the haunts of the art and music world, and the counterculture. Because of these roots, illicit drugs remained illegal for most of the last 100 years, while alcohol and tobacco were and are legal for most of the population. However, it should be understood that this legal status has little to do with the relative hazards of the different drugs. While illegal drugs are often not safe, legal status is not a good barometer of the risks associated with a specific drug.

Even today this misconception is perpetuated in public policy and even in some prevention programs. For example, the media campaign launched in the mid-1980s that included the famous TV sound bite "This is your brain on drugs" never mentioned alcohol or tobacco. Even some segments of the federal government seem more intent on addressing the "real drugs"—cocaine, marijuana, LSD, and so forth.[9] Recently, tobacco has received significant media attention in the national "Truth" campaign, funded by the national tobacco settlement of 1998. (See Chapter 3 for more details.) Because of the confusion about which substances are drugs, prevention specialists and drug educators, including many in government, now use the phrase *alcohol, tobacco, and other drugs* (ATOD) in place of the word *drug* to avoid this misunderstanding. The abbreviation ATOD will be used throughout this text.

Terminology also generates conflict when dealing with drug consumption. The term *drug abuse* has already been defined, and it is generally understood. However, the term implies that there are other patterns of consumption, and so we have the term **drug use**. It is possible to take a drug in a way that is not harmful, and in fact may be helpful (e.g., when one takes a medication prescribed by a physician). A drug is not categorically bad; harm comes by using a specific drug in a specific dosage, in a certain mood or mind-set, in specific environmental circumstances, with a specific predisposition to risk on the part of the consumer. In this context, illegality is irrelevant, except as it presents an additional risk.

The term *drug use* therefore suggests that some consumption of even illegal drugs may not be bad. For many people, and some segments of the U.S. government, this notion is not acceptable. This camp maintains that because all drugs (especially the illicit ones) are bad, all drug consumption is abuse. A variation of this viewpoint is that although adults may use alcohol, it is illegal for young people to do so. Therefore, drinking by adolescents, regardless of quantity or consequence, is labeled drug abuse.

This view of prevention then becomes an acid test for drug education materials and prevention curricula. If they use the term *drug use*, as distinct from *drug abuse*, they are ruled out of hand. Likewise, materials that focus on abuse as opposed to use are deemed unacceptable, regardless of their actual value in the real world.[10,11] Clearly, ideology has been allowed to cloud the issue. At least one agency in the U.S. government has questioned the scientific basis for rejecting all materials and programs that do not take a no-use approach but instead aim at reducing harm.[12]

The thoughtful educator recognizes that drugs of all kinds have a potential to do harm, and that young people grow up more successfully without nonmedical consumption of drugs. However, half truths and distortions, no matter how well intentioned, do not promote long-term success toward that end. There are times and places where abstinence is the right objective, and one that can be achieved. There are also times when the right objective is to delay onset, avoid the most destructive use, and help those who are already using to decrease intake (i.e., **harm reduction**). It is also appropriate and desirable, from ideological and prevention standpoints,[13] to teach and expect young people to obey the laws, in spite of the inconsistencies in public policy.

That said, it may be instructive to be aware of a "style sheet" of drug terminology that has been developed by federal agencies (see Hints & Tips box).[14] The suggested terms are more than an effort to be precise: In some cases they reflect the current political climate surrounding the war on drugs. Other terms are more evenhanded and well conceived.

At this time, government at all levels is heavily involved in funding drug abuse education and prevention. Because the U.S. government is a significant supporter of community activities in this regard, perhaps it is appropriate for the agencies involved to call the tune about the issues and terms just discussed. However, it is also important for educators and prevention specialists at the local level to understand the predominant attitudes and not allow them to inhibit creative and earnest efforts to stem the tide of casualties that drug abuse creates. Drug educators also have the task, requiring not a little courage, of trying to correct these widespread misconceptions about drug problems in our society.

Who Is the Target Group of Drug Education?

While it may be said that the tools used for drug education and prevention are blunt instruments, this is not because the problems have not been studied. Countless research projects conducted by government, universities, and community agencies have at least elucidated the nature of the problem.

What we know from research is that use of alcohol and other drugs tends to follow a curve beginning around sixth grade for most adolescents. (See **Figure 1.3.**) The curve gradually rises until about age 25 and then recedes from that point on. Relatively few adolescents in most communities

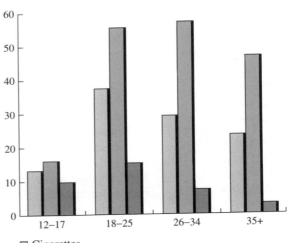

☐ Cigarettes
☐ Alcohol
■ Illicit drugs

Figure 1.3 ATOD Use by Age, 2000

Source: National Household Survey on Drug Abuse.

get seriously involved in illegal drugs, even though a majority may experiment with some of them, typically marijuana. Patterns of alcohol use by adolescents, particularly binge drinking, are of great concern, but binge drinking also tends to dramatically diminish starting in the mid-20s. The curve for tobacco starts at about the same time, but declines much more slowly: People continue to smoke until they suffer premature death from tobacco-related causes or until they otherwise quit smoking, usually much later in life than age 25. However, few people take up regular smoking after age 20; most people who become regular smokers do so by that age. These facts indicate that the logical target groups for the greatest emphasis on drug abuse prevention are children and adolescents.

However, another point should be made. The use of alcohol, tobacco, and other drugs is not randomly distributed among all youth. Research has shown patterns among users and nonusers and has led to a list of risk factors for drug abuse. The concept is that some young people are more likely than others to begin using drugs. They are called **high-risk youth**.

Numerous characteristics and circumstances that indicate increased likelihood for drug abuse have been identified. The most frequently cited set of traits, and those appearing in the text of the Federal Anti-Drug Abuse Act of 1986,[15] are presented in the FYI box. Some additional risk factors have been recognized, including difficulties in family management, being a latchkey child, hyperactivity and antisocial behavior, positive parental attitudes toward drug use, low commitment to school, rebelliousness, alienation, lack of social bonding, and having drug-using friends.[16,17]

In general, the characteristics are ones of economic disadvantage, social dysfunction, and unsupportive home and community environments. It is probable that the characteristics are not exclusive for drug abuse but are the hub of an array of problems, including violence, delinquency, early and inappropriate sexuality, school dropout, social isolation, and distancing from mainstream values and pursuits.

These high-risk characteristics seem entrenched and indomitable, and they result in problems over which society has had no resounding victories. However, a subset of risk research has identified the concept of **resilience**. A substantial proportion of youth possessing high-risk characteristics grow up unscathed, avoiding drug abuse problems, school failure, and incarceration. As adults they establish normal family and other social relationships and achieve success in employment pursuits. Much has been learned about how these resilient children manage to overcome significant disadvantages and how their experience could be translated into programs, policies, and interventions to benefit those who are not so resilient on their own.[18] The FYI box on page 11 outlines the "protective factors" that are influential in the lives of resilient children.

A corollary to the high-risk youth concept is that prevention programs need to focus more explicitly on youth at greatest risk. This concept has major implications for prevention programs. Until recently most prevention programs were directed at students as though they were homogeneous in their characteristics and needs. Furthermore, most prevention was unwittingly geared toward low-risk students—those youth least likely to experience serious problems. The educational thrust had been to concentrate on modifying the individual student's knowledge, attitudes, skills, and behaviors with respect to drugs. However, research on high-risk youth indicates this is only a partial solution.

The high-risk characteristics outlined earlier have little to do with knowledge, attitudes, and skills. Traditional classroom-based programs can be planned, implemented, and evaluated to increase our effectiveness in addressing educational needs. However, risk characteristics also must be addressed if prevention programs are to affect the most vul-

Youth at High Risk for Drug and Alcohol Abuse

A high-risk youth is an individual who is younger than 21 years and is at risk of becoming, or has become, a drug user or alcohol abuser and has one of the following characteristics:

- Is a school dropout
- Has experienced repeated failure in school
- Has become pregnant
- Is economically disadvantaged
- Is the child of a drug or alcohol abuser
- Is a victim of physical, sexual, or psychological abuse
- Has committed a violent or delinquent act
- Has experienced mental health problems
- Has attempted suicide
- Has experienced long-term physical pain due to injury

nerable. A whole new approach will be required, one akin to public health programs.

Because the drug problem in society has been defined as an educational problem and a criminal justice problem, a more holistic approach has not been taken; those fighting the drug war have been armed with only a small set of weapons. However, a public health approach has much to offer. While many state and national leaders promote the use of public health strategies to combat drug abuse, adoption on the local level is slow.

Public health professionals think in terms of **target groups,** a defined segment of the population that will be the focus of program strategies. The public health approach takes one further step by analyzing the context of the problem, using what is called the **public health model,** shown in **Figure 1.4.** (Other prevention models will be presented in later chapters.)

The model considers first the **host,** that is, members of the target group. Who is at risk? What are their characteristics and needs? What are their attitudes and practices relevant to this problem? What personal traits make them vulnerable? A second factor the model considers is the **agent,** in this case alcohol, tobacco, or other drugs. What is it about the drug that is hazardous or addictive? Is there any way it could be modified to reduce risk? Could it be made less available to the target group? The third factor is the **environment,** the social and physical surroundings that affect the development of drug problems. What is home life like, and how could it be altered to prevent the problem? Do media messages and portrayals promote the development of drug problems? What are school and community policies with respect to drugs? Are adequate

social and medical services available to address the precursor problems?

This model for attacking the drug problem is beginning to be used, but it is an uncomfortable fit with conventional school programs and services. However, if we are to effectively intervene with high-risk youth, a comprehensive strategy will be required. This approach is beginning to take place in many states and schools, with a proliferation of student assistance programs and family resource centers. Although these will be discussed more fully in Chapter 11, they are mentioned here as examples of innovations in the educational system that show promise of more effectively addressing the prevention needs of high-risk students.

Drug Use Surveillance

For most of our history, no national data were available on individual drug consumption. Data that were available were of three principal types: (1) figures on the wholesale distribution of alcohol and tobacco, from which could be calculated per capita consumption; (2) statistics on the consequences of drug abuse, such as the incidence rate of mortality from alcoholic cirrhosis; and (3) statistics from the criminal justice system, such as confiscation of drug caches or arrests for alcohol- and drug-related offenses.

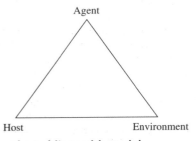

Agent

Host   Environment

Figure 1.4 **The Public Health Model**

Factors That Protect Against Drug Abuse
Constitutional Factors
• High activity level
• Low degree of excitability and distress
• High degree of sociability

Environmental Factors
• Fewer than four siblings
• At least two years between siblings
• Close bond with at least one caretaker
• Opportunity to develop special interest or hobby
• Required by circumstances to be helpful
• For girls: Needed to take care of siblings
• For boys: Firstborn, having a male role model, having rules in daily life, required to do chores

External Support
• Well liked by classmates
• At least one close friend
• Informal helping network
• Finding school a refuge from family problems
• Having a supportive teacher
• Participation in extracurricular activities

These indicators of the size of the drug problem are still used and provide helpful information, but they don't give us many details on use patterns in the population, and they are indirect measures of actual consumption.

In 1975, the U.S. government began supporting a large national survey of adolescent substance abuse. The survey has been repeated every year since then. Called Monitoring the Future, the survey has routinely received responses from 15,000 to 17,000 high school seniors regarding their behavior and attitudes about alcohol, illegal drugs, and tobacco. During the early 1990s, grades 8 and 10 were added to the survey.

While the actual levels of drug use reported may be disputed (i.e., because of underreporting or overreporting), the important finding is the trend plotted from 1975 to the present. Throughout this text, references will be made to the Monitoring the Future survey because it is considered to be the most valid and reliable national drug survey of the school population.

Another important national survey is the National Household Survey on Drug Abuse. It also is a survey of drug use behavior and attitudes. In contrast to Monitoring the Future, however, the National Household Survey gathers data on all age groups 12 and older, and it is done by in-person interviews as opposed to group administration of questionnaires.

Another well-known school drug survey is conducted by the Parents Resource Institute for Drug Education (PRIDE). Although this survey is not designed to be a representative sample of U.S. schoolchildren, data reported by the PRIDE survey are very similar to those in Monitoring the Future. An added feature is that the PRIDE survey gathers data on all grades from 4 to 12.

More recently, another source of data has been developed, the Youth Risk Behavior Survey. This survey gathers data on high school students. While it contains questions about alcohol, tobacco, and other drugs, it also includes items on other risk behavior such as sexuality, violence, suicide, diet, and exercise. Statistics are reported for the nation at large and for each participating state.

The final data source to which reference will be made is the Drug Abuse Warning Network (DAWN). DAWN began in the early 1970s and has evolved over the years. Currently, it contains two subsets. First, a representative sample of hospital emergency rooms is monitored each year to gather data on drug- and alcohol-related emergency room visits. Though not always true in the past, current statistics are representative of the United States as a whole. Second, medical examiners in 27 U.S. metropolitan areas report on alcohol- or other drug-related deaths. This subset is not representative of the United States as a whole.

Each of these surveys makes a unique contribution to illuminating various dimensions of America's drug problem. It is important for drug educators and prevention specialists to be familiar with these sources, periodically taking the measure of the problem and comparing local problems against those of the nation as a whole.

Summary

This chapter has attempted to lay the groundwork for the following chapters. As the book progresses through prevention history, drug information, school-based prevention theory and practice, intervention and treatment, evaluation, and public policy issues, the concepts discussed in this chapter provide a thread of continuity.

Scenario | Analysis and Response

Michelyn has to consider the worth of valid but radical moves versus her opportunity to influence programming and policy over the long term. It is clear that her proposals, in their current form, are not likely to get the support of her board. If she pushes too hard for change, she is at risk of being replaced by someone more malleable by the board. She decides that she wants to stay with the coalition and try to exert change more gradually.

Her counterproposal to the board is to carve out from the budget a category of funds that will be earmarked for new program strategies that have evidence of effectiveness from other places. Coalition partners will have the opportunity to tap these funds for projects that meet science-based criteria. These projects will be required to be carefully evaluated.

In the meantime, Michelyn plans to build better relationships with board members in order to establish credibility and more confidence in her leadership and expertise.

Learning Activities

1. Inventory the drug abuse prevention activities in your community. What programs are carried out by the school system, and what drug education curricula are used? Are other agencies involved in prevention? What is their contribution? Is there an effective community coalition? Who participates in it, and in what projects has it engaged?

2. Try to obtain budget data from your state public and mental health agencies on how many dollars are spent addressing alcohol and other drug problems. What is the relative distribution among prevention, intervention, and treatment?

3. Interview appropriate personnel involved with your school system's drug education and prevention program. Analyze their views concerning no-use programs versus harm reduction programs. Ask them about the use of science-based programs.

4. Select one of the indicators of high risk for drug abuse. Identify programs and activities sponsored by your local school and community that address the specific risk characteristic you have selected.

5. Search *www.health.org* on the Internet to obtain data reports from the various national drug use surveys. Call the National Clearinghouse for Alcohol and Drug Information (1-800-SAY-NO-TO) for additional information.

Notes

1. *National Drug Control Strategy* (Washington, DC: Office of National Drug Control Strategy, The White House, February 2000).
2. Donna E. Shalala, "Drug Trends in 1999 Among American Teens Are Mixed," presented at a press conference, Washington, DC, Old Executive Office Building, December 17, 1999.
3. "Drug Education Gets an F." *U.S. News & World Report,* October 13, 1986, 63, 64.
4. *Prevention in Perspective* (Washington, DC: National Association of State Alcohol and Drug Abuse Directors, January 1989).
5. Office for Substance Abuse Prevention, *The Future by Design: A Community Prevention System Framework* (Washington, DC: DHHS, 1990).
6. O. Ray and C. Ksir, *Drugs, Society, and Human Behavior* (St. Louis: Times Mirror/Mosby, 1990).
7. J. Helmer and T. Vietorisz, *Drug Use, the Labor Market and Class Conflict* (Washington, DC: The Drug Abuse Council, 1974).
8. D. F. Duncan and K. Rheinboldt, "Labor Markets and Drug Laws: A Statistical Test of a Radical Theory," paper presented at Academy of Criminal Justice Sciences, Oklahoma City, OK, March 13, 1980.
9. *The War on Drugs: Failure and Fantasy* (Washington, DC: American Public Health Association, September 1992).
10. Arlene B. Seal, "There Is No Choice!" *Campuses Without Drugs* 3, 3 (1990).
11. *Drug Prevention Curricula: A Guide to Selection and Implementation* (Washington, DC: Office of Educational Research and Improvement, U.S. Department of Education, 1988).
12. *Drug Abuse Prevention: Federal Efforts to Identify Exemplary Programs Need Stronger Design* (Washington, DC: U.S. General Accounting Office, Report to the Subcommittee on Select Education, Committee on Education and Labor, House of Representatives, August 1991).
13. Social Development Research Group, "The Social Development Strategy," University of Washington, School of Social Work, 1989.
14. Office for Substance Abuse Prevention, "Editorial Guidelines," *The OSAP Prevention Pipeline* 5, 4 (July/August 1992): inside back cover.
15. Office for Substance Abuse Prevention, *Communicating About Alcohol and Other Drugs: Strategies for Reaching Populations at Risk,* DHHS Publication No. (ADM) 90-1665 (Rockville, MD: DHHS, 1990), 12, 13.
16. J. D. Hawkins, D. M. Lishner, and R. F. Catalano, "Childhood Predictors and the Prevention of Adolescent Substance Abuse," in *Etiology of Drug Abuse: Implications for Prevention,* C. L. Jones and R. J. Battjes, eds., DHHS Publication No. (ADM) 87-1335 (Rockville, MD: DHHS, 1985).
17. J. D. Hawkins, D. M. Lishner, R. F. Catalano, and M. O. Howard, "Childhood Predictors of Adolescent Substance Abuse: Toward an Empirically Grounded Theory," *Journal of Children in Contemporary Society* 18 (1986): 11–48.
18. Emmy E. Werner, "Resilient Children." *Young Children,* November 1984, 68–72.

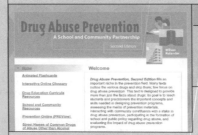

web resources

The Web site for this book offers many useful resources for educators, students, and professional counselors and is a great source for additional information. Visit the site at **http://healtheducation.jbpub.com/drugabuse/.**

Chapter Learning Objectives

Upon completion of this chapter, students will be able to:

1. Summarize the abuse of drugs at various times since the second half of the 19th century.

2. Describe changes in government policy concerning alcohol and other drug abuse that occurred in the first 20 years of the 20th century.

3. Compare the patterns of drug abuse from 1920 to 1960 with patterns after 1960.

4. Describe the changes regarding tobacco consumption that have occurred in the last 100 years.

5. Analyze the factors responsible for changes in tobacco consumption.

Scenario

Many preschools and kindergartens have "Grandparents Day," when children are invited to bring their grandparents and great grandparents to school. The primary purpose is for these adults to visit and observe and to feel a part of the lives of the children. However, a secondary purpose is for the children to have a "living history" lesson in which they can learn in a semi-structured way about life at the time when their grandparents were children.

Evie Dominguez is a young kindergarten teacher who is planning for the annual Grandparents Day program. In addition to establishing some basic learning skills in the kindergarten program, she wants to begin the children's education regarding drug abuse. Her strategy is to collect from library archives newspaper articles from the 1930s, 1940s, and 1950s that have to do with alcohol, tobacco, and illegal drugs. She wants to provide this material to the grandparents in advance, and to ask them to spend a few minutes reflecting on the stories and headlines from their own perspective of growing up at that time.

Chapter 2

Drug Abuse Problems: Background and Setting

Introduction

The biblical King Solomon said, "There is nothing new under the sun" (Ecclesiastes 1:9). Even though we sometimes think that drug problems didn't occur until the 1960s, history tells us that drugs have been used and abused for millennia. The Book of Genesis recounts Noah's drunkenness shortly after emerging from the ark.[1] Alcohol use has been part of most civilizations since ancient times. Writing around 850 B.C., Homer made reference in the *Iliad* and the *Odyssey* to the undesirable effects of alcohol.[2,3] Opium and marijuana use was also recorded in ancient Greece, China, India, and the Middle East.[4-6] Native people were using coca and tobacco when the first European explorers arrived in the New World, and this drug use predated the Europeans' arrival by hundreds of years.[7,8] It is believed that tobacco was used as incense in the religious ceremonies of the Mayan civilization (A.D. 470 to 620). (See **Figure 2.1.**) From that beginning, tobacco use gradually spread throughout Mexico and Central America.

Because of the long history and almost universal distribution of drug use in the human family, some would postulate that humans have an innate drive to find ways to alter their consciousness and perception of reality. This view is supported by the presence of mind-altering substances in the natural ecology and the presence in the nervous system of endogenous receptors for opium-like substances called **endorphins.**[9]

Oliver Wendell Holmes had a very low opinion of the drug therapy commonly practiced in his day, but he made an exception for opium, about which he said, "The Creator himself seems to prescribe, for we often see the scarlet poppy growing in

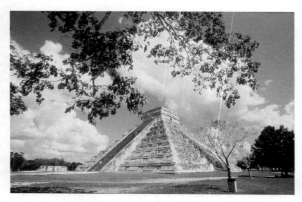

Figure 2.1 **Mayan Ruins**   Tobacco was used in worship practices of the Mayan people. (© Betts Anderson/Unicorn Stock Photos)

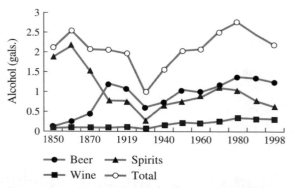

Figure 2.2 **Apparent U.S. Per Capita Consumption of Pure Alcohol, 1850–1998**

Source: G. D. William, F. S. Stinson, S. D. Brooks, D. Clem, and J. Noble, *Apparent Per Capita Alcohol Consumption: National, State, and Regional Trends, 1977–1989,* NIAAA Surveillance Report No. 20, DHHS Publication No. (ADM) 281-89-0001 (Washington, DC: U.S. Government Printing Office, 1991).

the cornfields, as if it were foreseen that wherever there is hunger to be fed there must also be pain to be soothed."[10] A different spin might be to lament our tendency to self-destruct in a variety of ways. We should not be surprised to find drug abuse in our communities; it is nothing new.

What *is* new is the wide diversity of abused substances. This is part and parcel of the science and technology explosion that began in the 19th century. Humanity has applied inventive ingenuity to every facet of living, and pharmacology, licit or otherwise, is no exception. One brash commentator described this as "better living through chemistry." Whether or not the remark is humorous, the consequences of modern-day drug abuse are, for many, detrimental indeed.

While lessons could be learned from studying drug abuse throughout history, across all cultures, this is beyond the scope and purpose of this book. Other references are available for the interested reader.[11–13] However, to understand the nature of our current problems, it is helpful to review the history of drug use and abuse over the past 200 years.

Drug Use in the 19th Century

Alcohol

During the 19th, 20th, and 21st centuries, no essential changes occurred in the nature of alcoholic beverages. However, their consumption and place

in society have changed a great deal. Many regulations have come and gone, and packaging and marketing have evolved in ways designed to influence consumption and public attitudes. However, the three basic forms of alcoholic beverages—beer, wine, and distilled spirits—have remained, though public preference (i.e., market share) for one type or another has changed. Distilled beverages were the most popular 150 years ago.[14] Today beer holds that title.[15] (See **Figure 2.2.**)

From 1800 to 2000, alcohol consumption waxed and waned. Figure 2.2 and other evidence indicate that per capita consumption was much higher in the early 1800s than it is today.[16,17] Also, alcohol drinking was once primarily restricted to men, particularly in American society. This gender gap is much less pronounced today.

Long before national alcohol prohibition, individual states enacted restrictions and sanctions on alcohol. During the 19th century, public attention was more focused on alcohol than on other drugs, in part because other drugs were fewer in number and used by less of the population. It was also because other substances (e.g., morphine) were not recognized as harmful, at least not right away. In fact, opiate drugs were prescribed by physicians as a cure for, or at least a preferable alternative to, alcoholism.[18] Paradoxically, alcohol abuse tends to be denied and overlooked in modern times, even though it may be the most socially harmful form of drug abuse.

Tobacco

Tobacco consumption in the 19th century was almost entirely in the form of pipe smoking and smokeless tobacco, since cigarettes were not widely available until the 20th century.[19] As with alcohol, tobacco use was predominantly a male habit. While the essential nature of tobacco has not changed, hazards were not apparent during the 19th century for several reasons. First, pipes and smokeless tobacco are less harmful than cigarettes. Second, people didn't usually live past the fifth decade, which wasn't long enough for them to experience the chronic diseases that result from smoking. Finally, it wasn't until the 20th century that medical science could specifically label many diseases and determine underlying causes. Even if someone's death was tobacco related, it would not have been recognized as such.

For these reasons, few voices were raised against tobacco until the middle of the 20th century. The few early voices that were raised were responding on the basis of ideology or **empirical concepts** of healthful living and temperance, rather than scientific evidence.[20]

These tranquil beginnings explain why tobacco is so entrenched in today's society. It has been a profitable crop for hundreds of years, and its consumption has long been legal. This status makes tobacco much more difficult to restrict and regulate than other drugs, such as marijuana, that have been outside of mainstream society until more recent times.

Opiate Narcotics

Opiate drugs have undergone "breakthroughs" not seen with alcohol and tobacco; that is, various new forms have appeared since 1800. At that time, opium was the principal drug in the narcotics category. Morphine was isolated from crude opium very early in the century, followed by codeine in the 1830s. Finally, in the late 1890s, heroin was developed and marketed.

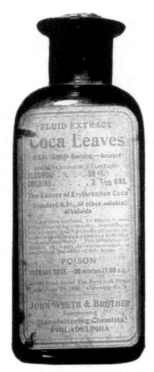

Figure 2.3 Patent Medicines Patent medicines provided unlimited access to many drugs that are now considered hazardous and in some cases have been made illegal.

These drugs were widely available with no restrictions. They were marketed through all of the retailing and advertising methods of the day. Perhaps the most prominent form was as an ingredient in **patent medicines**, which were in some ways equivalent to today's over-the-counter drugs. (See **Figure 2.3.**) They were obtained from a variety of legal sources other than physicians.

The patent medicine entrepreneurs wrote the book on false advertising and did not shrink from recommending their **nostrums** for any and all health problems, from the trivial to the terminal. The prevailing level of science literacy in the general population was not equal to the challenge. Even when states began to place legal restrictions on physicians who prescribed and dispensed opiates, patent medicines went unregulated.[21] Patent medicines generally contained opium (including codeine and morphine), alcohol, or both, and sometimes marijuana.

The comforting properties of those drugs guaranteed continued use with or without a cure of the original symptoms. This resulted in their indiscriminate and widespread use in the 19th century.[22,23]

Opiates were a central tool in medicine even though they could not be called curative. Even in the absence of specific acute pain, the opiates would make any problem seem better. Common applications included diarrhea, menstrual and menopausal discomfort, infant colic, and cough.[24] With the development of the hypodermic syringe in the middle of the century, the addictive property of the opiates was exacerbated.

The socioeconomic profile of opiate users was much different 150 years ago from what it is today. The typical user was a middle-aged white female from the upper echelons of society.[25] Today the user is more likely to be a lower-class adolescent male. This change is probably not caused by the characteristics of the drug as much as by changes that have taken place in society, particularly in the way opiates are regulated.

When the great railroads were being built across North America, opium was associated with imported Chinese laborers. In the same way, many myths surrounded cocaine and African Americans, particularly in the South. Society's attitudes toward drugs have been intertwined with xenophobia and nationalism.[26] Fear and suspicion of a group of people were transferred to the drug associated with the group, without much conscious awareness. These attitudes were repeated in the 20th century with marijuana.

The addictive properties of opium have long been recognized, though the consequences of use in the past were less severe because of its easy availability on the open market. However, the biochemical dynamics of addiction were not understood. It was thought that each new generation of opiate was an effective cure for dependency on the last. For example, morphine was promoted as a cure for opium addiction. The phenomenon of **cross-tolerance** was unrecognized. Because administering the next drug eliminated the withdrawal symptoms brought on by withholding the first, it was believed something of therapeutic value was accomplished. The disappointment may have been bitter when

the truth was first learned. However, the lesson was repeated with different pairs of drugs at different times in the 1800s. To a degree, it has been repeated again in our experience with heroin and methadone, beginning in the 1960s. (See additional discussion of methadone treatment in Chapter 12.)

In spite of the well-accepted medical value of opiates, their hazards became increasingly recognized; states thus began to place restrictions on consumption and distribution. It wasn't until the first decade of the 20th century that national restrictions were applied.

Cocaine

Cocaine was used long before 1800. Prior to about 1850, its use was limited to chewing coca leaves, derived from a shrub indigenous to the eastern side of the Andean Mountains of South America.[27] (See **Figure 2.4.**) Chewing coca leaves produces an effect not unlike the doses of caffeine found in coffee and cola drinks today; even though the habit is

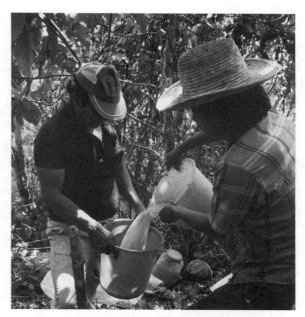

Figure 2.4 **Cocaine Production**   Coca shrubs, the source of cocaine, grow well in the mountains of South America. The leaves have been used for drug effects for hundreds of years. (AP/Wide World Photos)

endemic in the coca-growing regions, there is little evidence of individual or social problems due to such consumption.

While chewing tobacco leaves is quite common in North America, coca chewing has never entered the culture. About 1860, the active ingredient of coca leaves was isolated and named *cocaine*.[28] This technological advancement brought a dimension of hazard that was not present with chewing coca leaves.

Cocaine became a common ingredient of patent medicines and Coca-Cola (it has since been removed from the latter), and was used by the German military in the 1880s to combat fatigue. Sigmund Freud became a proponent of cocaine, recommending it for depression and nervous system disorders. Less than 10 years later, he and other physicians began to have doubts and reservations about cocaine because of its addictive properties and other side effects. The patent medicine industry continued to market various products that included cocaine for a wide variety of health problems. The U.S. government began to put restrictions on the use and sale of cocaine early in the 20th century, as it had done with opiates.

In summary, it might be said that drug problems were common during the 19th century, and it would be accurate to describe the situation in the late 1800s as a drug **epidemic**, perhaps more severe than the current one.[29] The consequences of that drug abuse were great for individuals, families, and society as a whole. Governments were unable, and mostly unwilling, to address the problems; consequently, the violence that we see today between drug users, dealers, and law enforcement agencies did not occur. Perhaps this is why public expressions of concern were more muted. Today's drug problem is a much harsher reality.

Drug Use in the Early 20th Century

Early in the new century, the medical profession was beginning to exercise much more restraint in prescribing opium and cocaine, and society was beginning to be much less favorably disposed to easy drug use. These changes happened before government controls were implemented; public

concern was the impetus for the new laws that would be passed. However, efforts in the 20th century to restrict the use of alcohol and drugs were an eclectic mixture of good and bad intentions, rational policy and zealous absurdity, public-spirited activism, and political and professional self-interest.

By the end of the 19th century, the patent medicine industry's abuses were beginning to wear thin with government leaders, the medical profession, and ordinary people in communities. However, two events precipitated the fall of the first domino in the war on drugs. Muckraking journalists began to investigate and attack the industry. The most prominent example was a series of articles, called "The Great American Fraud," written for *Collier's* magazine by Samuel Adams in 1905. The second was the 1906 publication of Upton Sinclair's *The Jungle*. The book was about the meat-packing industry rather than drugs, but it spurred the nation's outrage and accelerated the "progressive" role of government in regulating business and industry. Shortly afterward, the Pure Food and Drug Act (1906) was enacted.

Regarding drugs, the act's main objective was accurate labeling. While this did not prevent the sale or purchase of narcotics, cocaine, or any other drugs, it did affect the level of consumption. Large segments of the public ceased to buy many patent medicines once they knew their ingredients. Only later did the Pure Food and Drug Act require not only honest labeling but also safety and effectiveness. Many other state and federal laws were advanced to restrict the actual use of alcohol and other drugs.

The efforts toward this goal were squarely in the middle of the political arena, and many voices were ringing in the ears of policymakers. At the time, the medical and pharmacy professions were trying to organize to improve their image and status, create mechanisms for self-policing, and protect their professional autonomy. The fit between the interests of those professions and the public good was not perfect. For one thing, many unscrupulous physicians and pharmacists made significant profits by serving people who abused drugs; they were therefore resistant to any efforts that would threaten their livelihoods. Other professionals were more restrained and sensitive to the ethical issue of carelessly dispensing harmful and habit-forming drugs. However, they were opposed to government interference in professional practice and felt that patient care should not be the subject of legislation. There was also jockeying for predominance between the medical and the pharmacy professions, which gave another twist to the legislative and political proceedings.

Among the public, many were zealous regarding the temperance cause and viewed alcohol and drug abuse as morally wrong and physically degrading. Their position was not encumbered with facts, but was more an ideology. Interestingly enough, the temperance movement was not a monolithic unity: Some factions were singleminded about "demon rum" but not at all interested in other drugs. The temperance camp believed in marshaling the powers of government to bolster the moral frailty of humankind with respect to alcohol and drugs. Around the turn of the 20th century, temperance supporters were very optimistic about their cause; later in the century, the enthusiasm for legislated temperance waned considerably.

Then there were the "experts" who tried to find reasonable and effective solutions to the problems caused by excessive drug consumption. Early in the century, the behavioral or social sciences were virtually nonexistent, so little genuine research was brought to bear on drug problems. These experts were usually one of two types: (1) bureaucrats from various branches of government, such as the Departments of Agriculture, State, Treasury, or Commerce; or (2) physicians who provided patient care to alcoholics and addicts. These two groups often had their own agendas, and their ideas did not always lead in the same direction. Furthermore, many of the policy positions advanced were empirical and relied on trial and error rather than on a theoretical or research base.

Consequently, early efforts at drug use control can be characterized as a cat and mouse game. Whatever legislative tool was applied, someone would find a way to circumvent it—the public, professionals, business, the underworld—demonstrating the maxim "Nothing is foolproof, because

fools are so ingenious." This game has continued to be played out. Even though some lessons have been learned, and science has been increasingly utilized, progress has been slow. Changes in drug consumption seemed to occur in spite of any government intervention.

From 1900 to about 1920, use of narcotics, cocaine, and marijuana declined, according to the limited evidence available. However, public awareness of the dangers of drugs and political interest in the issue increased. The more the problem was discussed and debated, the bigger the problem appeared to become. Some of this excessive interest was propagated by opportunists in government or other leaders for their own personal advancement. Nevertheless, during this time the United States made a commitment to the "war on drugs," first with the Pure Food and Drug Act, then with the Harrison Act of 1914, and next with national prohibition, the Eighteenth Amendment of the Constitution, enacted in 1919.

The Harrison Narcotic Act was the first national effort to restrict the use of narcotics. Cocaine was also specified by the act. The Harrison Act was continuously strengthened over a period of years, even though there was little evidence that it ever accomplished its intended goal. In the early 1930s, prohibition of alcohol was overturned. This occurred because national leadership recognized the economic consequences caused by prohibition and believed that the benefits of prohibition did not justify the cost.

Illegal Drug Use: 1920 to 1960

During the period from 1920 to 1960, illegal drug use became largely confined to the fringes of society: lower-class urban neighborhoods, minority groups, and the avant garde in the art and music world. This point of view is accepted conventional wisdom, but may be only an unchallenged assumption. No credible statistics are available on the use of drugs in the nation as a whole until the 1970s; consequently, assertions about the extent and nature of drug use prior to the 1970s are based mostly on anecdotes and impressions. It is true that there was little public recognition of drug use as a problem in mainstream society. Also, traditional values (e.g., the work ethic, delaying gratification) were in the ascendancy; alternative lifestyles and life views were not readily tolerated in a largely unicultural period in the United States.

During the late 1930s to the end of World War II, the international narcotics trade was substantially disrupted by war in Europe, North Africa, and the Pacific. However, this was not permanent, and opium and marijuana suppliers soon found new producers, such as those in Mexico, that were out of the way of war. Soon after the declaration of peace, the narcotics trade resumed at full force.

Illegal Drug Use: 1960 to the Present

Following World War II, the nation got back to work with optimistic resolve, and many families lost sight of other values beyond materialism. With the dawn of the 1960s, the relative domestic tranquility of prior years gave way to dramatic social upheavals in gender and generational relationships, civil rights, and socioeconomic class differences. Paradoxically, the productivity of the 1950s made possible more leisure time and increased the educational opportunities necessary for the inception and articulation of ideas and philosophies that challenged the status quo. Drug use received relentless national attention and generated horror among parents, educators, and "the establishment." In addition, the nation became aware of substantial drug use by American troops fighting the Vietnam War. The excesses of drug consumption were probably exaggerated, but this was a reaction to the change from the postwar years that came before.

Although actual drug use in the 1960s may not have been as great as levels seen in the late 1970s, it shocked the country because it was a dramatic increase over past use, it was done openly with hubris and enthusiasm, it occurred on Main Street with middle-class youth, and it found the leaders in education and government totally unprepared to respond. (See **Figure 2.5.**) The public reaction to this development was exacerbated by all of the other social turmoil occurring simultaneously.

With the coming of the 1970s, the country became more sedate and composed: The Vietnam

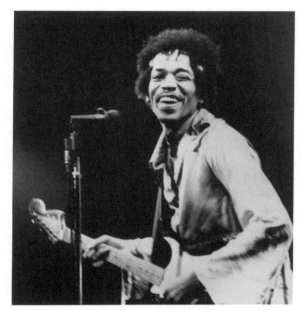

Figure 2.5 **Drugs and Popular Culture** Jimi Hendrix, and several other high-profile entertainers, died from drug overdoses at the beginning of the current drug abuse epidemic. (UPI/Bettmann)

War ended and healing began, grandiose social programs enacted in response to the 1960s protests continued to do their intended work, and the country set about fighting the threat of drug abuse. This fight took two forms. Beginning with the Nixon administration, a "get tough" law and order policy became politically irresistible and became a major influence in drug policy that has lasted to the present day. At the same time, educators groped in the theoretical dark, resulting in a parade of educational approaches with no research or evaluation data to support their use. This educational effort is discussed further in Chapter 7.

Beginning in 1975, the U.S. government began supporting the national survey of adolescent substance abuse known as Monitoring the Future (see Chapter 1). While the actual levels of drug use reported may be disputed (i.e., because of underreporting or overreporting), the important finding is the trend that the survey plots. Some of these data are shown in **Figure 2.6.** The survey shows that drug use was increasing until about 1980, declined

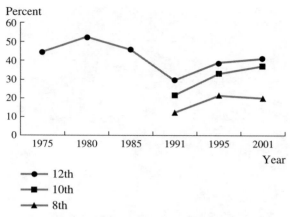

Percent

Figure 2.6 Past-Year Use of Illicit Drugs by 12th, 10th, and 8th Graders, United States, 1975–2001

Source: National Institute on Drug Abuse, Monitoring the Future Study, 2001.

through the early 1990s, and has increased slowly since. Cocaine use increased until about 1985, declined through about 1992, and has slightly increased since then. The latest figures (for 2001) show that drug use by high school seniors is slightly higher than it was in 1995. It is not possible to predict from available data what the trend in the future will be. The findings of Monitoring the Future are corroborated by the National Household Survey (see Chapter 1) of drug use in American households.

The bad news is that drug abuse seems to be undergoing a shift in our society, once again leaving Main Street and becoming concentrated among the poor and minority residents of inner-city slums. There is a subset of society that can be described as recreational drug users. They use drugs in a restrained manner so as not to interfere with careers and family relationships.[30,31] However, in general, for those who have a real and potential stake in the American Dream, drug abuse is becoming unattractive and untenable. For those who don't succeed in the educational system and live with social and economic disadvantages, drug abuse seems to have become endemic, if not epidemic.

In contrast to similar circumstances in the 1930s and 1940s, this time around laissez-faire reactions will not meet the challenge. Drug-related violence

touches every community, and the interdependence of all people within the economy and government programs forces us to pay attention. It remains to be seen if Americans will retain interest in the drug epidemic or whether apathy will develop, parallel to the apathy regarding immunization that has occurred with the elimination of the infectious disease epidemics of the 1940s and 1950s.

The Unique Case of Tobacco

The public treatment of tobacco during the last 100 years has been quite different from that given to alcohol and other drugs, largely because the association of the word *drug* with tobacco was rarely made prior to the 1960s. Even now, many people still do not think of tobacco as a drug. However, efforts to discourage tobacco use were not unknown in earlier times, though the motivation for such efforts may have been more ideological than medical.

Tobacco use was officially banned in many countries in the Middle East, Europe, and Asia during the 1600s.[32] Because of tobacco's popularity even in elite circles, the bans were ineffective and eventually ignored. In the late 1800s and early 1900s, grass-roots organizations sprouted in the United States. Called antitobacco leagues, they were patterned after the temperance and antisaloon leagues. There was strong public opposition to smoking by women and children, and many states enacted legislation to prohibit smoking altogether. The laws did not work and were eventually revoked, except for provisions to restrict the purchase of tobacco by young people.

However, no great official concern was ever directed toward tobacco as it was to other drugs. One reason is that tobacco has very American origins. While other drugs were associated with foreign influences thought to be somehow subversive or unwholesome, tobacco was never looked upon in that way. And even though people recognized that tobacco use often became habitual, it didn't seem to cause the individual and social damage attributed to other drugs. The deluge of evidence linking tobacco with disease and death did not begin until the second half of the 20th century.

For most of its history, tobacco was consumed primarily by chewing, snorting snuff, or by smoking pipes and cigars. Cigarette-like cigars were smoked prior to the arrival of Columbus, but they were the exception rather than the rule. Cigarettes did not become popular until the early 1900s, when they became the predominant form. This development occurred for several reasons. The technology for mass production of cigarettes became available, making possible large quantities at a small unit price. The cigarette was also small and contained a dose of nicotine that was closer to the wants of most consumers. Then, the variety of tobacco known as "bright" or "flue cured" was introduced; this tobacco was milder than burley and other types of tobacco and easier to smoke, especially for young initiates. In addition, public health officials aggressively tried to stop the public chewing of tobacco because spitting the juice was associated with the spread of tuberculosis; ironically, this campaign may have induced many people to switch to smoking. Finally, cigarettes were advertised far and wide, with appeals to pleasure, sophistication, and the idea that "everybody is doing it."

All of these influences led to a startling rise in cigarette smoking beginning in the 1920s and continuing into the 1960s, as illustrated in **Figure 2.7**.[33] Although there were some isolated bits of biomedical research that might have caused concern,[34,35]

for most of that period the rise in tobacco consumption was almost entirely unopposed. Only in the last 40 years have we recognized that cigarette smoking is the most harmful way to use tobacco because of the deep and prolonged inhalation of smoke.

Perhaps the most important development that kicked off the current antitobacco campaign was a large-scale **epidemiological study** conducted in the 1950s and 1960s by Dr. E. Cuyler Hammond, with sponsorship by the American Cancer Society.[36] This and other research led to the 1964 report of the Surgeon General's Advisory Committee on Smoking and Health.[37] For the first time, the U.S. government took the unequivocal position that smoking was responsible for heart disease, lung cancer, and other diseases and that it shortened the life of smokers. Since 1964, the government, private agencies, and medical and public health organizations increasingly have brought pressure to bear on limiting tobacco consumption.

At the same time, the tobacco industry has dug in its heels, resisting and finding ways to circumvent the antitobacco forces. For example, in the early 1970s cigarette advertising was banned from television. However, many public events, such as auto races and other sports events, are heavily sponsored by tobacco companies. (See **Figure 2.8**.) Even though there are no actual radio and TV tobacco ads, cigarette logos and a prosmoking message are

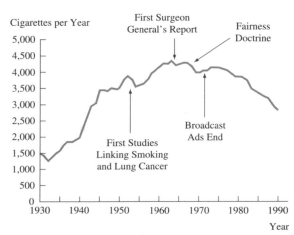

Figure 2.7 **U.S. Per Capita Cigarette Consumption, 18 Years Old and Over**

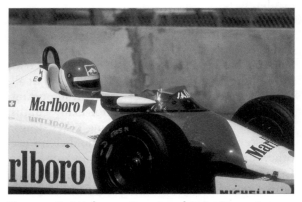

Figure 2.8 **A Tobacco-Sponsored Auto Race**   In spite of a television advertising ban, tobacco products are still promoted via broadcasts of tobacco-sponsored sporting events. (© Robert Ginn/Unicorn Stock Photos)

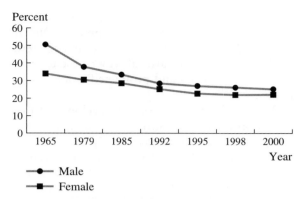

Percent

Figure 2.9 **Smoking Prevalences for Men and Women Aged 18 and Older, 1965–2000**

Source: National Health Interview Survey.

communicated to millions of viewers, including children.[38]

The Surgeon General's report had only a temporary effect on decreasing smoking. Many people quit on hearing the news about the report, but within a few months most relapsed and went back to smoking. However, over the last 30 years the undeniable trend has been a decreasing number and rate of adult smokers,[39] as illustrated in **Figure 2.9.** Millions of people have quit; many more millions have not started. This progress is a result of an array of strategies that have been brought to bear on the problem. These strategies are described in detail in Chapter 3.

Nevertheless, smoking is still a major drug problem in America. Twenty-five percent of adults[40] and 19% of high school seniors[41] smoke regularly. Smoking has been held responsible for as much as 10% of the cost of illness[42] and at least 18% of all deaths,[43] and tobacco is considered an important **gateway drug.**[44] In other words, for many youths cigarettes are the first step to using other drugs. Adolescents who don't smoke are unlikely to use other drugs, such as marijuana and cocaine. Conversely, youth who smoke cigarettes are much more likely than their nonsmoking peers to go on to using other drugs.

One of the things that accelerated the antitobacco movement was the revelation of the hazards of **secondhand smoke.**[45] Many smokers were willing

to risk the health hazards of smoking for themselves because of the perceived benefits that they received in the short run or because they found smoking cessation too difficult. However, when it became well known that smoke could hurt those in proximity, including children, smoking became socially incorrect. Cigarette smoking now carries a social stigma, and this negative social pressure has been one of the most important factors motivating people to quit in the last 20 years.

The antitobacco campaign will continue in the future. Key initiatives will include school-based instruction, more limits on marketing and promotion, financial incentives through health insurance mechanisms to reward nonsmoking, litigation against tobacco companies for smoking-related illness and death, more access to smoking cessation materials and technology, increased purchase prices through taxation, further limits to smoking in public, and further limits to young people's access to tobacco products.

Alcohol Since Prohibition

With the repeal of national prohibition, the right to control alcohol consumption was left up to the individual states. Some states continued their own prohibition laws or permitted "local option" referendums that would decide the "wet or dry" issue on a county or city level. Other than these and other legal controls, such as drunk-driving laws, alcohol was not earnestly addressed as a drug problem until the 1970s. During the 1970s, some educational approaches (e.g., "responsible use") and public policies (e.g., lowering the minimum drinking age) actually made things worse.

Alcohol consumption decreased during the Prohibition years, but rose at the time of repeal. The trend since about 1930 has been one of continuous increases in per capita consumption, up until about 1980.[46] Since 1980, alcohol consumption has consistently declined, as shown in Figure 2.2.

Alcohol increasingly has been recognized as a drug, and as perhaps the most serious drug problem we have. After years of almost exclusive focus on illegal drugs, alcohol is finally getting its due:

Laws are getting tougher, ever-greater restrictions are being placed on marketing and sales, taxes are being increased, and more and more educational resources are being directed toward reducing alcohol abuse.

Summary

Distinct from other animals, humans are characterized by being relentless seekers of new understanding of life and the world around them. This bent might be epitomized by Boorstin's comment, "All the world is still an America."[47] One hopes that discoveries are for our betterment, but some are directed to making the life we have more instantly pleasurable. There will undoubtedly be drug use and abuse in the future, and there will also be new drugs and new patterns of use. The intent of this book is to prepare professionals with tools that are suitable for meaningful prevention activities in the present and for future challenges as well. The history that has been recounted here should help guide the way.

Scenario | Analysis and Response

Ms. Dominguez is quite surprised at what she finds in doing the newspaper search. She had assumed that drug use was a modern phenomenon, but instead learned that there is a rich and complex history surrounding alcohol, tobacco, and other drugs. The thoughts and comments of the grandparents were animated and insightful, and brought encouragement to the children that they too could pass through the hazards of drug abuse and grow up to have happy lives.

Learning Activities

1. Visit a local museum and try to find exhibits of patent medicines. From the exhibit, learn the ingredients of the medicine and for what it was used.
2. Go to the library and find articles and photos on the Prohibition era. Include a search of newspaper records.
3. Write a short biography of Harry J. Anslinger, focusing particularly on his career in federal drug control.
4. View a copy of *Reefer Madness* from a local video shop. Critique the video in light of your current knowledge of marijuana.
5. Interview someone who was a college student in the 1960s. Find out his or her experiences with and memories of drug and alcohol use during those years. Compare his or her account with your own experience.
6. Audit copies of magazines from the 1940s, 1950s, 1960s, 1970s, 1980s, and 1990s. Observe and document the changes that took place in cigarette advertising.

Notes

1. Gen. 9:20, 21.
2. Homer, *Iliad*, VI, 261.
3. Homer, *Odyssey*, XIV, 464.
4. T. Nicholson, "The Primary Prevention of Illicit Drug Problems: An Argument for Decriminalization and Legalization," *Journal of Primary Prevention* 12, 4 (1992): 275–288.
5. J. M. Scott, *The White Poppy: A History of Opium* (New York: Funk & Wagnalls, 1969).
6. S. H. Snyder, "What Have We Forgotten About Pot?" *New York Times Magazine*, December 13, 1970.
7. Peter T. White, "Coca: An Ancient Indian Herb Turns Deadly," *National Geographic* January 1989, 3–97.
8. Egon Caesar Corti, *A History of Smoking* (London: George G. Harrap, 1931).
9. Ashley Grossman, "Endorphins: Opiates for the Masses," *Medicine and Science in Sports and Exercise* 17, 1 (1985): 101–105.
10. Oliver Wendell Holmes, "Currents and Counter-currents in Medical Science," quoted in *Familiar Medical Quotations*, Maurice B. Strauss, ed. (Boston: Little, Brown, 1968), 124.
11. R. E. Schultes and A. Hofmann, *Plants of the Gods* (New York: McGraw-Hill, 1979).
12. N. Taylor, *Plant Drugs That Changed the World* (New York: Dodd, Mead, 1965).
13. G. C. Stewart, "A History of the Medicinal Use of Tobacco, 1492–1860," *Medical History* 11 (1967): 228–268.
14. M. Keller and C. Gurioli, *Statistics on Consumption of Alcohol and on Alcoholism* (New Brunswick, NJ: Rutgers Center of Alcohol Studies, 1976).

15. Thomas M. Nephew, Gerald D. Williams, et al., *Apparent Per Capita Alcohol Consumption: National, State, and Regional Trends, 1977–97*, Surveillance Report 51 (Washington, DC: U.S. Department of Health and Human Services, 1999).

16. Keller and Gurioli, *Statistics on Consumption of Alcohol and Alcoholism*.

17. W. J. Rorabaugh, *The Alcoholic Republic: An American Tradition* (New York: Oxford University Press, 1979).

18. Edward Brecher, *Licit and Illicit Drugs* (Boston: Little, Brown, 1972).

19. J. E. Brooks, *The Mighty Leaf* (Boston: Little, Brown, 1952), 274–275.

20. Ellen G. White, *The Ministry of Healing* (Mountain View, CA: Pacific Press Publishing Association, 1905), 326–330.

21. David F. Musto, *The American Disease: Origins of Narcotic Control* (New York: Oxford University Press, 1987), 9.

22. James A. Inciardi, "Over-the-Counter Drugs: Epidemiology, Adverse Reactions, Overdose Deaths, and Mass Media Promotion," *Addictive Diseases: An International Journal* 3 (1977): 253–272.

23. James A. Inciardi, *The War on Drugs II* (Mountain View, CA: Mayfield Publishing, 1992), 2, 3.

24. Brecher, *Licit and Illicit Drugs*.

25. Ibid.

26. J. Helmer and T. Vietorisz, *Drug Use, the Labor Market and Class Conflict* (Washington, DC: The Drug Abuse Council, 1974).

27. White, "Coca."

28. Grossman, "Endorphins."

29. David F. Musto, prepared testimony delivered before the House Select Committee on Narcotics Abuse and Control, Washington, DC, September 29, 1988.

30. J. Reneau, T. Nicholson, J. White, and D. Duncan, "The General Well-Being of Recreational Drug Users: A Survey on the WWW," *International Journal of Drug Policy* 11 (2000): 315–323.

31. T. Nicholson, J. White, and D. Duncan, "A Survey of Adult Recreational Drug Use Via the World Wide Web: The DRUGNET Study," *Journal of Psychoactive Drugs* 31, 4 (1999): 415–422.

32. Brecher, *Licit and Illicit Drugs*, 212.

33. Ibid., 230.

34. Moses Barron, reported to Minnesota State Medical Society, August 25, 1921, cited in E. Brecher and R. Brecher, *The*

Consumers Union Report on Smoking and the Public Interest (Mount Vernon, NY: Consumers Union, 1963), 13–14.

35. M. Johnston Lennox, "Tobacco Smoking and Nicotine," *Lancet* 243 (December 19, 1942): 742.

36. E. C. Hammond and D. Horn, "Smoking and Death Rates— Report on Forty-four Months of Follow-Up of 187,783 Men. II. Death Rates by Cause," *Journal of the American Medical Association* 166, 11 (March 15, 1958): 1294–1308.

37. U.S. Department of Health, Education, and Welfare, *Smoking and Health: Report of the Advisory Committee to the Surgeon General of the Public Health Service,* PHS Publication No. 1103 (Washington, DC: Government Printing Office, 1964).

38. A. Blum, "Circumvention of the Television Ban on Tobacco Advertising," *New England Journal of Medicine* 324, 13 (March 28, 1991): 913–917.

39. K. E. Warner, "Effects of the Antismoking Campaign: An Update," *American Journal of Public Health* 79, 2 (February 1989): 144–151.

40. Centers for Disease Control and Prevention, "Cigarette Smoking Among Adults—United States, 1997," *Morbidity and Mortality Weekly Report,* November 5, 1999.

41. "Drug Trends in 1999 Among American Teens Are Mixed," press release, U.S. Department of Health and Human Services, December 17, 1999.

42. U.S. Office of Technology Assessment, *Smoking-Related Deaths and Financial Costs* (Washington, DC: OTA, September 1985).

43. Estimates of tobacco-related mortality range from 390,000 to 500,000. Annual deaths in the United States were 2,404,598 in 1990. Tobacco-related deaths are between 16% and 21%.

44. R. R. Clayton and C. G. Leukefeld, "The Prevention of Drug Use Among Youth: Implications of 'Legalization,' " *Journal of Primary Prevention* 12, 4 (1992): 389–392.

45. U.S. Department of Health and Human Services, *The Health Consequences of Involuntary Smoking: A Report of the Surgeon General,* DHHS Publication No. (CDC) 87-8398 (Rockville, MD: DHHS, 1986).

46. Rorabaugh, *The Alcoholic Republic.*

47. Daniel J. Boorstin, *The Discoverers* (New York: Random House, 1983), vxi.

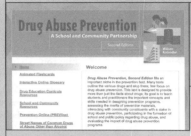

Chapter Learning Objectives

Upon completion of this chapter, students will be able to:

1. Compare the various types of alcoholic beverages and summarize their capacity to intoxicate.

2. Describe patterns of alcohol consumption in the population over time.

3. Compare and contrast the consequences of moderate versus excessive alcohol consumption.

4. Explain and illustrate challenges to the prevention of alcohol abuse.

5. Outline the health and other consequences of using tobacco products.

6. Contrast the efforts to prevent smoking with the counterefforts of the tobacco industry.

7. Explain the rationale for the national Tobacco Master Settlement Agreement of 1998.

8. Outline the provisions of the settlement and describe the implementation.

Scenario

The Smythe County Anti-Drug Coalition consists of dedicated and concerned parents, school personnel, law enforcement officers, clergy, and representatives of the media and business communities. The coalition has good representation from the community, but Smythe County is a small, rural community, and the resources available for programs are few. The coalition wants to maximize its impact on drug problems, especially among young people, and is debating how best to invest its budget.

Some in the coalition believe there should be a focus on the entire drug problem, including alcohol, tobacco, and other drugs. Others think a focus on the most important issue is the right approach, but are not sure what *is* the most important issue, or how it can be determined.

How should the coalition proceed? What factors should be considered, and what steps should be taken in making this important decision?

Chapter 3

Alcohol and Tobacco: Fugitives from the War on Drugs

Introduction

The status of a chemical substance with respect to state and federal drug laws is not very revealing of the nature of a drug's effects or potential for addiction or other harm. This is because the drug laws are influenced by political and bureaucratic considerations, not just science. Valid or not, society has chosen to make some drugs illegal for possession and personal consumption while others are entirely legal, or prohibited only to the young. The authors have decided to emphasize alcohol and tobacco as the most serious and damaging drug problems, regardless of these substances' current legal status. This chapter treats alcohol and tobacco exclusively. The chapters to follow discuss caffeine, over-the-counter and prescription drugs, and illegal drugs, including narcotics, stimulants, sedatives and hypnotics, and hallucinogens.

The reader should recognize that what is presented in this and the next two chapters is not an exhaustive discussion of the body of knowledge on drugs of abuse. Many excellent books are available that provide precisely that.[1,2] The purpose of this book is to teach drug abuse prevention, not drugs. Although being knowledgeable concerning drug facts will support effective drug education and prevention, it is only a limited prerequisite. Furthermore, the authors want to reinforce the concept that effective drug education is not just about teaching drug information. Educators and prevention specialists must have an adequate knowledge base of drug information to feel confident in their drug education efforts and to not be intimidated by perceptions that adolescents have superior knowledge in this regard. However, drug facts are the least important component of drug education, and therefore this and the next chapters give only highlights. We have tried to include what we believe is the basic minimum information required for those aspiring to be effective drug educators.

Alcohol

If one were to intersect frequency of use with the magnitude of undesirable consequences, alcohol would be pinpointed as society's most serious drug problem. That is, alcohol is among the most widely and heavily used drugs, and it does more harm than all other drugs. On the other hand, its moderate use enhances the quality of life for many people, marking special events such as weddings and graduations, playing a prominent role in religious traditions, and bringing pleasure and sociable relaxation to lives beset with boredom and anxiety. This is the great paradox of drug education.

Alcohol comes in three principal forms: beer, wine, and distilled spirits. Differences between these beverages are illustrated in **Figure 3.1**. While the alcohol content of these forms varies, it is important to understand that in standard serving sizes they have very similar amounts of pure alcohol. This is because beer and wine, which have lower percentages of alcohol, are served in larger quantities, whereas distilled beverages, which have greater concentrations of alcohol, are served in smaller amounts. This puts to rest the notion that beer and wine are somehow less dangerous or harmful than liquor. Many parents mistakenly are less concerned about their teenager's drinking because it is "only" beer. In fact, beer is responsible for more alcohol-related auto crashes than the other forms of alcohol.[3]

Things get more complex when variations in the three basic alcoholic beverage types enter into the discussion. While most beer has about 4% or 5% alcohol content, malt liquor has up to 8%. Yet malt liquor may be sold in the same size can as beer. Drinking 12 ounces of malt liquor can deliver 100% more alcohol than a similar can of beer. Recently, malt liquor has been marketed in containers as large as 64 ounces; a 40-ounce bottle of malt liquor can be purchased for as little as $2.00.[4]

A more common example of variation is the wine cooler. First introduced in the early 1980s, by 1986, wine coolers accounted for 25% of all U.S. wine sales.[5] Wine coolers were innovations because they are easy to drink and flavored more like soft drinks. The cynical among us might suspect that this was designed by the producers to appeal to consumers, such as youngsters, who did not like the taste of conventional alcoholic beverages. According to a national survey done by *Weekly Reader*, only 27% of students in grades 4

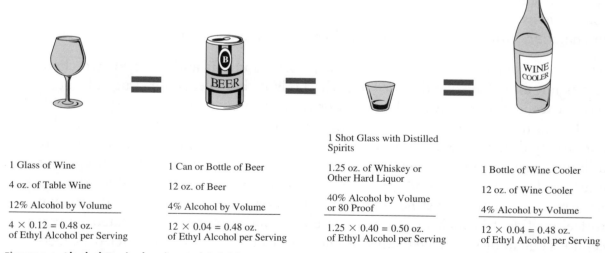

1 Glass of Wine	1 Can or Bottle of Beer	1 Shot Glass with Distilled Spirits	1 Bottle of Wine Cooler
4 oz. of Table Wine	12 oz. of Beer	1.25 oz. of Whiskey or Other Hard Liquor	12 oz. of Wine Cooler
12% Alcohol by Volume	4% Alcohol by Volume	40% Alcohol by Volume or 80 Proof	4% Alcohol by Volume
$4 \times 0.12 = 0.48$ oz. of Ethyl Alcohol per Serving	$12 \times 0.04 = 0.48$ oz. of Ethyl Alcohol per Serving	$1.25 \times 0.40 = 0.50$ oz. of Ethyl Alcohol per Serving	$12 \times 0.04 = 0.48$ oz. of Ethyl Alcohol per Serving

Figure 3.1 Alcohol Equivalencies and Drinking Note: Of course, the above calculations would not apply if a dessert wine were consumed in place of table wine, if a higher-alcohol-content beer or a "lite beer" were drunk instead of regular beer, or if higher-proof distilled spirits were used in place of 80-proof liquor.

to 6 identified wine coolers as drugs;[6] a national survey done in 1991 found that 42% of junior and senior high students who drank identified wine coolers as their favorite drink.[7] The survey also projected that this age group drank 35% of all wine coolers sold in the United States. The 2000–2001 PRIDE survey reported that 49% of high school students had consumed wine coolers in the previous year, 1 percentage point less than had consumed beer.

The second concern about wine coolers is that some may be as high as 9% alcohol by volume. At that level, drinking a 12-ounce wine cooler is not like drinking a can of beer but more like drinking 12 ounces of malt liquor. Given that many young people don't even recognize that these beverages are alcoholic, this becomes a significant concern for parents and drug educators.

More recent additions to alcohol product variation are hard cider, hard cola, and hard lemonade. Many believe that these so-called alcopops (sweet, fruit-flavored, malt-based drinks) appeal more to teenagers than to adults and that teens are more likely to consume them. The products come in hip, bright, and colorful youth-oriented packaging. The labels resemble nonalcoholic lemonade, fruit punches, and soft drinks—all popular with teens—and often do not disclose the alcohol content.[8]

Given that all types of alcoholic beverages are potentially hazardous, the critical issue is this: How much is a person drinking, and how often does he or she drink? The type of beverage is only a secondary concern.

Another issue is alcohol consumption by young people. In many European countries, children commonly drink alcohol in family settings and typically experience no negative consequences. However, in our society, adults have traditionally forbidden children to drink, particularly since the repeal of national alcohol prohibition. Even without legal restraints, social attitudes have supported this restriction. The rationale is that alcohol consumption is adult behavior; children and adolescents are emotionally and developmentally not capable of responsible drinking. The maturity and self-restraint required for the safe use of alcohol are not found in inexperienced and impulsive youth. Furthermore, teens do not practice moderate social drinking; they drink to get drunk. This view sounds more like ideology than fact, and it is hard to document. Table 3.1 shows statistics from the 2000 National Institute of Drug Abuse's National Household Survey on Drug Abuse.[9] The figures show that 12- to 17-year-olds drink less frequently than older groups. However, this doesn't answer the question about whether they drink heavier when they do drink. Table 3.1 shows that 10.4% of teens binge drank in the past month, compared with 37.8% of 18- to 25-year-olds and 30.3% of 26- to 34-year-olds. The 2001 Monitoring the Future survey determined that 16.6%, 39.9%, and 53.2% of 8th, 10th, and 12th graders, respectively, had been drunk in the last year. Several studies have shown that current and heavy drinking tend to increase through about age 22 and decline afterward.[10]

	Table 3.1		
		Drinking Frequency by Age, 2000		

Age	Lifetime (%)	Past Year (%)	Past Month (%)	Past-Month Binge (%)
12–17	41.7	33.0	16.4	10.4
18–25	84.0	74.5	56.8	37.8
26–34	89.2	75.1	58.3	30.3
35+	85.0	61.0	46.8	16.4

Source: National Household Survey of Drug Abuse, 2000.

Thus, it is true that many young people drink large quantities, and they do so frequently. Prior to the late 1980s, minimum drinking ages varied among the states from as low as 16 to as high as 21. During the 1970s there was a national movement to lower the minimum drinking age. This was driven by youth activism, commercial interests, the 26th amendment to the Constitution having given voting privileges to 18-year-olds, and the platitude that if 18-year-olds could die in Vietnam, they ought to be able to buy a brew at their local tavern. It was also supported by the state of the art in prevention at that time, which believed that keeping alcohol consumption forbidden to those under 21 created an aura of forbidden fruit that made alcohol even more appealing as a symbol of adulthood and created much more destructive drinking practices on the part of adolescents.

The natural experiment that ensued consisted of most states lowering the minimum drinking age, followed several years later by a reversal of the trend. By the late 1980s, every state in the United States had raised the drinking age to 21. Epidemiologists learned that when the drinking age was lowered, youth did more drinking, as indicated by more of them being killed or injured in highway crashes. When the drinking age was raised to 21, the highway fatality rates declined. Estimates are that the 21-year-old minimum legal drinking age saves about 1,000 youths from highway fatalities each year in the United States.

Although the minimum drinking age of 21 is not entirely effective, teens drink less than they would if the age limit were lower. Given the facts that most Americans support the current drinking age, that the 21-year minimum saves lives, and that it is the law of the land, the authors believe that prevention programs should encourage nondrinking lifestyles for those under 21. In some circumstances, other alternatives may also be appropriate, such as postponing first use of alcohol or diminishing excessive drinking.

Trends in Alcohol Consumption

During the 1980s and early 1990s, alcohol consumption declined consistently, year by year. However, since 1995 there has been virtually no

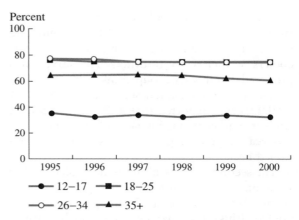

Figure 3.2 **Past-Year Use of Alcohol by Age, 1995–2000**

Source: National Household Survey on Drug Abuse.

change in reported alcohol use. (See **Figure 3.2.**) This is demonstrated by the Monitoring the Future survey and the National Household Survey on Drug Abuse. Liver cirrhosis mortality and alcohol-related traffic fatalities have continued to decline. (See **Figures 3.3** and **3.4.**) On the other hand, the prevalence of binge drinking by people in their early 20s has increased in recent years. (See **Figure 3.5.**)

It is difficult to attribute the changes in ATOD use prevalence. When the trends are going in the desired direction, the tendency is to take credit for the progress, citing the efforts of various prevention strategies. However, when the trends are stagnant or moving in the wrong direction, it is easier to blame other factors rather than to consider that perhaps our prevention strategies are not working. In reality, ATOD use is influenced by a variety of known and unknown factors. Some of the known factors we *can* influence (e.g., greater public awareness about the hazards of heavy drinking, increased attention to alcohol in school-based prevention programs, greater interest in healthful living in general) and some we cannot (e.g., the aging of the population—older people drink less).

It has been conjectured that women are drinking more than in the past, as an outgrowth of feminism and women's liberation; evidence does not support such a trend. However, among women who do drink, there seems to be more binge drinking

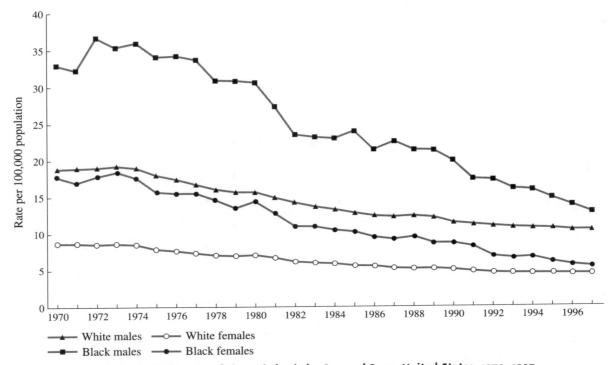

Figure 3.3 Age-Adjusted Death Rates of Liver Cirrhosis by Sex and Race, United States, 1970–1997

Source: F. Saadatmand, F. S. Stinson, B. F. Grant, and M. C. Dufour, *Liver Cirrhosis Mortality in the United States, 1970–97*, Surveillance Report 54 (Rockville, MD: NIAAA, Division of Biometry and Epidemiology, Alcohol Epidemiologic Data System, December 2000).

by those in their early 20s.[11] (See **Figure 3.6.**) Geographic differences in alcohol consumption have also been noted. There is great variation from state to state and from country to country. However, the consumption figures must be interpreted with care; not all alcohol sold in an area is purchased by residents. Tourists may buy more alcohol than others, and consumers may travel from one state to another to take advantage of a lower tax rate. Nevertheless, people in some places do seem to drink more than others. (See **Figure 3.7** and Table 3.2.)

Patterns in drinking can also be found by racial groups. Overall drinking levels are higher for whites than African Americans, but African Americans tend to have more drinking-related problems, perhaps because of interactions with other differences unrelated to drinking (e.g., socioeconomic status). It is unknown whether African Americans differ from whites in biological vulnerability to alcohol.

Among the different Hispanic groups in the United States, there is much diversity in alcohol consumption. Drinking among Hispanics is also influenced by the degree of acculturation: As people become more like the dominant American culture, their drinking patterns become more like those of the general population. However, Hispanic men drink more than other white men, while Hispanic women drink less than other white women. The prevalence of alcohol-related problems is higher among Hispanic men than among African American or other white men.

Among racial groups, Asian Americans have the lowest rate of alcohol consumption and alcohol-related problems. Among American Indians and Alaska Natives, drinking varies by group (or tribe), so generalizations are not possible: Some groups have very high rates of consumption and problems, whereas others have very high rates of abstaining from alcohol.

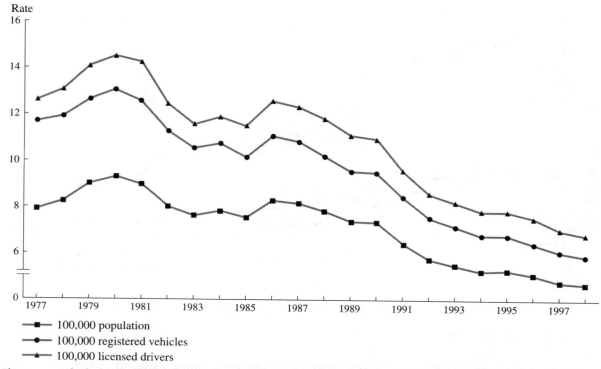

Figure 3.4 **Alcohol-Related Traffic Fatality Rates per 100,000 Population, Registered Vehicles, and Licensed Drivers, United States, 1977–1998**

Source: H. Yi, F. S. Stinson, G. D. Williams, and M. C. Dufour, *Trends in Alcohol-Related Fatal Traffic Crashes, United States, 1977–98*, Surveillance Report 53 (Rockville, MD: NIAAA, Division of Biometry and Epidemiology, Alcohol Epidemiologic Data System, December 2000).

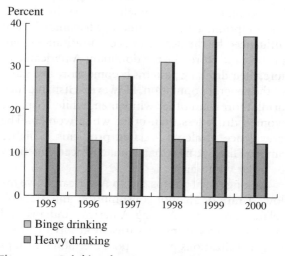

Figure 3.5 **Drinking by 18- to 25-Year-Olds, 1995–2000**

Source: National Household Survey of Drug Abuse.

The Dynamics of Alcohol Consumption

When alcohol is swallowed, normal digestive functions begin taking place immediately. Alcohol enters the bloodstream in a matter of minutes, being absorbed first from the stomach and then from the small intestines. Absorption is accelerated if the stomach is empty or if a carbonated beverage accompanies the alcohol. As alcohol enters the circulatory system, its presence is measured by **blood alcohol level (BAL)**. In some states, a BAL of 0.1% (one-tenth of 1%) means the driver is legally drunk. However, a growing number of states, currently 34 (see **Figure 3.8**), and other countries (e.g., Canada) maintain a legal limit of 0.08%. Public support is increasing for implementing a limit of 0.00% for drivers under the legal drinking age.[12]

Figure 3.9 presents approximate BALs by number of drinks consumed and the weight of the

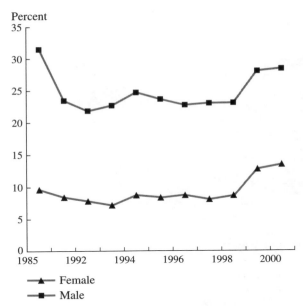

Percent

Female
Male

Figure 3.6 Binge Drinking by Gender, 1985–2000
Source: National Household Survey on Drug Abuse.

Table 3.2

Spirits Consumption (Pure Alcohol) in Selected Countries, 1999

Nation	Liters per Person
Russia	6.5
Latvia	5.6
Romania	4.7
Slovak Republic	4.3
Thailand	3.1
China	3.0
Japan	2.5
France	2.4
Germany	2.0
United States	1.9
Canada	1.8
United Kingdom	1.5
Mexico	0.7
Italy	0.5
Turkey	0.4
Argentina	0.3

Source: Productschap voor Gedistilleerde Dranken, *World Drink Trends*, *2000* (Henley on Thames, UK: NTC Publication, 2000).

drinker. It illustrates that the more drinks a person consumes within a given period of time, the higher the BAL and the level of intoxication. The other variable is body weight. A small person will register a higher BAL than a larger person in response to an identical amount of alcohol because a greater proportional dose goes to the brain of the smaller person. Because the average woman is smaller than the average man, women will usually show signs of intoxication before men when they drink the same amount. Other biochemical differences between men and women also account for women's lesser ability than men to tolerate alcohol.

In addition to how much alcohol is consumed, the speed of consumption, and the size of a person, other factors affect BAL and the amount of intoxication caused by drinking. These factors include whether drinking is done with food or on an empty stomach. Food in the stomach competes with alcohol for absorption and tends to slow the entrance of alcohol into the bloodstream. In addition, eating helps a person feel full, giving a signal that the person has had enough.

Another important factor that influences intoxication is illness. When a person's energy and vitality are decreased due to sickness, he or she will often have less resilience to counteract the effects of alcohol. Drinking and driving will help to illustrate. If a person drinks alcohol, it will interfere with his or her vision, reflexes, reaction time, and judgment, all of which are necessary for safe driving. Illness alone may dull the driver in those same ways. Together, alcohol and sickness make driving even more dangerous. This situation may be compounded by the sick person taking medication, which may exaggerate the dulling effects that alcohol has on driving.

Several other factors may also come into play. Evidence indicates that some people have a qualitatively different early experience to alcohol. This biological characteristic may be a marker that they are at high risk for alcohol abuse problems.[13] A person's mood and expectation of what drinking will do to or for him or her also affect the nature and degree of intoxication.[14] That is, attitudes about a particular drinking situation may interact with the simple drug effects of alcohol.

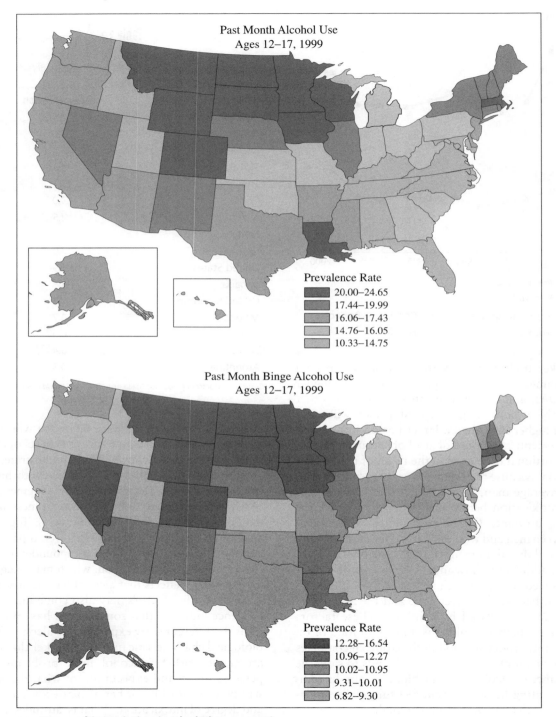

Figure 3.7 Geographic Variation in Alcohol Consumption, 1999

Source: National Household Survey on Drug Abuse.

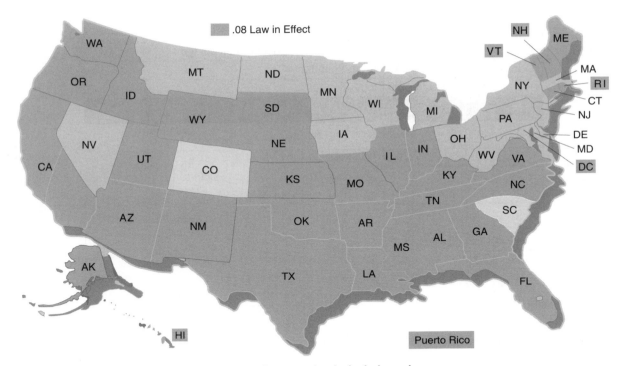

Figure 3.8 States with an Intoxication Limit of 0.08% Blood Alcohol Level, 2002

Source: National Commission Against Drunk Driving.

As BAL rises, a person will experience a range of physical and psychological changes stemming from the fact that alcohol is a central nervous system depressant. Changes begin with a slight mood elevation and a feeling of warmth and relaxation. Usual social inhibitions are lowered, enabling the person to talk, dance, or otherwise participate in activities with other people much more freely. Impairment of judgment soon begins. At about this time, as drinking continues and BAL rises, reaction time increases and muscle coordination decreases. All of this occurs after about two drinks for most people. Although the drinker is not drunk as usually understood, he or she should not drive for at least an hour after drinking that amount and reaching this level of intoxication. Other activities, such as operating machinery, also pose significantly increased risk. (See **Figure 3.10**.)

If drinking continues, BAL continues to rise. The drinker loses ambulatory balance, and speech, vision, and hearing become slightly impaired. As BAL escalates, these losses become more evident and magnified. Judgment becomes more severely impaired, the drinker finds it difficult to move without assistance, and his or her sensory perceptions are extremely distorted or limited. If a person is not drinking at a very fast pace, BAL gradually rises until the person becomes unconscious, causing the drinking bout to cease. Once this occurs, BAL begins to drop as alcohol is metabolized and eliminated from the system. However, there is still danger because the excessive alcohol intake can cause vomiting even after the person has passed out; the person may aspirate vomited material into his or her lungs. While this is rare, it is potentially deadly.

If a person is drinking rapidly, enough alcohol can be consumed prior to passing out so that the BAL becomes high enough to cause a fatal overdose. Death occurs because the nervous system mechanism that regulates respiration is shut down by the intoxication, leading to respiratory arrest.

Women										
	Approximate Blood Alcohol Percentage									
Drinks	Body Weight in Pounds									
	90	100	120	140	160	180	200	220	240	
0	.00	.00	.00	.00	.00	.00	.00	.00	.00	Only Safe Driving Limit
1	.05	.05	.04	.03	.03	.03	.02	.02	.02	Impairment Begins
2	.10	.09	.08	.07	.06	.05	.05	.04	.04	Driving Skills Significantly Affected
3	.15	.14	.11	.10	.09	.08	.07	.06	.06	
4	.20	.18	.15	.13	.11	.10	.09	.08	.08	Possible Criminal Penalties
5	.25	.23	.19	.16	.14	.13	.11	.10	.09	
6	.30	.27	.23	.19	.17	.15	.14	.12	.11	Legally Intoxicated
7	.35	.32	.27	.23	.20	.18	.16	.14	.13	
8	.40	.36	.30	.26	.23	.20	.18	.17	.15	
9	.45	.41	.34	.29	.26	.23	.20	.19	.17	Criminal Penalties
10	.51	.45	.38	.32	.28	.25	.23	.21	.19	

Subtract .01% for each 40 minutes of drinking.
One drink is 1.25 oz. of 80 proof liquor, 12 oz. of beer, or 5 oz. of table wine.

Men									
	Approximate Blood Alcohol Percentage								
Drinks	Body Weight in Pounds								
	100	120	140	160	180	200	220	240	
0	.00	.00	.00	.00	.00	.00	.00	.00	Only Safe Driving Limit
1	.04	.03	.03	.02	.02	.02	.02	.02	Impairment Begins
2	.08	.06	.05	.05	.04	.04	.03	.03	Driving Skills Significantly Affected
3	.11	.09	.08	.07	.06	.06	.05	.05	
4	.15	.12	.11	.09	.08	.08	.07	.06	Possible Criminal Penalties
5	.19	.16	.13	.12	.11	.09	.09	.08	
6	.23	.19	.16	.14	.13	.11	.10	.09	
7	.26	.22	.19	.16	.15	.13	.12	.11	Legally Intoxicated
8	.30	.25	.21	.19	.17	.15	.14	.13	
9	.34	.28	.24	.21	.19	.17	.15	.14	Criminal Penalties
10	.38	.31	.27	.23	.21	.19	.17	.16	

Subtract .01% for each 40 minutes of drinking.
One drink is 1.25 oz. of 80 proof liquor, 12 oz. of beer, or 5 oz. of table wine.

Figure 3.9 **Estimated Blood Alcohol Level by Number of Drinks, Body Weight, and Gender**

Source: National Commission Against Drunk Driving.

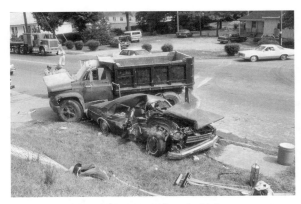

Figure 3.10 A Crash Scene Drunk driving accounts for about 40% of highway accidents and is a leading cause of death. *(© D&I MacDonald/Unicorn Stock Photos)*

Several lessons can be learned from this continuum of intoxication. The first is that impairment occurs before a person feels drunk. Changes may be subtle, yet small changes can significantly increase various safety hazards. The second lesson is that someone else's intoxication level is very difficult to assess.[15] Society expects police officers, bartenders and waitresses, and friends to be able to intervene, preventing someone from either drinking excessively or driving after drinking. However, only when a person is severely impaired—usually well above the legal limit for drinking and driving—is it easy for most people to accurately recognize the signs of dangerous intoxication. (See **Figure 3.11.**)

A third lesson is that "safe drinking," which seeks to avoid long-term consequences and the immediate hazards of too much alcohol, cannot be guided by a person's subjective feelings and impressions while he or she is drinking. Safe drinking guidelines must be based on a specific number of drinks within a specific period of time under a specific set of circumstances for a drinker having a specific set of biological and social characteristics. A series of prevention programs called "Talking About Alcohol and Drugs" approaches responsible drinking in this way. However, the task of responsible drinking is always confounded by the individual's loss of judgment and higher brain functions. Consequently, safe drinking must be promoted and structured in a comprehensive way. Not only does an individual require education and other

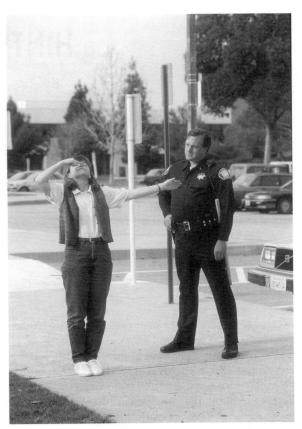

Figure 3.11 Roadside Sobriety Test Many communities are mounting programs such as roadside sobriety tests to reduce drunk driving. *(© David Young-Wolff/PhotoEdit)*

resource inputs, but he or she must also have a range of social and legal supports to encourage moderation and discourage irresponsible behavior.

There are many consequences for excessive drinking, which will be reviewed in the next section. However, it is important to recognize that drinking may bring modest but genuine benefits to many people. Moderate amounts of alcohol can reduce stress, tension, and anxiety,[16] and low levels of drinking can reduce the risk of death from heart disease.[17,18] Moderate drinkers are also less likely than abstainers to be hospitalized.[19,20] The apparent benefits of drinking have been disputed because when moderate drinkers and abstainers are compared on the basis of health status indicators alone, there may be those in the abstainers group who

Alcohol　　**39**

HINTS & TIPS

Moderate Drinking Guidelines

1. No more than one drink per day for most women; no more than two drinks per day for most men. (A drink is defined as 12 ounces of beer, or 5 ounces of wine, or 1.5 ounces of 80-proof distilled spirits.)
2. Those in the following circumstances should not drink:
   - Women pregnant or trying to conceive
   - People planning to drive or engage in other activities requiring attention and skill
   - People taking medication
   - Recovering alcoholics
   - Persons under the age of 21
3. Certain medical conditions, such as stomach ulcer, may also preclude drinking alcohol.
4. The guidelines provide for less drinking by women than men. Reasons include smaller body size, lower levels of a stomach enzyme that breaks down alcohol, and proportionately more body fat and less body water, causing alcohol to become more concentrated in female drinkers. It is also recommended that elderly people drink no more than one drink per day because of changes in body fat content that are part of normal aging.

Source: National Institute on Alcohol Abuse and Alcoholism, "Moderate Drinking," *Alcohol Alert* 16, April 1992.

are current abstainers because of serious health problems. This situation causes a serious flaw in the comparison. However, several studies have examined this issue and found that the health advantage enjoyed by moderate drinkers cannot be totally explained by "sick quitters."[21]

These benefits may be offset by the potential risks of moderate drinking, including certain types of strokes, motor vehicle crashes, harmful interactions with medications, certain types of cancers, birth defects, and the risk that moderate drinking will lead to chronic, excessive consumption.[22]

In summary, it may be said that from a public health or medical perspective, moderate drinking is not harmful for most adults. That is not to say that those who don't drink should start. Many valid reasons exist for someone to choose abstinence; about a third of American adults have made that choice. However, those who do drink moderately should not necessarily be worried.

The critical issue for those who do drink is to determine what moderate drinking is. The U.S. Department of Agriculture and the U.S. Department of Health and Human Services have jointly developed a set of guidelines, presented in the Hints & Tips box. Promoting the guidelines requires some optimism. Most people who drink do not abuse alcohol, even without knowing any particular formal guidelines. Those people who do abuse alcohol are perhaps less responsive to external guidelines, even if they know them. However, there may be a small proportion of current drinkers, translating into a large number of people, who take a prudent approach to life in general and would be ready to heed new information regarding their drinking. More important, establishing and proclaiming the guidelines sets the stage for a gradual change in attitudes about social drinking. As those attitudes move in the direction of greater restraint, they will provide more support to the drinking choices made by individuals. More attention to the consequences of alcohol abuse might also help bring about this change.

Consequences of Alcohol Abuse

As mentioned earlier, about one-third of adults in the United States choose not to drink. Among those who do drink, most don't drink excessively. It is estimated that 10% of drinkers consume about 50% of the alcohol sold; the other 50% of alcohol sold is drunk by the remaining 90% of drinkers.[23] It is therefore a minority of people that experiences or causes most alcohol-related problems.

However, because this small percentage adds up to millions of drinkers, and because the consequences of alcohol abuse always affect many others beyond the drinker, great harm is done to individuals, families, and the society.

By itself, greater individual and public awareness of consequences of alcohol abuse is not sufficient to substantially affect drinking behavior. It can, however, play a role in a comprehensive behavior change program. Educators and prevention specialists need to be familiar with alcohol-related problems and pass the information on to their classes and target groups. It is important to emphasize again that the consequences discussed in this section are not from *any* alcohol consumption, but from *excessive* drinking and drunkenness.

From a societal perspective, alcohol-related death may not be the greatest alcohol-related problem. It is nevertheless significant. Of all deaths in the United States, 3%, or about 103,000 per year, are attributed to alcohol.[24] This number is a conservative estimate because many alcohol-related deaths may be unrecognized or unreported. Specific alcohol-related causes of death include chronic liver disease and cirrhosis; motor vehicle crashes; other types of accidents, such as drowning and fires; suicides; street homicide; and domestic violence. The average victim of these deaths loses 26 years of potential life.[25] About 18% of alcoholics die by suicide. One survey found that men who drink two or more drinks per day are twice as likely to die before age 65 as those who drink 12 or fewer drinks a year.[26]

In addition to mortality, much illness is caused by alcohol abuse. Estimates are that one-fourth of hospitalized patients have alcohol-related problems.[27] Average medical expenses in a family with an alcoholic are often 10 times higher than those for other families; those expenses decline dramatically after the alcoholic enters treatment and begins successful recovery. Some of the specific health problems closely linked to alcohol abuse include liver diseases; inflammation of the esophagus and peptic ulcer; pancreatitis; deficiency and abnormal metabolism of vitamins, minerals, proteins, carbohydrates, and fats; cardiovascular disorders; increased susceptibility to infection; increased risk for cancers of the liver, esophagus, nasopharynx, and larynx; and brain damage.

The surprising thing about the diseases associated with alcohol abuse is that the cause often goes unrecognized: Health professionals fail to distinguish that drinking contributed to the primary diagnosis.[28] This suggests a need for more alcohol education for health professionals. The federal plan for health promotion, Healthy People 2010, has set as an objective the screening and counseling of a greater number of problem drinkers for alcohol abuse by the end of the decade.[29]

The most obvious alcohol-related illness is alcohol dependence, or **alcoholism**. Estimates are that 10.5 million U.S. residents are alcoholics, while an additional 7.2 million drink heavily enough that they will experience serious consequences in the future.[30] Alcoholism presents an array of undesirable secondary problems, including medical problems, criminal behavior, employment problems, financial difficulties, family and relationship problems, and mental disorders. Alcoholism is discussed further in Chapter 12.

Another common and well-known result of alcohol abuse is highway auto crashes. Driving performance drops off dramatically after BAL exceeds about 0.08%. This is illustrated in **Figure 3.12**, which shows the risk of auto crash fatality. The risk of a fatal auto crash at a BAL of 0.10% is eight times higher than normal.[31] Drunk driving also results in many nonfatal injuries. Auto crashes are the number one cause of potential years of life lost prior to age 65. Evidence also indicates that alcohol-related crashes result in death or serious injury more frequently than crashes where alcohol is not involved.[32] In auto crashes that involve pedestrians, motorcycles, or bicycles, the walkers or riders are frequently intoxicated.

Many studies show an association between excessive drinking and injuries due to falls, fires, and drownings. While the evidence strongly suggests that alcohol contributes to these important causes of death and injury, a cause-and-effect relationship has not yet been demonstrated. Similarly, there is a lot of circumstantial evidence linking alcohol abuse with suicide, spouse abuse, child abuse, homicide, and other violent crime. However, a cause-and-effect

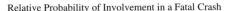
Relative Probability of Involvement in a Fatal Crash

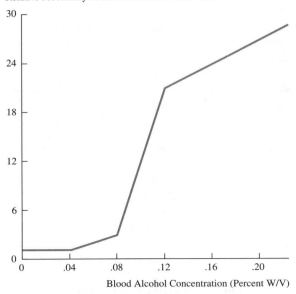

Blood Alcohol Concentration (Percent W/V)

Figure 3.12 **Probability of Involvement in Fatal Crashes for Drivers with Blood Alcohol Concentrations at Given Levels**

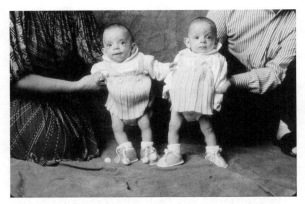

Figure 3.13 **Children with Fetal Alcohol Syndrome**
Fetal alcohol syndrome may cause facial disfigurement in addition to brain and other internal abnormalities.

(© George Steinmetz)

relationship has not yet been proved. If such a relationship were demonstrated, the mechanism would be that alcohol removes inhibitions sufficiently to permit the manifestation of destructive or dysfunctional impulses, or that alcohol makes certain people aggressive and violent as a direct drug effect.

Perhaps the alcohol abuse consequences that receive the least attention in society are fetal alcohol syndrome (FAS) and fetal alcohol effects (FAE). Over the last 10 years, the media have disseminated a lot of information about babies suffering the effects of their mother's crack use during pregnancy. While that may be a significant problem, it is far less common than FAS/FAE. Approximately 9,000 children, 1 in 454, are born with FAS each year in the United States.[33] Another 36,000 suffer from FAE.[34] There is much variation and uncertainty regarding the true prevalence of FAS/FAE because it is often not diagnosed; however, it is known that rates of FAS/FAE are higher in children born to African American and Native American women.

Fetal alcohol syndrome is characterized by growth deficiency, facial and cranial abnormalities, central nervous system dysfunctions, and organ system malformations. (See **Figure 3.13**.) It is one of the leading causes of mental retardation. FAE is similar, with the abnormalities being milder and less frequent. Some of the defects of FAS/FAE, particularly the facial features, may be corrected or show improvement over time. However, the cognitive deficiencies seem least subject to improvement.

Fetal alcohol syndrome is caused entirely by mothers drinking during pregnancy, and therefore is 100% preventable. While many mothers have consumed alcohol during pregnancy with no apparent harm to their offspring, the consensus in the medical community is that the threshold between safe and unsafe drinking for pregnant women is unknown, and therefore women are urged to abstain entirely during the gestation period, and even when they are trying to get pregnant. (See **Figure 3.14**.)

It is possible to attach cost estimates to alcohol-related premature death, disease, accidental property losses, legal expenses, treatment costs, productivity losses, expenses in the criminal justice system, and social services. In 1998, the National Institute of Alcohol Abuse and Alcoholism estimated that the economic costs of alcohol abuse were $148 billion in 1992 and $165 billion by 1995,

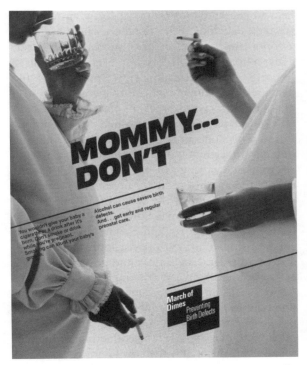

Figure 3.14 A Drug and Pregnancy Poster Culturally sensitive efforts may help reduce drinking during pregnancy. (Courtesy March of Dimes Birth Defects Foundation)

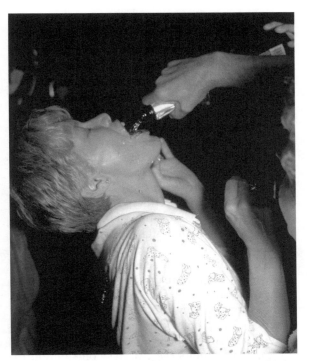

Figure 3.15 A College Drinking Party Abusive drinking is a prominent aspect of social life on most college campuses. (©Jeff Greenberg/PhotoEdit)

which was $640 for every man, woman, and child in the United States, or approximately $22 for every gallon of alcoholic beverages sold.[35] These costs become even more compelling when it is recognized that they are greater than the revenues generated by excise taxes on alcohol.[36] While this may be the least important undesirable consequence of alcohol abuse, it demonstrates a tremendous drain on individual and social resources.

One final concern about alcohol that might catch the attention of students is the impact of drinking on school performance. Although some students at all performance levels use and abuse alcohol, students who drink the most have poorer grade point averages. One study found that good students drank less than a third as much as poor students.[37] Furthermore, it has been reported that alcohol abuse is often the cause of college dropout. Given the fact that drinking tends to peak between the ages of 18 and 22, this association has great

significance for college campuses everywhere. (See **Figure 3.15**.)

Challenges to the Prevention of Alcohol Abuse

Young people recognize that alcohol abuse is a serious problem. Educators recognize that alcohol abuse is a serious problem. Alcoholics recognize that alcohol abuse—at least other people's—is a serious problem. Even the alcohol industry recognizes that alcohol abuse is a serious problem! With this universal recognition, it is fair to ask, "Why can't the problem be solved?"

The answer may be found at many different levels. At the personal level, many people are simply uninformed about the hazards of excessive alcohol drinking, how much is safe, and times when drinking is not safe. There is a continuous need to raise public awareness in this regard. Even when aware of the hazards, many drinkers believe that their personal drinking is normal, appropriate, and harmless, even when it is not. This **denial** response is also experienced by those close to the drinker, such as family members, friends, and coworkers. Human nature being what it is, finding and adhering to a balance between the benefits of alcohol consumption and its dangers are difficult for many people.

Philosophical differences between many alternative views exist. Some people feel that drinking, and even at times drinking to intoxication (occasional binging), brings exhilaration and vitality to life and would therefore only caution others about drinking and driving. Others take a much more conservative, temperate approach, feeling that any drinking to excess is harmful and should be avoided, not only for themselves, but for the community at large. On a different dimension, some people are much more libertarian in sentiment and believe that people should be free to drink any way they want, as long as they don't endanger anyone else. Others feel that society has an investment in every citizen, who should be protected. If excess drinking impairs or limits the citizen's contribution to society, or increases the cost of maintaining him or her in society, the government has an interest in discouraging such drinking.

These alternate points of view are value judgments that cannot be proved or disproved. The best we can hope for is consensus. Because opinions on these issues vary so much, it is difficult to mount an effective prevention campaign: Everyone is marching to a different beat. It may be that the ebb and flow of alcohol and drug abuse that occurs over a period of decades is simply a reflection of the degree of society's consensus regarding the appropriate use of alcohol and how drinking should be addressed by the community.

This lack of unanimity has implications for those in the business of drug abuse prevention. Although directly targeting individual drinking behavior may be important, it is also important to organize communities through citizens' groups, coalitions, task forces, and so forth, with the intent of not only implementing activities but also generating discussion and consensus concerning the basic question "What do we want to do about alcohol drinking in our community?" Consensus on this issue would help to generate more support for environmental strategies such as restrictions on where and how alcohol can be sold, or price increases on beverages. This approach has not been widely used because, as a process, it is slow and difficult and because professionals are more attracted to neat and straightforward program plans with measurable objectives to be accomplished in a given timeframe. This concept of developing consensus and forging partnerships is discussed further in Chapter 9.

Another challenge to prevention efforts is the energy the alcohol industry invests in promoting drinking. This takes the form of TV and radio advertising; ads in magazines and newspapers; sponsorship of sports and cultural events; sponsorship of civic organizations; lobbying of local, state, and federal legislators and government officials; and aggressive marketing campaigns. (See **Figure 3.16**.) In a broader context, alcohol promotion is just a specific example of the conflict between public health concerns and economic interests; other examples include the production and sale of tobacco products and the consideration of safety factors versus cost in the making of automobiles.

At least three points of contention exist between the alcohol industry and the public health interests of society: (1) advertising directed at those under 21; (2) advertising that distorts the place of alcohol in life, suggesting that life is incomplete without drinking, and that success, enjoyment,

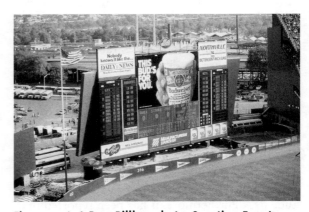

Figure 3.16 A Beer Billboard at a Sporting Event
Alcohol advertising has a pervasive presence in sports arenas and stadiums. (© Richard Hutchings/PhotoEdit)

affluence, popularity, and sexuality all will be limited without drinking; and (3) advertising and marketing designed to increase consumption of alcohol to levels potentially harmful in the short or long term. It is not difficult to find numerous examples of all three. Because the alcoholic beverage producers have great economic power, drug abuse prevention specialists face a daunting challenge in trying to reduce the harm done by alcohol consumption. This topic is addressed further in Chapter 14.

Tobacco

As discussed in Chapter 2, tobacco has a long history in the United States. It has been part of American society from the very beginning. Because of its place in both the urban and rural mainstream, it has only recently been called a drug. Although the barrage of medical science warning of the hazards of tobacco use began in the 1940s and 1950s, it wasn't until the late 1970s that tobacco was consistently linked with the word *drug*. Even the scientific community was initially reluctant to say that tobacco was addicting; instead, the preferred term was **habituating**. This attitude was later to change.[38]

The tobacco industry has fought against grouping tobacco with drugs. *Drug* conjures up images that are repugnant and loathsome to polite society; marketers want to avoid any social connotations surrounding their product that would hurt sales. In Kentucky, the authors' home state, tobacco use is still not addressed as aggressively as in other states, because of the power of the state's tobacco industry.

However, tobacco certainly meets the requirements for being labeled a drug. It contains numerous chemical substances that alter many internal functions, including brain activity. One of the chemicals, **nicotine**, is powerfully addictive. With sufficient exposure, tobacco has devastating effects on health. It is also closely associated with use of other drugs, such as alcohol and marijuana.

In the 1960s, law enforcement agents often proclaimed that marijuana use almost always led the user to harder, more dangerous drugs. This thinking was based on their observation that heroin addicts usually had a history of using marijuana earlier in their lives. The assumption was made that after a period of using marijuana, the drug would no longer satisfy; users would have a craving for something stronger. Although widely believed, this concept was not valid. However, in the late 1970s, the term *gateway drug* was coined, and became more and more associated with tobacco and alcohol.

It is now understood that early use of tobacco is one of the best indications that adolescents are now using or will use alcohol and the illegal drugs in the future. Young people who are smoking in middle school and high school are much more likely to also use other drugs, and young people who don't smoke are much less likely to use any other drugs.[39] Tobacco's addictive properties, the health consequences associated with tobacco use, the burdensome costs of unnecessary medical expenses and productivity losses, and tobacco's role as a principal gateway drug all provide compelling reasons for intensive prevention efforts targeting tobacco.

Tobacco Products

Smoking cigarettes is the predominant way tobacco is used today. However, pipes and cigars are popular, especially in different cultures. Chewing tobacco is quite common as well. Less common but not unknown is drinking tobacco prepared as a liquid, snuffing (inhaling through the nose) powdered tobacco, using tobacco enemas or rectal suppositories, applying tobacco preparations to the skin, and licking a paste-like tobacco preparation called ambil.[40] These alternate consumption methods have similarities and differences. The more exotic ways just mentioned often combine tobacco with other chemical substances, such as herbs with hallucinogenic properties. In addition, they may deliver a much larger dose of nicotine than is commonly taken in mainstream Western society. The larger doses may bring about more exaggerated acute effects, but have less of the long-term damage experienced by typical cigarette smokers.

Tobacco smoking brings additional hazards because burning and high temperatures induce chemical changes that make tobacco even more carcinogenic (i.e., cancer causing). Also, smoking pulls the carcinogens into the lungs, where they cause the single greatest worldwide health consequence of tobacco use: lung cancer. For a number of years, the tobacco industry has been experimenting with a "smokeless" cigarette in an effort to reduce lung cancer.

Trends in Tobacco Consumption

In modern society, the greatest prevention focus regarding tobacco has been on cigarette smoking. Pipes and cigars are much less popular, although cigar use increased in popularity during the 1990s. Chewing tobacco and snuff have seen a resurgence in recent years, particularly in rural areas and on athletic playing fields, but still are used to only a limited extent. Between 1964 and 1986, 17- to 19-year-old American males increased their use of snuff by a factor of four.[41] Table 3.3 presents statistics on cigarette smoking in the United States in 2001. **Figure 3.17** shows consumption of the various types of tobacco products by teens and young adults.

Cigarette smoking has dramatically declined since the mid-1960s. Whereas in 1965, 50% of adult men smoked cigarettes,[42] in 1999 only 25.7% did.[43] Nearly half of all living adults who have ever smoked have quit.[44] It has been estimated that between 1965 and 1985, three-quarters of a million deaths were avoided because of people quitting smoking or fewer people starting.

Women have traditionally smoked less frequently than men. Since World War II, the divide between male and female smoking has gradually decreased, so that now about 22% of women are current smokers, just a little fewer than men. Smoking by African Americans is similar to the rate for whites, whereas Hispanics tend to smoke less.[45] Smoking is also more common in the midsection of the country and in the South than it is in the West and the Northeast. The other demographic change has been that smoking is increasingly being concentrated among persons of low income and less education.[46]

The good news is that smoking declined among young people throughout the 1980s and into the 1990s. **Figure 3.18** shows a general decline in smoking among teens from 1995 to 2001. This suggests

Table 3.3

Cigarette Smoking by Age, Gender, and Frequency, United States, 2001

Age and Gender	Ever Smoked (%)	Past Month (%)
12–17		
Female	33.9	13.6
Male	33.6	12.4
18–25		
Female	66.2	35.7
Male	71.9	42.7
26+		
Female	65.5	22.1
Male	78.2	26.4
Total (12+)		
Female	62.5	23.0
Male	72.3	27.1

Source: National Household Survey on Drug Abuse, 2001.

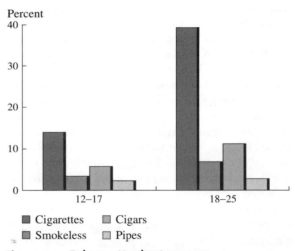

Figure 3.17 Tobacco Use by Age, 2001
Source: National Household Survey on Drug Abuse, 2001.

that the proportion of smokers in the population in the future will continue to decline. The U.S. Public Health Service has established a goal of only 12% of adults being smokers by the year 2010.[47] Unfortunately, there is a 20-year delay between the initiation of smoking and the most serious health consequences of smoking. Consequently, the curve

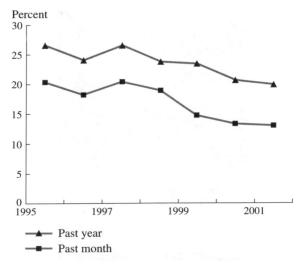

Figure 3.18 Smoking, Ages 12 to 17, 1995–2001
Source: National Household Survey on Drug Abuse.

Legend:
- ▲ Past year
- ■ Past month

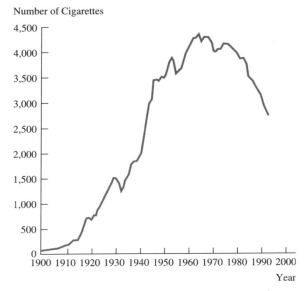

Figure 3.19 U.S. Per Capita Cigarette Consumption, 1900–1991*

*1991 provisional data.

Source: D. R. Shopland, T. F. Pechacek, and J. W. Cullen, "Toward a Tobacco-Free Society," *Seminars in Oncology,* 17 (1990): 402–412.

in the prevalence of smoking (see **Figure 3.19**) will be followed 20 years later by a similarly shaped curve in the incidence of smoking-related death and disease. One illustration of this phenomenon can be seen by looking at cancer deaths. Smoking is the principal cause of lung cancer. Even though smoking has been declining for quite some time, lung cancer deaths have only recently started to decline. The current deaths and diseases are due to smoking in the past. Therefore, it will be a period of years before mortality starts to decline.

How Tobacco Affects the Body

Tobacco smoke contains over 4,000 distinct chemicals, including 43 known to cause cancer.[48] This biochemical knowledge is of great importance to basic medical scientists, but of little practical value for educators and prevention specialists. It is sufficient for the latter group to understand that there are three basic substances found in tobacco smoke.

The first is nicotine, which causes addiction and induces detrimental effects on the cardiovascular system. Smokers actually pace their smoking to maintain a certain blood level of nicotine: If the level is too low, they experience craving and withdrawal symptoms; if it is too high, they have a

toxic reaction that may include nausea, tremors, and nervousness. Smokeless tobacco delivers amounts of nicotine equal to those received from cigarettes. Some smokeless users keep tobacco in their mouths even while they sleep to maintain the desired blood level of nicotine. **Figure 3.20** displays the immediate effects of nicotine.

The next substance is **tar**. Tar is actually composed of numerous substances, but for simplicity's sake it can be said that tar is the tobacco constituent responsible for causing cancer. Because tar is produced by the burning of tobacco and is partly gaseous, it is technically not found in smokeless tobacco. However, there is a counterpart to tar in smokeless tobacco, which also causes cancer. (See **Figure 3.21**.)

Carbon monoxide is the final substance, released only when tobacco is smoked. It is a by-product of combustion (burning) and interferes with the work of red blood cells in delivering oxygen to cells throughout the body. It also damages the walls of blood vessels, accelerating **atherosclerosis**. This contributes to a double whammy: oxygen deficiency

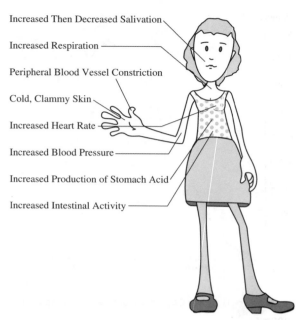

Increased Then Decreased Salivation

Increased Respiration

Peripheral Blood Vessel Constriction

Cold, Clammy Skin

Increased Heart Rate

Increased Blood Pressure

Increased Production of Stomach Acid

Increased Intestinal Activity

Figure 3.20 The Physiological Effects of Nicotine

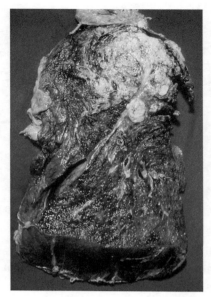

Figure 3.21 Blackened Lung Tar is the principal culprit in tobacco's link to lung cancer. (© Gordon T. Hewlett)

caused by red blood cell impairment in combination with restricted circulation brought on by nicotine. In the short run, this combination causes shortness of breath and limited endurance. In the long run it contributes to the development of heart and circulatory disease.

Health Consequences of Smoking and Other Tobacco Use

The list of specific assaults to health mounted by tobacco on the human body is long. The U.S. Surgeon General has issued annual reports on the health consequences of tobacco use since 1964. A simple summary of these reports might be that tobacco does no good for any part of the body—almost no portion of the body goes unscathed. Recounting all the specific diseases related to tobacco amounts to overkill; highlights are probably sufficient to provoke a desire to quit or to help discourage initiation of use.

In this age of budget deficits and handwringing over health care costs, it should be noted that tobacco use is very costly for society. Tobacco use in the United States has a tab of $75 billion in medical costs and $82 billion in productivity losses per year, an amount greater than the excise taxes levied.[49] Tobacco use accounts for about 5% of the national cost of illness. In 1999, about 22 billion packs of cigarettes were sold in the United States; economic costs per pack averaged $7.18.[50]

Perhaps the first concern regarding tobacco is its deadliness. While estimates vary, the U.S. Surgeon General has stated that about 442,000 deaths per year are attributable to smoking.[51] In the United States and similarly developed countries, smoking is responsible for about 24% of deaths in men and 6% of deaths in women.[52] In the United States this amounts to one in every six deaths overall. Tobacco use also kills many people in developing countries. This year, about 4 million people will die from tobacco worldwide. By 2030, the figure is projected to rise to 10 million per year. If current smoking patterns continue, about 500 million people alive now will die from tobacco-related causes.[53] The problem seems to be getting worse in developing countries. For example, smoking among Chinese men increased from 40% in the 1950s to 63% in 1996. Worldwide, 82% of smokers live in developing countries.[54]

Table 3.4		
Annual Smoking-Attributable Mortality, United States, 1995–1999		
Disease	Deaths
Cancer	155,761
Cardiovascular disease	148,605
Respiratory conditions	98,007
Perinatal conditions	1,006
Burn deaths	966
Secondhand smoke deaths	38,053
Total	**442,398**

Source: U.S. Centers for Disease Control and Prevention, 2002.

Although there are many causes for these excess and unnecessary deaths, lung cancer and heart disease are the biggest contributors. About 80% of lung cancers are thought to be due to smoking. Heart disease is exacerbated by a wide variety of factors, such as high blood pressure and elevated cholesterol; smoking is only one of many causative factors. Additional diseases related to tobacco use include emphysema and chronic bronchitis; stroke; infant mortality; burn deaths; and cancers of the mouth, esophagus, pharynx, larynx, pancreas, cervix, kidney, and urinary bladder. Those who die from tobacco-related illnesses between the ages of 35 and 69 lose an average of 23 years of life.[55] It is no surprise that smoking has been labeled the most preventable cause of death. (See Table 3.4.)

Other health problems associated with smoking include premature aging of the skin, recession of the gums, periodontal disease, and low-birth-weight babies due to mothers smoking during pregnancy. (See **Figure 3.22**.)

While cigarette smoking is the most harmful form of tobacco use, pipes and cigars may have identical consequences, though pipe and cigar smokers seem to smoke less and inhale less deeply. Users of smokeless tobacco suffer the effects of nicotine to the same degree as smokers. They do not inhale carbon monoxide, but they do absorb chemicals that promote cancers of the mouth and throat. In addition, smokeless tobacco promotes receding gums and gingivitis, and the nicotine causes elevated blood pressure and blood lipids (i.e., fat and cholesterol).

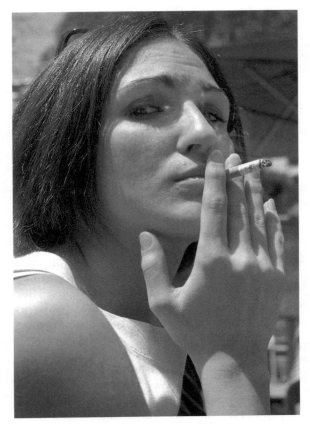

Figure 3.22 **Does Smoking Enhance Beauty?** Cigarette smoking is advertised as glamorous, but it has been shown to accelerate the wrinkling and aging of skin. (© David Young-Wolff/PhotoEdit)

These hazards are very well known, even by smokers. However, some smokers believe that if they have smoked for a long time it is too late for them—the damage already done would make quitting smoking a futile effort. Others think that if they have smoked for a long time and haven't yet been seriously ill, then they must be immune to the effects of tobacco. The truth is that the hazards of smoking don't occur on the same timetable for everyone. One person will suffer effects sooner; another will suffer them later. Given enough time, however, every smoker, snuffer, or chewer will experience health losses due to tobacco. All tobacco users should understand that it is always to their benefit to quit, no matter how long their habit has continued.[56]

All of the serious health concerns just discussed have had an impact on adults; this knowledge has motivated millions of smokers to quit. However, knowledge is not enough for many people. Knowledge may motivate, but smoking is addictive, and more than knowledge about health hazards is required for many people to quit successfully. Strategies for quitting smoking are discussed more thoroughly in Chapter 12. However, there is another limitation to the value of promoting awareness of tobacco's health hazards.

Much of drug education, including tobacco education, has been based on the **information model**, which assumes that people are rational and do not want to suffer harm; therefore, if you tell them about the dangers of some behavior, they will avoid it. This works to a limited degree with adults, but much less so with children and adolescents. Young people have a normal sense of invulnerability: They believe death and disease happen only to old people. Presenting the health hazards of smoking has little personal relevance to most youth. Furthermore, young people may even be enticed by danger. Being told that something is dangerous may be appealing for some. Besides, they know other kids who smoke, and none of these friends or acquaintances has ever had a smoking-related illness. They don't expect to smoke permanently, and certainly not long enough to get all those diseases they've heard about.

Experience has taught us that adolescents are much more motivated by the immediate, short-term consequences of smoking. These consequences include limited endurance in sports, bad breath, yellow teeth, smelly hair, and the perception that people like them do not smoke. In the long run these issues may seem trivial, but they are often influential with teens. The flip side is that many teen girls smoke because they believe it will help them control their weight. This false perception has been nurtured by tobacco ads (e.g., Virginia Slims) and popular lore. In any event, tobacco prevention programs targeting adolescents must prominently feature these short-term effects of smoking. Other issues important in preventing teens from initiating smoking are discussed in Chapter 14.

Secondhand Smoke

For many years, secondhand smoke was a subject of much speculation. People asked, "If breathing smoke through a cigarette is dangerous to health, how safe is it to breathe smoke from someone else's cigarette?" Speculation turned into growing evidence that there was in fact a health risk. In 1987 the U.S. Surgeon General officially declared, "Involuntary smoking is a cause of disease, including lung cancer, in healthy nonsmokers."[57] It has been found that sidestream smoke, which comes from the burning end of a cigarette, is even more carcinogenic than mainstream smoke, which courses though the cigarette's mouthpiece. Children whose parents smoke cigarettes take more sick days each school year than children of nonsmokers. Spouses of smokers are more likely to get lung cancer than spouses of nonsmokers. Currently, secondhand smoke is considered the third most important preventable cause of death in the United States (after primary smoking and alcohol abuse). It is estimated that secondhand smoking causes about 38,000 deaths per year (see Table 3.4.)

The toxicity of and damage done by ambient cigarette smoke is not debated by any legitimate scientist. The tobacco industry, however, true to form, disputes and discounts the evidence. An additional issue is exposure. Sustaining harm from secondhand smoke only comes after sufficient intensity and time of exposure. Casual and infrequent contact with tobacco smoke is unlikely to inflict any damage, although it may be temporarily irritating or unpleasant. However, continuous exposure over a long period of time almost inevitably inflicts harm. Such exposure is likely to occur in two places: at work or at home. Public transportation used to be another site of exposure until smoking was banned on trains, planes, and buses. Not much can be done by government agencies about home exposure—that domain is left to the responsibility and sensibility of family members.

Worksite smoking is a different story. It has been said that smoking causes statistics. It also causes litigation. Employers are in a legal double bind: They are compelled by fair employment standards to protect the right of smokers to smoke, especially if these workers were smokers when hired and had previously been allowed to smoke at work; they are also required by other government regulations to protect the health rights of nonsmokers. Efforts have been made in both directions. For example, companies are providing designated smoking areas for smokers; this is particularly true in the tobacco states of the southeast United States. Many other employers are banning on-premise smoking altogether: Workers may only smoke outdoors, not in the company buildings.

Bans are being enacted for several reasons. More and more, they are being demanded by nonsmoking employees, and there is the threat of civil suits brought by nonsmoking workers against companies. Also, smokers have more health insurance claims and costlier medical bills; these costs are increasingly being carried by business and industry. Finally, smoking bans are a powerful way to encourage people to quit smoking because the hassles imposed on the smoker may be an incentive to quit. Many employers are seeking to cultivate a nonsmoking workforce to lower overhead and increase productivity.

From a prevention perspective, the most important consequence of the attention directed to the hazards of secondhand smoke is that it has changed the social climate for smoking. In the days of innocence, smoking was macho and modern, but also mundane. No one wondered, "Do you mind if I smoke?" Now there is always the nagging thought, "Maybe my smoking is offensive to others." Smoking has become akin to bad breath and body odor and is socially incorrect in many circles.[58] Many smokers who are not primarily motivated by concerns for their own health are now trying to quit for social reasons.

Challenges to the Prevention of Tobacco Use

While striking progress has been made against tobacco consumption in our society, it remains a huge drug problem. Several factors make prevention of tobacco use difficult. First is the addictive nature of tobacco. In spite of what the tobacco industry executives say, nicotine is an addictive drug. (See **Figure 3.23**.) Most early users of tobacco, be it smoking or smokeless, do it because of peer pressure, as a way to exert their independence, or

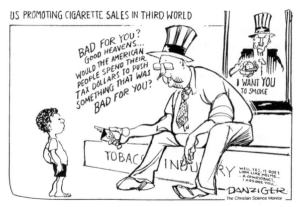

Figure 3.23 Cartoonist Taunts the Tobacco Industry Tobacco companies actively market cigarettes in foreign countries. Many Americans object to the assistance these countries receive from U.S. government trade representatives. (Drawing by Jeff Danziger in *The Christian Science Monitor,* © 1989.)

because they think it is sophisticated. However, it is not their conscious desire to become lifelong, permanent users; they expect that their use will only be for a short-term period. Once they get past the initial difficulty of using, they soon become addicted and, in spite of their desires, find it difficult to quit. Most adult smokers say they wish they had never started and would quit if they could. It is important for prevention programs to make adolescents understand the addictive nature of nicotine.

Another barrier to the prevention of tobacco use is the counterforce of the tobacco industry. Tobacco is the most heavily advertised product in our society, with an annual advertising budget in excess of $5 billion.[59] This advertising takes the form of magazine and newspaper print ads, distribution of promotional items (e.g., t-shirts), point-of-purchase displays, and sponsorship of sports (e.g., Winston Cup Racing, Virginia Slims Tennis Tournament) and cultural events (e.g., Kool Jazz Festival). Billboard tobacco advertising was prohibited by federal law in the late 1990s.

Many in the field of public health and drug abuse prevention find this deluge of cigarette promotion outrageous and consider it another form of drug pushing. The position of the tobacco industry is that it produces a legal product and therefore has the same rights as any other corporation to advertise as it sees fit. The industry denies that advertising influences anyone to smoke in the first place and claims it only modifies brand selection. Ostensibly, a smoker switches to another brand because of advertising, but doesn't start smoking in the first place because of ads.

After the initiation of the Joe Camel campaign, Camel's share of the children's cigarette market increased from 0.5% to 32.8%.[60] Part of the increase may have been due to brand selection among existing smokers, but to say that none of these children were first-time smokers or that the powerful images of the campaign did not facilitate their initiation into smoking is not credible.

In surveys of adolescents who were asked why they started smoking, advertising is given as a reason, but it is less important than parent and peer influences. However, given the severity of the tobacco problem, even minor factors should be addressed. Advertising has an impact, and it is a factor we can influence through public policy, something we can't do with peer or parental influence. (Advertising is treated more extensively in Chapter 14.)

This dilemma raises the side issue of whether tobacco companies target children and youth with their campaigns. The companies say no, yet the images portrayed in campaigns certainly appeal to youth. Past studies found that over 90% of sixth graders could identify Joe Camel, and more youth could associate Joe Camel with cigarettes than could adults.[61] Models in ads are usually young people doing activities that seem exciting to adolescents. Cigarette ads have been banned from television since 1971. However, the industry has been ingenious in getting its images before the television audience—for example, embedded in video footage at sporting events of all kinds.

The other reality, certainly known by tobacco companies, is that if the industry is going to stay in business, those who quit smoking or die must be replaced. These new recruits come from the ranks of teenagers. If teens can be enticed to smoke, they often will become regular customers for many years to come.

Aside from concern with the magnitude and nature of this massive campaign, there are several related issues. It has been recognized for some time that tobacco advertisers control the coverage that magazines devote to smoking and health.[62] In feature stories on good health practices, both *Time* and *Newsweek* have failed to mention smoking as a health hazard: Not surprisingly, the issues in which the features appeared carried many full-page ads for cigarettes.[63] In a study of women's magazines that carried cigarette ads, it was found that almost no coverage was given to the smoking and health issue over a ten-year period. In contrast, women's magazines that didn't advertise cigarettes, such as *Good Housekeeping* and *Seventeen*, included significantly more articles on smoking and health.[64] What this means is that the American public is not receiving full information about the health consequences of smoking. Self-censorship on the part of magazines has led to restricted dissemination of the truth about smoking and health.

This problem becomes even more significant because the tobacco companies are diversified conglomerates that produce and market a variety of other consumer goods, such as food, candy, soft drinks, and alcoholic beverages. Therefore, they can wield power beyond just the value of tobacco ads. A typical scenario follows: A magazine is considering a story on smoking and health. The tobacco company threatens to cancel not only the cigarette ads but also the ads for other products sold by the conglomerate. The magazine succumbs to the threat of losing perhaps millions of dollars in revenue, and so cancels the story. Incidents such as this scenario have occurred.[65]

Because of all these issues, there have been serious calls for the outright ban of tobacco advertising.[66] The tobacco industry has condemned such a suggestion by citing First Amendment rights to free speech and highlighting the economic contributions of the industry through jobs and tax revenue. In this fight they have an unnatural ally—the labor unions of tobacco workers and tobacco farmers. The free speech issue is a red herring: The Constitution does not unequivocally guarantee commercial speech.[67] However, the industry has great power and political influence. It has successfully impeded or at least delayed a wide variety of prevention policy initiatives such as public smoking restrictions,[68] and raising cigarette taxes.

Three events have taken place that are significant in the tobacco campaign. In 1994, the U.S. Congress passed the Synar Amendment (named after Oklahoma Congressman Mike Synar). This legislation stipulated that states must take specific steps to reduce youth access to tobacco. States have relied on millions of federal dollars to help fund their programs in prevention and treatment. The Synar Amendment attached stipulations for receiving these funds. States must prohibit tobacco sales to youth under the age of 18. They must monitor retail tobacco outlets and document that 20% or fewer are selling tobacco to minors. Even though all states now prohibit tobacco sales to minors, surveys show that many retailers continue to make these illegal sales. States enacted policies to comply with the Synar Amendment. Examples include banning cigarette vending machines, conducting youth sting operations to discover illegal sales, and requiring the presentation of IDs by young people making tobacco purchases.

More far-reaching than the Synar Amendment was the 1995 proposal by the U.S. Food and Drug Administration (FDA) to officially declare tobacco a drug, and therefore subject to regulation by the FDA. The FDA has further proposed that

- Age verification be required for tobacco purchases by youth
- Cigarette vending machines be prohibited
- Free samples and single cigarette sales be prohibited
- Tobacco advertising near schools be banned
- Advertising in magazines with more than 15% youth readership be black-and-white text only
- Sale or giveaway of cigarette promotional items be prohibited
- Brand-name sponsorship of sporting or entertainment events be prohibited (corporate-name sponsorship would still be permitted)
- The industry be required to fund ($150 million) a public education campaign to prevent kids from smoking

These initiatives were bitterly opposed by the tobacco industry, politicians with tobacco constituents, retailers, and those who benefit from tobacco advertising dollars. In spite of the support of then-President Bill Clinton and several other former presidents, previous surgeon generals, all of the national health-related professional organizations (e.g., AMA), and many important religious and civic organizations, the FDA proposal has never been implemented. Its very existence was truly remarkable. Only 10 years ago such a proposal would have been politically impossible, but a sea change in public attitudes has occurred that is challenging the traditional dominance of the tobacco industry.

In 1998, the attorneys general of the states came to a historic agreement with the tobacco companies. A couple of years earlier, several states had separately brought suit against the tobacco companies, with the purpose of recouping the cost of using state health care dollars (primarily Medicaid funds) to treat sick smokers. These states documented that taxpayers were carrying a large financial burden because of the medical expenses associated with smoking, and asked the courts for some relief from the tobacco companies. Once the original suits were successful, an avalanche of new suits began, with all the states wanting to participate. Rather than fight 50 separate court battles, the major tobacco companies negotiated a national settlement agreement with the attorneys general of each state.

In what was called the Master Settlement Agreement, the tobacco companies agreed to transfer $246 billion over a 25-year period to compensate states for the Medicaid treatment expenses associated with smoking. There were no restrictions on how the funds could be spent by the states, although the expectation was that funds would be invested in tobacco use prevention and smoking cessation. In addition, the companies agreed to eliminate their billboards and advertising in sports arenas, to no longer use cartoon characters in their marketing material, to not market to young people, and to make millions of pages of internal company documents available to the public. (These documents have been studied thoroughly by researchers, and show much about the marketing strategies of the companies, what they knew about the health consequences of tobacco use, and when they knew it.) Finally, the companies agreed to provide $300 million for five years to support a public education effort to reduce youth tobacco use. This led to the founding of the American Legacy Foundation, which is responsible for the "Truth" mass media campaign, and other initiatives.

Four years after the Master Settlement Agreement, there is much disappointment in the ranks of public health. Only a small portion of the billions of dollars provided by the agreement are actually being used for tobacco-related programs. Most states are using the money for other programs and to balance their budgets. One positive outcome of the settlement is that the tobacco companies have raised prices to help defray their settlement costs. Price increases generally will lead to declines in smoking, particularly among youth.

Summary

Both alcohol and tobacco are widely used drugs in our society. While the prevalence of use and abuse of these drugs decreased in the late 1980s and early 1990s, in recent years progress has stagnated. Both of these drugs extract a huge health and economic cost in the United States and the rest of the world. Deaths associated with smoking number more than all deaths caused by alcohol, AIDS, illegal drugs, traffic accidents, fires, homicides, and suicides combined. It is hard to find more compelling public health problems than those caused by the abuse of alcohol and tobacco.

Both the tobacco and alcohol industries have great power and political influence and have successfully impeded or at least delayed a variety of prevention policy initiatives, such as public smoking restrictions and increased alcohol taxes. Achieving the national objective of reducing adult smoking to 12% by the year 2010 is going to be a dogged fight, if the past is any indication. The objective probably will be met sooner or later. The level of optimism regarding achieving a more reasonable use of alcohol in our society is considerably more muted. Prevention specialists have much work to do in raising awareness and sensitivity to America's two worst drug problems.

Scenario | Analysis and Response

Coalitions have to live in the real world. They have to function with the resources at hand and the level of expertise among the membership. Leaders of coalitions have to gently lead: They can't go from lesson 1 to lesson 25 without covering the ground in between. It is common for directors and program coordinators employed by coalitions to have the advantage of formal training in prevention science and to be familiar with the material discussed in this chapter. However, they have to bring the coalition along at the members' own pace.

For many reasons, large portions of the general public think marijuana and cocaine are America's real drug problems. The material in this chapter should demonstrate otherwise. However, the coalition's director may have to compromise to retain the support of the members. It will be important to conduct local assessments of drug use and to continually highlight the consequences of the various drugs of abuse.

Little by little, most communities are focusing more and more on alcohol and tobacco: Smythe County will probably do the same, though progress will be at their own pace.

Learning Activities

1. Research your local community concerning restrictions on the times and places where packaged alcoholic beverages may be sold. Determine if the restrictions are the same for all types of beverages.
2. Gather statistics on your local campus or a nearby school system concerning the trend over the last five years with respect to use of alcoholic beverages and tobacco products.
3. Go to a store and systematically chart a cross section of beer brands, noting the placement and graphic design of warning labels. Assess the ease with which consumers can recognize and read the warning labels.
4. Interview a physician or other professional employed in an emergency room to determine his or her perspective on alcohol-related

emergency room visits. Find out the frequency and nature of such visits, and how the alcohol abuse is addressed beyond the medical emergency.

5. Interview a sample of cigarette smokers to find out how long they have smoked, why they started, how they feel about smoking now, and what it would take for them to stop.

6. Peruse your local campus and surrounding community to find out what the current restrictions on smoking in public places are.

Notes

1. Oakley Ray and Charles Ksir, *Drugs, Society, and Human Behavior,* 9th ed. (Columbus, OH: McGraw-Hill, 2001).

2. Glen Hanson, Peter Venturelli, and Annette E. Fleckenstein, *Drugs and Society,* 6th ed. (Boston: Jones and Bartlett, 2000).

3. Dale Berger and John Snortum, "Alcoholic Beverage Preference of Drinking and Driving Violators," *Journal for Studies on Alcohol* 46 (1985): 232–239.

4. Marin Institute for Prevention of Alcohol and Other Drug Problems, "Bigger Containers of Potent Beer Brew Big Trouble in Inner City Communities," *Advocacy Action Alert,* March 1, 1993.

5. R. A. Steffens, F. S. Stinson, C. G. Freel, and D. Clem, *Apparent Per Capita Alcohol Consumption: National, State, and Regional Trends, 1977–1986,* Surveillance Report No. 10 (Rockville, MD: National Institute on Alcohol Abuse and Alcoholism, 1988).

6. American Public Health Association, "Policy Statement 9213(PP): Advertising and Promotion of Alcohol and Tobacco Products to Youth," *American Journal of Public Health* 83 (March 1998): 468–472.

7. U.S. Department of Health and Human Services, Office of the Inspector General, *Youth and Alcohol: A National Survey* (Washington, DC: DHHS, 1991).

8. George Hacker, "National Poll Shows 'Alcopop' Drinks Lure Teens: Groups Demand Government Investigate 'Starter Suds,'" press release, Center for Science in the Public Interest, May 9, 2001.

9. Substance Abuse and Mental Health Services Administration, *Summary of Findings from the 2000 National Household Survey on Drug Abuse,* DHHS Publication No. (SMA) 01-3549 (Rockville, MD: DHHS, 2001).

10. U.S. Department of Health and Human Services, *Seventh Special Report to the U.S. Congress on Alcohol and Health,* DHHS Publication No. (ADM) 90-1656 (Rockville, MD: DHHS, 1990), 28.

11. P. Mercer and K. Khavari, "Are Women Drinking More Like Men? An Empirical Examination of the Convergence Hypothesis," *Alcoholism: Clinical and Experimental Research* 14 (May/June, 1990): 461–466.

12. National Highway Traffic Safety Administration, *0.08 BAL Illegal Per Se Level: State Legislative Fact Sheet* (Washington, DC: Department of Transportation, 1996).

13. Joachim Knop, "Premorbid Assessment of Young Men at High Risk for Alcoholism," in *Recent Developments in Alcoholism,* Vol. 3, Marc Galanter, ed. (New York: Plenum Press, 1983).

14. S. A. Brown, "Adolescent Alcohol Expectancies and Risk for Alcohol Abuse," *Addiction and Recovery* 105 (1990): 16–19.

15. James W. Langenbucher and Peter E. Nathan, "Psychology, Public Policy, and the Evidence for Alcohol Intoxication," *American Psychologist,* October 1983, 1070–1077.

16. C. Baum-Baicker, "The Psychological Benefits of Moderate Alcohol Consumption: A Review of the Literature," *Drug and Alcohol Dependence* 15 (1985): 305–322.

17. R. D. Moore and T. A. Pearson, "Moderate Alcohol Consumption and Coronary Artery Disease: A Review," *Medicine* 65 (1986): 242–267.

18. P. Boffetta and L. Garfinkel, "Alcohol Drinking and Mortality Among Men Enrolled in an American Cancer Society Prospective Study," *Epidemiology* 1 (1990): 342–348.

19. A. L. Klatsky and A. B. Friedman, "Alcohol Use and Cardiovascular Disease: The Kaiser-Permanente Experience," *Circulation* 64, Suppl. III (1981): 32–41.

20. M. P. Longnecker and B. MacMahon, "Associations Between Alcoholic Beverage Consumption and Hospitalization, 1983 National Health Interview Survey," *American Journal of Public Health* 78 (1988): 153–156.

21. Boffetta and Garfinkel, "Alcohol Drinking and Mortality"; A. L. Klatsky, M. A. Armstrong, and G. D. Friedman, "Risk of Cardiovascular Mortality in Alcohol Drinkers, Ex-Drinkers, and Nondrinkers," *American Journal of Cardiology* 66 (1990): 1237–1242.

22. National Institute on Alcohol Abuse and Alcoholism, "Moderate Drinking," *Alcohol Alert* 16, April 1992.

23. U.S. Department of Health and Human Services, *Sixth Special Report to the U.S. Congress on Alcohol and Health,* DHHS Publication No. (ADM) 87-1519 (Rockville, MD: DHHS, 1987), 3.

24. U.S. Department of Health and Human Services, *Seventh Special Report.*

25. Centers for Disease Control, "Alcohol-Related Mortality and Years of Potential Life Lost—United States, 1987," *Morbidity and Mortality Weekly Report* 39, 11 (March 23, 1990): 175.

26. National Institute on Alcohol Abuse and Alcoholism, "National Mortality Followback Survey," presented by

Mary Dufour at the American Public Health Association meeting, New York, October 1, 1990.

27. U.S. Department of Health and Human Services, *Seventh Special Report,* xxii.

28. Ibid., 21.

29. U.S. Department of Health and Human Services, *Healthy People 2010,* 2nd ed. (Washington, DC: U.S. Government Printing Office, 2000).

30. U.S. Department of Health and Human Services, *Seventh Special Report,* ix.

31. Ibid., 164.

32. Ibid., 165.

33. Ibid., 140.

34. H. J. Harwood and D. M. Napolitano, "Economic Implications of the Fetal Alcohol Syndrome," *Alcohol Health and Research World* 10, 1 (Fall 1985): 41.

35. National Institutes of Health, "Economic Costs of Alcohol and Drug Abuse Estimated at $246 Billion in the United States," press release, May 13, 1998.

36. W. C. Manning, E. B. Keeler, J. P. Newhouse, E. M. Sloss, and J. Wasserman, "The Taxes of Sin: Do Smokers and Drinkers Pay Their Way?" *Journal of the American Medical Association* 261 (1989): 1604–1609.

37. "Study Shows Heaviest College Drinkers Earn Lowest GPAs," *Prevention Forum* (Fall 1992), 18.

38. U.S. Department of Health and Human Services, *The Health Consequences of Smoking: Nicotine Addiction. A Report of the Surgeon General* (Rockville, MD: DHHS, 1988), 10.

39. D. Kandel and K. Yamaguchi, "From Beer to Crack: Developmental Patterns of Drug Involvement," *American Journal of Public Health* 83 (1993): 851–855.

40. U.S. Department of Health and Human Services, *Smoking and Health in the Americas,* DHHS Publication No. (CDC) 92-8419 (Atlanta, GA: Centers for Disease Control and Prevention, 1992).

41. U.S. Department of Health and Human Services, *Reducing the Health Consequences of Smoking: 25 Years of Progress. A Report of the Surgeon General,* DHHS Publication No. (CDC) 89-8411 (Atlanta, GA: Centers for Disease Control, 1989).

42. Ibid.

43. Public Health Service, *Health, United States, 2001, with Urban and Rural Health Chartbook* (Washington, DC: U.S. Government Printing Office, 2001).

44. Centers for Disease Control and Prevention, "Cigarette Smoking Among Adults—United States, 2000," *Morbidity and Mortality Weekly Report* 51, 29 (2002): 642–645.

45. Public Health Service, *Health, United States, 2001.*

46. U.S. Department of Health and Human Services, *Healthy People 2010,* 2nd ed.

47. Centers for Disease Control and Prevention, "Cigarette Smoking Among Adults."

48. U.S. Department of Health and Human Services, *Reducing the Health Consequences of Smoking,* 21.

49. Centers for Disease Control and Prevention, "Annual Smoking-Attributable Mortality, Years of Potential Life Lost, and Economic Costs—United States, 1995–1999,"

Morbidity and Mortality Weekly Report 51, 4 (2002): 300–303.

50. Ibid.

51. Ibid.

52. R. Peto, A. D. Lopez, J. Boreham, M. Thun, and C. Health, "Mortality from Tobacco in Developed Countries: Indirect Estimation from National Vital Statistics," *Lancet* 339 (May 23, 1992): 1268–1278.

53. Frank J. Chaloupka, *Curbing the Epidemic: Governments and the Economics of Tobacco Control* (Washington, DC: The World Bank, 1999).

54. Ibid.

55. Peto, Lopez, Boreham, Thun, and Health, "Mortality from Tobacco."

56. Centers for Disease Control and Prevention, "The Surgeon General's 1990 Report on the Health Benefits of Smoking Cessation (Executive Summary)" *Morbidity and Mortality Weekly Report* 39, RR-12 (1990): 1–12.

57. U.S. Department of Health and Human Services, *The Health Consequences of Involuntary Smoking. A Report of the Surgeon General*, DHHS Publication No. (CDC) 87-8398 (Atlanta, GA: Centers for Disease Control, 1987).

58. U.S. Department of Health and Human Services, *Reducing the Health Consequences of Smoking.*

59. Federal Trade Commission, January 27, 1992.

60. J. D. DiFranza, J. W. Richards, P. M. Paulman, et al., "RJR Nabisco's Cartoon Camel Promotes Camel Cigarettes to Children," *Journal of the American Medical Association* 266 (1991): 3149.

61. Ibid.; P. M. Fischer, M. P. Schwartz, J. W. Richards, et al., "Brand Logo Recognition by Children Aged 3 to 6 Years— Mickey Mouse and Old Joe Camel," *Journal of the American Medical Association* 266 (1991): 3145.

62. K. E. Warner, "Cigarette Advertising and Media Coverage of Smoking and Health," *New England Journal of Medicine* 312 (February 7, 1985): 384–388.

63. Ibid.

64. E. M. Whelan, M. J. Sheridan, K. A. Meister, and B. A. Mosher, "Analysis of Coverage of Tobacco Hazards in Women's Magazines," *Journal of Public Health Policy* 2 (1981): 28–35.

65. Fischer et al., "Brand Logo Recognition."

66. L. A. White, "Total Ban on Cigarette Advertising: Is It Constitutional?" *ACSH News and Views* 5 (1984): 4–7.

67. Ibid.

68. L. White, "Telling the Tobacco Companies to Butt Out— A Profile of the Proposition P Campaign," *ACSH News and Views* 5 (1984): 9–11.

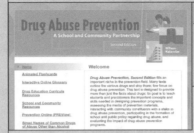

web resources

The Web site for this book offers many useful resources for educators, students, and professional counselors and is a great source for additional information. Visit the site at **http://healtheducation.jbpub.com/drugabuse/.**

Chapter Learning Objectives

Upon completion of this chapter, students will be able to:

1. Compare and contrast prescription drugs with over-the-counter drugs.

2. Weigh the advantages and disadvantages of steroid use in athletics.

3. Explain when caffeine may be hazardous and describe the nature of the hazards.

4. Recall several examples of inhalants and explain why it is impossible to eliminate the supply of those drugs.

5. Name the potential hazards of inhalant drugs.

Scenario

The Greenton school system has been approached by a large soft drink company that wants to negotiate an exclusive contract for the sale of the company's products in the school. The agreement would require the exclusive sale of company soft drinks in the cafeteria and in vending machines. In addition, the company would have the right to put up ads in hallways, on school buses, and on the school's closed-circuit television system. In return, the school would receive hundreds of thousands of dollars in an annual contract fee, with possible additional bonuses based on sales.

The superintendent and the school board are debating this proposal and are very attracted to the positive impact it could have on the school system's finances. The money would provide for a lot of "extras" not well funded by the state and local education taxes.

Alice Phelps is the middle school health educator and has become aware of this pending decision on the part of the school board. What counsel should she give to the principal and the board?

Chapter 4

Other Drugs, Mostly Legal

Introduction

To dispel the confusion about whether alcohol and tobacco are drugs, the term *alcohol, tobacco, and other drugs (ATOD)* has evolved. This term clearly designates alcohol and tobacco as drugs. This chapter discusses other drugs that are of concern to prevention specialists and health educators but are less restricted and of less interest to the criminal justice system than the drugs discussed in Chapter 5. Nevertheless, these drugs are potentially hazardous and should be a legitimate component of drug education. Over-the-counter and prescription drugs are considered first.

It is important to understand how drugs are named. A chemist gives a drug its **chemical name** by using words and numbers that describe its molecular structure—for example, 4-chloro-*N*-furfuryl-5-sulfamoylanthranilic acid. (See **Figure 4.1.**) Once it is recognized that the drug has valuable applications, it is given a standardized **generic name**; the previous example is called furosemide. Finally, when a drug is ready to be marketed, the pharmaceutical company that developed it gives it a **brand name,** which is legally protected. Furosemide's brand name is Lasix.

The brand name and the drug itself are the private property of the pharmaceutical company for 17 years. At the end of that time, other companies may legally sell the drug, using the generic, but not the brand, name. The generic version usually is cheaper because the second company does not have research and development expenses. However, not all generic drugs are **biologically equivalent** to their brand-name counterparts, particularly in the case of drugs given in very small doses, such as digitalis or thyroid hormone. People should ask their physician or pharmacist if

H-Chloro-N-Furfuryl-5-Sulfamoylanthranilic Acid

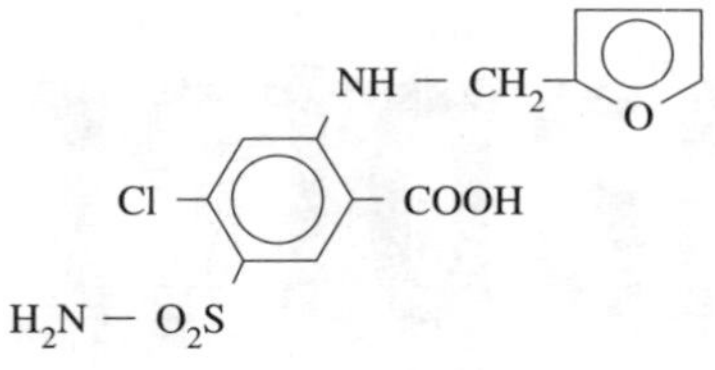

Furosemide
(Lasix)

Figure 4.1 **A Drug Chemical Structure**

a generic drug form is available and whether it is recommended. Biological equivalency is sometimes an issue with prescription drugs, but rarely with over-the-counter (OTC) drugs; generic OTC drugs are usually just as effective as brand-name OTC drugs.

Over-the-Counter Drugs

Medications were unregulated in the 19th century. No government controls were in place, so anyone, regardless of their scientific and medical expertise, could produce, market, and dispense drugs. This practice began to change in the 20th century. Certain drugs were regarded as potent and hazardous enough to warrant controls. This belief led to the prescription drug designation, which required physicians to approve patients' purchases of these drugs from licensed pharmacists. Other drugs were considered to be much less hazardous and so did not require any legal controls on purchasing. This category became known as over-the-counter drugs.

Over the years, amendments to the Pure Food and Drug Act of 1906 have more stringently regulated OTC drugs. First came a requirement for accuracy in labeling. Next came a requirement that these drugs be safe. Finally, in the early 1960s, OTC drugs were required to be effective, that is, to have the benefits they claimed to have. The variety and number of OTC drugs are enormous, and health officials have only limited resources to monitor their manufacture and sale. Consequently, there have been instances where OTC drugs were marketed and only later determined to be either unsafe

or ineffective. By and large, these drugs are safe if taken appropriately; their effectiveness is much less certain.

OTC drugs are designed for the temporary relief of uncomplicated symptoms or to otherwise address simple health concerns that do not require professional care. They are popular because people can manage minor health problems independently and avoid the expense of a physician visit. However, their popularity is also heightened by aggressive advertising (see the FYI box on page 61). OTC drug marketers use sophisticated techniques to promote their products. Some of these techniques may be deceptive or misleading. They can create awareness for products that might not be perceived as needed in the absence of advertising. Examples include assertions that good health requires a daily laxative and daily vitamins, that early morning social relationships are intolerable without a mouthwash because of "morning breath," and that women emit offensive odors if they do not use a vaginal deodorant. A discussion of advertising should be included, along with specific information about OTC drugs, in school drug education. Students should learn to analyze specific advertising appeals by identifying (1) the motive behind the ad, (2) the source of the ad, (3) the qualifications of the speaker or researcher cited, (4) the adequacy of the information provided, and (5) the congruency between the health content in the ad and known science.[1]

It is possible to identify more than 20 unique categories of OTC drugs. The most important are analgesics, cold and cough remedies, vitamin and mineral supplements, antihistamines and allergy products, laxatives, and antacids.

Analgesics

Analgesics, or pain relievers, come in five basic forms: aspirin, acetaminophen, ibuprofen, ketoprofen, and naproxen sodium. Ibuprofen was a prescription drug (e.g., Motrin) until 1981, when it was approved for OTC use with brand names such as Advil and Nuprin. Ketoprofen was a prescription drug for arthritis, introduced in the mid-1980s. Recently it was approved for OTC use at a lower dose. Orudis is one of the brand names used for ketoprofen. Naproxen was a prescription drug (e.g., Naprosyn) from 1976 until January 1994, when the FDA approved its use as an OTC pain reliever. All of these drugs are equally effective for lowering fevers and relieving dull pain, including headaches, toothaches, and menstrual cramps. In addition, in large doses aspirin reduces the joint inflammation common to arthritis. Furthermore, aspirin is recommended for some middle-aged and older people to combat the circulatory system's tendency to form blood clots. Recommended dosage varies, but is typically one tablet per day or every other day.

As with all drugs, analgesics should be used with caution. In large or frequent doses, aspirin may irritate the stomach and cause the stomach lining to bleed. Aspirin should not be given to children with flu-like symptoms: fever, malaise, head and other body aches, and upper respiratory congestion. Aspirin use by children and adolescents in such circumstances has been associated with Reye's syndrome, a rare but serious disorder that can damage the brain, liver, and kidneys.

On the other hand, acetaminophen and ibuprofen may be toxic to the liver and kidneys, while naproxen may cause gastrointestinal bleeding and ulceration. Prolonged, frequent use of any analgesic drugs should be medically supervised.

Cold and Cough Remedies

Because upper respiratory viral infections are very common, and because medical science can do nothing to cure them, OTC drugs that relieve symptoms are very popular. There are only two cautions regarding these drugs. First, cold symptoms are the body's way of recovering from an infection. Drugs that suppress the symptoms place an extra burden on the body, thereby possibly prolonging convalescence. When possible, the home remedies of warm fluids and extra rest are preferable.

The other caution has to do with the way cold remedies are formulated. Because many symptoms occur with colds (e.g., fever, headache, sore throat, runny or congested nose), the drugs often include chemicals for all possible cold symptoms. For example, one product is marketed as "The Nighttime Sniffling, Sneezing, Coughing, Aching, Stuffy Head, Fever, So You Can Rest Medicine." However, people don't always have all possible

symptoms, so they should take only drugs that are designed for their symptoms and avoid unnecessary use of other chemicals. Often it is helpful to discuss symptoms with a pharmacist and ask for a recommendation for suitable drugs.

It should be noted that adolescents' abuse of cough medicines is common in most communities. Some cough medicines contain alcohol and codeine and, taken in large enough amounts, can cause mood-altering effects. In isolation this effect is not a significant problem, but parents and stores that sell cough medicines should be aware of it.

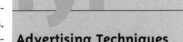

Vitamin and Mineral Supplements

Americans spend more on vitamins and minerals than on any other category of OTC drug. (See **Figure 4.2.**) There are times when these products

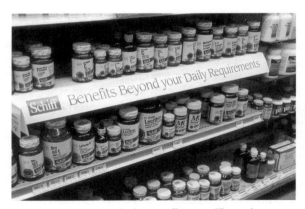

Figure 4.2 Display Shelves in "Natural" Food Store
Many Americans rely on vitamin and mineral food supplements and believe they cannot be healthy without them. (© Michael Newman/PhotoEdit)

Herbs and Folk Medicine

They Worked Their Own Remedy: An Interview with Mrs. Janie Hunter

We doesn't go to no doctor. My daddy used to cook medicine—herbs medicine: seamuckle, pine top, lison molasses, shoemaker root, ground moss, peachtree leaf, big-root, red oak bark, terrywuk.

Now when my children have fever I boil lison molasses; squeeze little lemon juice in it. Once they go to bed it strike that fever right away. That something very good.

And you hear about children have worm? We get something called jimsey weed. You put it in a cloth and beat it. And when you done beat it, you squeeze the juice out of it, and you put four, five drop of turpentine in it, give children that to drink. You give a dose of castor oil behind 'em. You don't have to take 'em to no doctor.

If anybody fall down and break bone, my daddy get a towel and pour some water in the basin—put half a bottle of white vinegar in it. He hot the towel and bathe the leg in some mud. Go in the creek and get some mud, band that whole leg up in mud. Couple days you be walking. That knits it right back together.

For a cut, to stop 'em from bleeding, Daddy just get a big spoonful of sugar and throw 'em in there. He say once a cut stop bleeding it's not dangerous. Spider webs grow up in the house and you get that and tie 'em on. Web grow right in there.

If you get sores you get something you call St. John out in the field. And you see those little bump grow on a gum tree; you get them and you burn them two together and just tie 'em right on that wound. That heals right up.

When my little boy got a nail stuck in his feet, I got a basin of hot water with physic salt and let him hold he feet down in that—draw the poison out. Then I tie a piece of butts meat on it. His foot get better.

You hear about some little thing run back in its hole—fiddler crab? We use that for whooping cough. Catch the crab, boil 'em up with something else—I can't call the name—and strain 'em through a white cloth. Give that for drink. It'll cure the running whoop.

All this from old people time when they hardly been any doctor. People couldn't afford doctor, so they had to have and guess. Those old people dead now, but they worked their own remedy and their own remedy came out good.

Source: Guy Carawan, *Ain't You Got a Right to the Tree of Life?* (New York: Simon and Schuster, 1966).

are useful and may be important: during pregnancy (e.g., folic acid) and lactation; with certain diseases that cause nutritional deficiencies; for people who do not eat a well-balanced diet (e.g., weight-conscious teenage girls); when a deficiency disease is diagnosed (e.g., anemia); and when calcium supplements are needed to prevent osteoporosis.

However, many people believe that vitamin and mineral supplements can have benefits beyond maintaining normal health. Recent claims include that vitamins can prevent cataracts, increase IQ, and prevent heart disease and cancer. In this regard, there has been particular interest in antioxidant vitamins, such as vitamin E. Furthermore, some people believe that an adequate amount of vitamins and minerals cannot be obtained from food because of soil depletion on farms and food-processing methods.

The weight of scientific evidence indicates that, with the exceptions noted earlier, the required amounts of vitamins and minerals to support good health can be readily obtained from a well-balanced diet. If people are not getting the minimum amounts of vitamins they need from food, supplements are valuable. However, there is conflicting evidence concerning the value of supplements beyond the recommended levels. The authors believe that people should be encouraged and taught to eat wisely rather than rely on pills to supplement a poor diet. Healthy eating should be promoted with environmental and social changes that reinforce and enable such behavior. It may be that recommendations for vitamin intake will be increased in the near future, but, for the time being, let the buyer beware.

Antihistamines and Allergy Products

Like colds, allergies are also very common. Similarly, medical science has no quick fix for allergies. Many OTC and prescription products will relieve typical symptoms such as itchy, watery, or puffy eyes, runny nose, and headache. (See **Figure 4.3.**) Just as with cold remedies, people should be careful about taking unnecessary ingredients. Also, allergy products often contain **antihistamines**, which may cause drowsiness. Great caution is appropriate when driving or operating machinery while these drugs are being used.

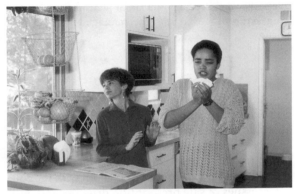

Figure 4.3 Facial Allergy Symptoms Are Very Apparent and Common What drugs do you take when you feel like this? (© David Young-Wolff/PhotoEdit)

Laxatives

It seems as though Americans have an obsession with the regularity of their bowels. They believe that the intestinal tract should respond in a consistent, mechanistic way, but that constipation should be expected as a normal part of everyday life. However, the truth is that constipation should be a rare problem. It is usually caused by inadequate fluid intake, sedentary living, and insufficient amounts of dietary fiber. Chronic constipation eventually leads to hemorrhoids, caused by excessive straining with bowel movements. Both of these problems can be avoided by drinking six to eight glasses of fluid each day, getting regular, vigorous exercise, and eating foods with generous amounts of fiber (e.g., fruits, vegetables, whole grains). When constipation and hemorrhoids do occur, OTC drugs may be temporarily helpful, but the individual should make changes in his or her lifestyle for long-term prevention. (See **Figure 4.4.**)

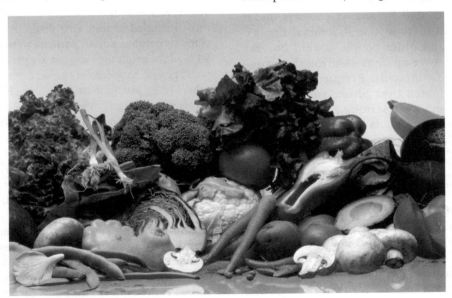

Figure 4.4 High-Fiber Foods Eating generous quantities of these foods would make laxatives unnecessary for most people. (© PhotoDisc)

1. Never take OTC drugs for a prolonged period of time without seeking counsel from a medical professional.
2. When you are prescribed drugs, be sure to mention to the physician any OTC drugs you take on a regular basis.
3. Avoid combination drugs with chemicals for symptoms you don't have.
4. Read the label on the package to determine appropriate dosage and any conditions (e.g., pregnancy) that indicate the drug should not be used. Comply with the directions.
5. Keep OTC drugs out of the reach of children.
6. Note the expiration date after which the drug is no longer reliable.
7. Seek the counsel of a physician or pharmacist regarding symptoms that may be managed with OTC drugs.

Antacids

An occasional binge brings relief to the austerity of a disciplined, healthy lifestyle. Unfortunately, many people overeat and overdrink more than occasionally. Not surprisingly, upset stomach is very common; in adults, it usually results from excesses. Antacids will relieve discomfort, but prudence indicates that if you don't want an upset stomach then you should not eat or drink too much.

One concern with antacids is that they may disguise pain caused by **angina pectoris**, heart disease, or disorders in the abdominal organs. Middle-aged and older people should be very careful not to cover up signs of serious heart disease with OTC antacids. Frequent heartburn should be evaluated by a physician to rule out heart disease or other serious problems in the gastrointestinal system. (See the Hints & Tips box entitled "General Guidelines for Safe Use of OTC Drugs.")

Prescription Drugs

In this age of medical technology, prescription drugs have taken center stage in the health care system. In the past, people spoke with awe about the "wonder drugs." Certainly, advances in the pharmacological treatment of pain and disease are a wonder to behold, especially to those people who remember life prior to the development of those drugs. However, some of the luster of these wonder drugs disappeared when people realized that they don't solve every problem, they can have disagreeable side effects, and their cost prohibits their purchase by many people. Nevertheless, prescription drugs are part of everyone's life sooner or later. In drug education, we are concerned both with the consumer issues of safe prescription drug use and with the potential for abuse of prescription drugs.

In 1999, medications were prescribed to patients by physicians about 1.1 billion times in the United States; in 66% of outpatient medical visits, treatment included at least one drug.[2] Although physicians sometimes advise patients to use OTC drugs, 84% of the drugs they suggest are prescription drugs. Some physician specialists prescribe more drugs than others (e.g., psychiatrists use more; orthopedic surgeons use the least). Medical use of drugs increases with age; elderly patients are more likely to get prescriptions and more likely to get more than one prescription at a time. Table 4.1 presents some of the most commonly used prescription drugs.

Because prescription drugs generally are used under the direction of a physician or other health professional, it is less important for the average person to learn detailed information about them than is the case with OTC drugs. People *do* need to learn the general principles for safe and effective use of prescription drugs, however. These principles are presented in the Hints & Tips box entitled "General Guidelines for Safe Use of Prescription Drugs."

Talk to your physician, give information, and ask questions.
- Is the drug really necessary?
- How should the drug be taken and for how long?
- Should any foods be avoided?
- Is it safe to drink alcohol while using the drug?
- Are there any side effects? What should I do if they occur?
- Can a generic drug be taken?

- Tell the physician if cost will prevent you from purchasing the drug.
- Tell the physician what other drugs you are using.
- Comply with the physician's directions.
- Ask the pharmacist questions that you forgot to ask the physician.
- Devise a system to organize daily intake of different drugs.

[Table 4.1]	
Ten Drugs Most Commonly Used in Outpatient Medical Care	
Drug Brand Name	**Therapeutic Use**
Claritin	Antihistamine
Lasix	Diuretic
Prednisone	Steroid replacement, anti-inflammatory
Synthroid	Thyroid hormone replacement
Lipitor	Cholesterol-lowering agent
Premarin	Estrogen replacement
Prilosec	Anti-acid ulcer treatment
Tylenol	Pain reliever
Amoxicillin	Antibiotic
Celebrex	Anti-inflammatory

Source: National Center for Health Statistics, 2001.

Some drugs may be abused because they have mind- and mood-altering properties. This can occur with drugs obtained legally from one or more physicians or illegally from the black market (see the FYI box). The prevalence of this form of drug abuse is illustrated in **Figure 4.5**. There is no guarantee that drugs purchased on the street contain the ingredients that the buyer thinks they contain. However, abusers of prescription drugs consume drugs made by pharmaceutical companies.

If the user's mind is clear, a drug can be taken with certainty of dosage. In contrast, users of street drugs have no way of knowing how large a dose they are getting. Similarly, prescription drugs contain no impurities, whereas street drugs may have other substances mixed in that carry additional hazards.

Preventing adolescent abuse of prescription drugs is similar to the strategy used for other drugs. Parent training in combination with pharmacy networking can create an environment that helps deter prescription drug abuse. Parent training is needed because prescription and OTC drugs initially come from the home medicine cabinet. Likewise, computer networking of pharmacies makes it more difficult for people to fill multiple prescriptions of the same drug. Technology proliferation makes this a likely part of the future.

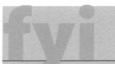

OxyContin

In the last few years there has been a sudden and dramatic increase in the use and trafficking in OxyContin, a prescription pain reliever. The generic ingredient of OxyContin is oxycodone, a synthetic narcotic. Oxycodone is found in other medications, such as Percocet, but OxyContin has a much higher dose. The drug has become the drug of choice in many rural communities and has become the principal drug problem addressed by many rural police departments.

Source: Office of National Drug Control Policy, 2001.

A Perspective on Coffee Growing

We grew coffee on my farm. The land was in itself a little too high for coffee, and it was hard work to keep it going; we were never rich on the farm. But a coffee-plantation is a thing that gets hold of you and does not let you go, and there is always something to do on it: you are generally just a little behind with your work.

Coffee growing is a long job. It does not all come out as you imagine, when, yourself young and hopeful, in the streaming rain, you carry the boxes of your shining young coffee-plants from the nurseries, and, with the whole number of farm-hands in the field, watch the plants set in the regular rows of holes in the wet ground where they are to grow, and then have them thickly shaded against the sun, with branches broken from the bush, since obscurity is the privilege of young things. It is four or five years [un]til the trees come into bearing, and in the meantime you will get drought on the land, or diseases, and the bold weeds will grow up thick in the fields.... You plant a little over six hundred trees to the acre, and I had six hundred acres of land with coffee; my oxen dragged the cultivators up and down the fields, between the rows of trees, many thousand miles, patiently, awaiting coming bounties.

Source: Excerpted from Isak Dinesen, *Out of Africa* (Random House, 1938).

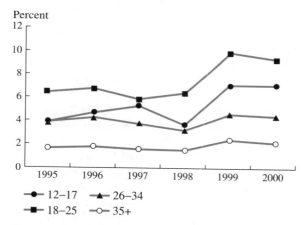

Figure 4.5 **Nonmedical Psychotherapeutic Drug Abuse by Age, 1995–2000**

Source: National Household Survey on Drug Abuse.

Caffeine

Caffeine may be the most widely used drug (see **Figure 4.6**); it is certainly more available than tobacco or alcohol and is consumed by people of all ages. People have consumed caffeine via coffee and tea for centuries. (See **Figure 4.7** and the Viewpoints box.) Caffeinated soft drinks have been sold for over 100 years, and over-the-counter products with caffeine have been produced for perhaps 50 years. Today's consumers are buying less coffee, more tea, and much more caffeinated soft drinks. A recent trend, however, is a growing interest in the so-called gourmet coffees. It is as yet unknown how these changes have affected overall caffeine consumption, but it seems clear that society at the beginning of the 21st century is sold on the benefits of caffeine. It is appropriate to wonder what the consequences are of such remarkable consumption of this drug.

Caffeine is a stimulant that causes increased alertness, decreased fatigue, and sharper concentration—this pick-me-up effect is the principal factor motivating its consumption. (See **Figure 4.8**.) Ray has insightfully observed that the popularity of this effect is congruent with values in Western society.[3] Whereas some cultures have a placid and contemplative approach to daily life, Westerners have places to go and things to see—in a hurry. They are driven to succeed, achieve, compete, accumulate, and experience; in short, they want more of everything. Caffeine is an enabler in this regard. It is a striking paradox that a soft drink comparatively high in caffeine is named Mello Yello!

Beyond this influence on mood and energy level, caffeine also increases heart rate, blood pressure,

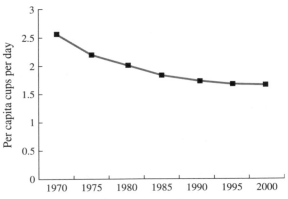

Figure 4.6 U.S. Coffee Consumption

Source: National Coffee Association, 2000.

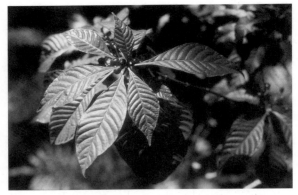

Figure 4.7 Growing Coffee Plants   Coffee has been an important crop in Africa and South America for decades. (© Fred Reisch/Unicorn Stock Photos)

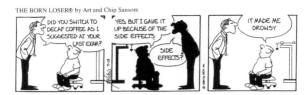

Figure 4.8 Caffeine Enables Mainstream Lifestyle

Reprinted by permission of Newspaper Enterprise Association.

respiration, blood glucose level, and urine production. However, these effects occur only in "naive users"—first-time or infrequent users.[4] The regular consumer of caffeine develops tolerance, and all of these effects disappear. Caffeine also increases blood fats, even in habitual users, but doesn't influence cholesterol.[5]

Caffeine may cause sleep disturbances and jittery nerves but, with regular use, tolerance develops, and these effects fade. However, people who consume large doses of caffeine experience withdrawal symptoms if they do not receive the accustomed dose. Symptoms may include headache, irritability, and restlessness.

While caffeine is consumed for its stimulating properties, it is little known that the effects seem to apply most to simple activities and tasks. More complex tasks that require high-level thinking, skill, and concentration are less enhanced by caffeine. Furthermore, the common belief that caffeine can reverse the stupor of alcohol intoxication is simply incorrect.

Caffeine also constricts (reduces the diameter of) the blood vessels that run through tissues covering the brain. This effect makes caffeine useful in relieving **migraine headaches**, which are caused by the swelling of those blood vessels.

In the recent past, caffeine consumption was cited as a risk factor for heart disease, cancer, **fibrocystic breast disease**, high blood pressure, and birth defects. Current medical opinion is that caffeine is not related to these conditions.[6]

During pregnancy, the kidneys and liver clear caffeine more slowly, raising the concern that any hazardous effects of caffeine might be exaggerated. However, there is no association between caffeine consumption and **congenital malformations**.[7] Caffeine does seem to present a risk for prenatal growth retardation, even in full-term pregnancies.[8] The mechanism for arrested fetal weight gain is not clear, but it is prudent to use caffeine sparingly, if at all, during pregnancy.

Caffeine stimulates acid production in the stomach, but it is uncertain if this is the sole reason why coffee drinkers often experience heartburn. There is no evidence to prove that caffeine causes stomach or intestinal ulcers.[9] However, this irritating effect is sufficient reason to eliminate caffeine from an ulcer patient's diet. Other substances in coffee may cause heartburn, so drinking decaffeinated coffee does not solve the problem.

Table 4.2		
Caffeine Content of Beverages and Foods		
Item	Average (mg)	Range (mg)
Coffee (5-oz. cup)		
Brewed, drip method	115	60–180
Brewed, percolator	80	40–170
Instant	65	30–120
Decaffeinated, brewed	3	2–5
Decaffeinated, instant	2	1–5
Tea (5-oz. cup)		
Brewed, major U.S. brands	40	20–90
Brewed, imported brands	60	25–110
Instant	30	25–50
Iced (12-oz. glass)	70	67–76
Cocoa beverage (5-oz. cup)	4	2–20
Chocolate milk beverage (8 oz.)	5	2–7
Milk chocolate (1 oz.)	6	1–15
Dark chocolate, semisweet (1 oz.)	20	5–35
Baker's chocolate (1 oz.)	26	26
Chocolate-flavored syrup (1 oz.)	4	4

Source: Food and Drug Administration.

Table 4.3	
Caffeine Content of Soft Drinks	
	Milligrams per 12 Ounces
Regular	
Cola, Pepper type	30–46
Decaffeinated cola, Pepper type	0.18
Cherry cola	36–46
Lemon-lime (clear)	0
Orange	0
Root beer	0
Ginger ale	0
Tonic water	0
Diet Drinks	
Diet cola, Pepper type	36–46
Decaffeinated diet cola, Pepper type	0–0.2
Diet cherry cola	30–46
Diet lemon-lime	0
Diet root beer	0
Club soda, seltzer, sparkling water	0

Source: National Soft Drink Association.

Recent evidence shows a relationship between **premenstrual syndrome** (**PMS**) and caffeine.[10] As caffeine consumption rises, so does the incidence of PMS. Although it is too early to conclude a causal relationship, it is possible that restricting caffeine may eliminate, or at least minimize, PMS. Without question, other psychological and biochemical factors are involved.

The cautions regarding caffeine are balanced by its beneficial impact on productivity at work or school, safety (e.g., in driving), and in treating certain headaches. Tables 4.2, 4.3, and 4.4 show the caffeine contents of common beverages, foods, and drugs. The limit of moderate caffeine intake is about three cups of coffee or five soft drinks per day.

The final concern regarding caffeine is not medical but psychosocial. Cola drinks are one of the most popular beverages among teenagers. Parents and teachers may wonder whether the volatile emotional state of adolescence might be less marked without the mood-altering properties of caffeine. However, caffeine is strongly ingrained in teen culture, and most parents feel a prohibition would not be worth the effort.

Steroids

The body produces steroid **hormones** that promote growth, healing, and the development and maintenance of gender characteristics. Steroids, called adrenocortical hormones or corticosteroids, have been used for a long time in conventional medical practice. However, some steroids have been altered to accentuate body-building (anabolic) effects and minimize gender-promoting (androgenic) effects; these derivatives are thus called *anabolic steroids*. When the word *steroids* is used in the context of drug abuse, anabolic steroids are what is meant. Anabolic steroids also have androgenic effects, which cause the greatest concern for users.

Table 4.4	
Caffeine Content of Drugs (Milligrams)	
Prescription Drugs	
Cafergot (migraine headaches)	100.0
Norgesic Forte (muscle relaxant)	60.0
Norgesic (muscle relaxant)	30.0
Fiorinal (tension headache)	40.0
Fioricet (headache pain relief)	40.0
Darvon compound (pain relief)	32.4
Synalgos-DC (pain relief)	30.0
Nonprescription Drugs	
Alertness Tablets	
No Doz	100.0
Vivarin	200.0
Pain Relief	
Anacin, Maximum Strength Anacin	32.0
Vanquish	33.0
Excedrin	65.0
Midol	32.4
Diuretics	
Aqua-Ban	100.0
Cold/Allergy Remedies	
Coryban-D capsules	30.0

Source: Food and Drug Administration.

Steroids are used by athletes, both male and female, to promote strength, power, speed, and aggressiveness. Russian athletes began this practice in the 1950s. There is evidence that steroids enhance athletic performance in these ways,[11] but only in the context of a complete training regimen of diet and exercise. The competitive edge provided by steroids alone is marginal. However, at the highest levels of athletics, small differences separate competitors. (See **Figure 4.9.**)

Many athletes feel pressure to use steroids because they believe all of their competitors are using them. (See **Figure 4.10.**) Many other drugs also are used to enhance athletic performance, including human growth hormones, amphetamines, caffeine, and analgesics/anesthetics. There is a philosophical debate on this issue: Should athletics be pure (i.e., without drugs) or should all new tech-

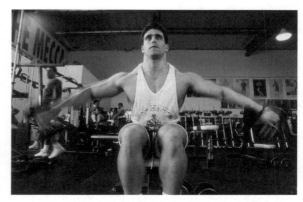

Figure 4.9 Body Builder Many adolescents believe that steroids can do this for them. (© Bill Aron/PhotoEdit)

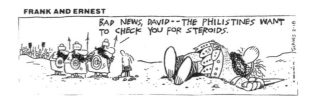

Figure 4.10 Cartoon Illustrating Extent of Steroid Use

Reprinted by permission of Newspaper Enterprise Association.

nologies (e.g., improved shoe design, lightweight materials, and drugs) be allowed?

Anabolic steroids are used most by professional athletes and those performing at international amateur events. However, their use has filtered down to the college and high school ranks. At the high school level, it is unlikely that they are a significant influence in athletics because so many other variables, such as age, size, and inexperience, affect competition. Some adolescents reportedly use steroids not for athletic success but for the muscular appearance attributed to use of the drugs.

Over the past 10 years, athletic organizations have enacted and actively enforced prohibitions on steroid use. The Olympic sprinter Ben Johnson is the most famous athlete to be affected by these restrictive policies. The magnitude of change in athletes' steroid use as a result of testing is unknown. However, Monitoring the Future has gathered data on students' steroid use since 1989. These data show a decline through 1993, with a slight increase in 1994. In 1995, 2.3% of seniors reported ever having used steroids.

Use of steroids may result in many side effects, including elevated cholesterol and blood pressure, deepening of the voice, changes in pattern of hair growth (e.g., baldness, increased body hair), acne, masculine traits in females, and psychological dependency. Most of the evidence about the harmful consequences of steroid use comes from experience with medical applications, not direct studies of athletic use. Most athletes do not take steroids continuously for a long period of time, but they may take doses much larger than those used in medical practice.

A variety of problems are attributed to steroids, including premature arrest of skeletal growth in teen users, cardiovascular disease, liver damage, mental disorders, cancer, and violent behavior ("roid rage"). These risks might be more tolerable when specific disease treatment is necessary, but athletics implies a condition of health. While there is legitimate reason for concern, especially with adolescent users, there is no unequivocal evidence that steroids are in fact harmful.[12] The hazard is that adolescents who use steroids usually get them from illicit suppliers rather than from medical sources, and there is always uncertainty and risk associated with street drugs. Furthermore, if steroids are injected, all the hazards of intravenous (IV) drug use (e.g., AIDS, hepatitis) are present.

Steroids are used because of two central themes in our society: (1) Self-esteem is based on external appearance and (2) one must win at all costs. These themes are virtually unquestioned and unchallenged by the mainstream. Steroids will be used as long as these attitudes are embraced by a significant segment of the population. It would seem that the motives that drive steroid use call for prevention strategies different from those employed to combat alcohol, tobacco, marijuana, and cocaine use.

Inhalants

Inhalants include a wide variety of **volatile chemicals** such as airplane glue, paint, gasoline, nail polish remover, correction fluid, and nitrates. (See **Figure 4.11**.) In a world filled with chemical technology, there is no end to the list of inhalable substances with mind-altering properties. This form of drug abuse is impossible to prohibit by supply-side interventions because the inhalable drugs are found in every home, school, store, church, and workplace.

The consumption pattern of inhalants is unique because younger students use them more than older students—the opposite of what is found with other drugs. Table 4.5 provides data on inhalant use by grade level. It is uncertain whether the greater use of inhalants than other drugs by eighth graders is just situational (i.e., eighth graders have access to

[**Table 4.5**]

Past-Year Use of Inhalants by Grade Level, 1996–2001

Grade	1996	1997	1998	1999	2000	2001
8	12.2%	11.8%	11.1%	10.3%	9.4%	9.1%
10	9.5	8.7	8.0	7.2	7.3	6.6
12	7.6	6.7	6.2	5.6	5.9	4.5

Source: Monitoring the Future, 2001.

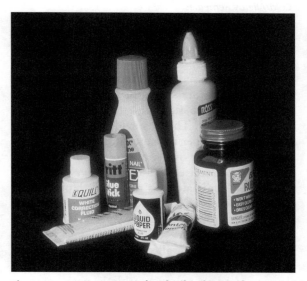

Figure 4.11 Assortment of Volatile Chemicals
Substances that can be used as inhalant drugs come in an endless variety and are found almost everywhere.
(© Bill Aron/PhotoEdit)

inhalants but not to other drugs) or whether older students become more attracted to drugs that are popular in adult society.

Because there is so much diversity among potential inhalants, it is difficult to identify a summary list of effects or consequences. Immediate symptoms might include euphoria, tremors, drooling, impaired speech, nausea, breathing problems, blurred vision, chills, sweating, faintness, anxiety, depression, and paranoia. In the long run, inhalant use can damage the nervous system, lungs, heart, and liver, and may cause death.

Summary

This chapter provided an overview of OTC and prescription drugs, caffeine, steroids, and inhalants. The first two are of great concern from the perspective of consumer health, as well as for their potential for addiction and abuse. Most people who become users of these drugs are introduced to them early in life and continue use throughout adulthood. If misused, these drugs can be extremely dangerous. Inhalants deserve concern because they are readily available, and most people are unaware of their risks if misused. Because there is no legitimate reason to consume inhalants, their use can only be described as misuse or abuse.

Although steroids are used by only a small percentage of youth, the hazards may be great. What remains unclear are the consequences and actual benefits of steroid use. Therefore, it is appropriate for all of these drugs to be addressed in school and community education programs.

Scenario | Analysis and Response

There is no question that a national trend exists of schools entering into marketing contracts with soft drink companies, and that many schools generate huge amounts of money for their budgets in this manner. It is hard to argue with this potential bonanza when so many schools are struggling to provide services within their budgetary limits.

On the other hand, what are the consequences of children and adolescents consuming even more caffeinated soft drinks? Will this contribute to behavioral

or discipline problems? Schools are not going to change teen culture by refusing to serve these soft drinks, but at least they won't be part of the problem. An additional concern with soft drinks, not caffeine per se, is their high calorie content. In a society where the proportion of obese youth is increasing every year, promoting the availability of high-calorie soft drinks is not a wise response.

What solutions could Ms. Phelps propose to the school board?

Learning Activities

1. Using a copy of the *Physician's Desk Reference* (PDR) or a similar reference book, identify 10 drugs that are available generically. Visit a pharmacy and compare the prices of the brand-name drugs with the generic drugs. Ask the pharmacist if all of the generic drugs are recommended or biologically equivalent.

2. Do an inventory of your home medicine cabinet. Identify all OTC and prescription drugs on hand. Determine if any of them has passed its expiration date. See if you can recall the exact dosage for each drug and any precautions or warnings. If you have any brand-name prescriptions, determine from a pharmacy if they are available generically.

3. Interview a coach or athletic trainer at your university or a local high school. Find out if he or she thinks steroids are being used and ask his or her opinion regarding the risks versus the benefits of their use. Also, determine if testing is done to detect steroid use.

4. Survey a group of peers to find out how much caffeine they use, what sources of caffeine are consumed, why they use caffeine, whether they have had any problems with caffeine, and whether they are concerned about their caffeine consumption.

5. Identify inhalant drugs sold in containers as commercial products. Determine if there are any warnings on the products' labels and what the natures of those warnings are. Suggest ways that parents could be made more aware of the attendant hazards of inhalants.

Notes

1. W. E. Schaller and C. R. Carroll, *Health, Quackery and the Consumer* (Philadelphia: W. B. Saunders, 1976), 39.

2. Donald K. Cherry, Catharine W. Burt, and David A. Woodwell, *National Ambulatory Medical Care Survey: 1999 Summary,* Advance Data No. 322 (Hyattsville, MD: National Center for Health Statistics, July 17, 2001).

3. O. Ray, *Drugs, Society and Human Behavior,* 3d ed. (St. Louis: C. V. Mosby, 1983), 454.

4. P. W. Curatolo and D. Robertson, "The Health Consequences of Caffeine," *Annals of Internal Medicine* 98 (part 1) (1983): 641–652.

5. Ibid.

6. Ibid.

7. L. Dlugosz and M. B. Bracken, "Reproductive Effects of Caffeine: A Review and Theoretical Analysis," *Epidemiologic Reviews* 14 (1992): 83–100.

8. L. Fenster, B. Eskenazi, G. C. Windham, and S. H. Swan, "Caffeine Consumption During Pregnancy and Fetal Growth," *American Journal of Public Health* 81, 4 (1991): 458–461.

9. Curatolo and Robertson, "The Health Consequences of Caffeine."

10. A. M. Rossignol and H. Bonnlander, "Caffeine-Containing Beverages, Total Fluid Consumption, and Premenstrual Syndrome," *American Journal of Public Health* 80, 9 (1990): 1106–1110.

11. J. R. DiPalma and G. J. DiGregorio, *Basic Pharmacology in Medicine,* 3d ed. (New York: McGraw-Hill, 1990), 533.

12. National Institute on Drug Abuse, *Anabolic Steroid Abuse,* DHHS Publication No. (ADM) 91-1720 (Rockville, MD: DHHS, Public Health Service, 1990), 142–164.

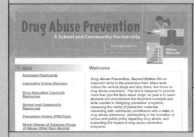

web resources

The Web site for this book offers many useful resources for educators, students, and professional counselors and is a great source for additional information. Visit the site at **http://healtheducation.jbpub.com/drugabuse/.**

Chapter Learning Objectives

Upon completion of this chapter, students will be able to:

1. Differentiate between amphetamines and cocaine and their forms, uses, effects, and hazards.

2. Assess the various hazards of narcotics and distinguish between direct hazards of the drug and hazards brought about by society's control policies.

3. Compare the effects and hazards of barbiturates with those of benzodiazepine drugs.

4. Contrast the hazards of marijuana and hallucinogenic drugs with those of stimulants, depressants, and narcotics.

5. Explain and give examples of club drugs.

Scenario

Some segments of society, notably the U.S. federal government, are fighting a war on drugs, mostly having the illegal drugs in the crosshairs. The Office of National Drug Control Policy, the lead agency in the war on drugs, has outlined a connection between terrorism and drugs: Those who use illegal drugs are supporting terrorism. The logic is that many terrorists are drug traffickers, using the proceeds to fund terrorist activities. In addition, many of the countries in Asia and the Middle East that aid and condone terrorists are also major world suppliers of illegal drugs.

Is this a legitimate connection to make? Is it an effective way to discourage drug abuse?

Chapter 5

Other Drugs, Mostly Illegal

Introduction

This chapter focuses on the drugs that many people mistakenly believe cause the worst drug problems. The authors feel that, as a group, these drugs get far more attention than they deserve. Often they are highlighted more than alcohol and tobacco in education programs; until recently they were exclusively targeted in national media antidrug campaigns, and they are certainly the main focus of the criminal justice system's effort to regulate and restrict drug use. These emphases are misguided, except in some inner-city neighborhoods.

Nevertheless, there is no question that these drugs are devastating to some people who use them and are the cause of much family and societal harm. Society's problem with illegal drugs is not trivial, and educators should do what they can to circumvent the personal and societal damage inflicted by these drugs. This chapter provides a knowledge base for that task. Material on education and prevention strategies is located in Chapters 7 through 10.

Stimulants

It is common to group together a number of drugs that excite or facilitate consciousness and heightened nervous system activity. These so-called stimulants include caffeine, nicotine, amphetamines, cocaine, and some of the club drugs. Caffeine and nicotine have been discussed in Chapter 4 and Chapter 3, respectively. Club drugs are discussed briefly in a later section of this chapter. Amphetamines and cocaine are similar enough to justify close comparison and contrast.

[**Table 5.1**]

Past-Year Use of Cocaine and Amphetamines by 8th, 10th, and 12th Graders, 1996–2001

	Grade	1996	1997	1998	1999	2000	2001
Cocaine							
	8	3.0%	2.8%	3.1%	2.7%	2.6%	2.5%
	10	4.2	4.7	4.7	4.9	4.4	3.6
	12	4.9	5.5	5.7	6.2	5.0	4.8
Amphetamines							
	8	9.1	8.1	7.2	6.9	6.5	6.7
	10	12.4	12.1	10.7	10.4	11.1	11.7
	12	9.5	10.2	10.1	10.2	10.5	10.9

Source: Monitoring the Future survey.

Background

As discussed in Chapter 2, cocaine has been used for centuries. In its extracted and concentrated form, it has been used in medical practice for more than 100 years, principally as a **local anesthetic**. Today it is used infrequently for anesthesia. Cocaine has made its greatest mark in illicit drug trafficking. Cocaine use by adolescents and adults did not change much during the 1990s. The Monitoring the Future survey (see Chapter 1) found that in 2001, 8.2% of high school seniors reported any lifetime use of cocaine, up from 6.0% in 1995. Similarly, 2.1% reported using the drug in the month prior to the survey, up from 1.3% in 1992. Only 0.1% of seniors reported daily cocaine use in 2001. Cocaine and amphetamine use by other age groups is reported in Table 5.1 and **Figure 5.1.**

Amphetamines were first developed in the 1920s. They have been used by military officials in many countries to maintain the vigilance and reduce the combat fatigue of pilots and other soldiers. Amphetamines were widely used in the treatment of asthma (with inhalers) because they are effective in dilating the lungs' airways, but they were found to be habit-forming, and abuse was common. OTC amphetamine inhalers are now banned in the United States.

Amphetamines also can cause loss of appetite, thus influencing eating behaviors. The effect of amphetamines is limited because tolerance is quickly developed (in three to six weeks). Because the

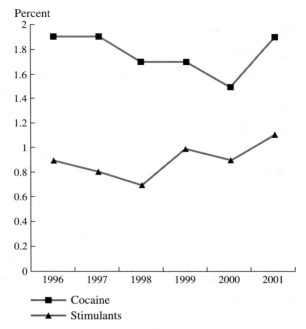

Figure 5.1 Past-Year Use of Cocaine and Other Stimulants, Age 12 and Older, 1996–2001

Source: National Household Survey on Drug Abuse.

mood-altering effects of these drugs are so appealing, users are tempted to increase their dosage to maintain the effects. This habitual use may continue regardless of the effects on appetite. Meanwhile, failure to change diet and exercise habits means there will be no permanent change in body weight. Prescription amphetamines are

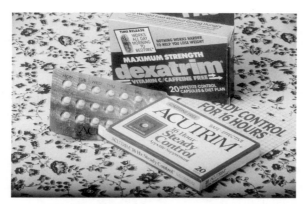

Figure 5.2 OTC Diet Pills Amphetamines have been largely replaced by these products for weight loss. (© Tony Freeman/PhotoEdit)

still on the market (e.g., Dexedrine, Dextrostat) and are primarily used for attention deficit hyperactivity disorder and narcolepsy. They are also sometimes prescribed for weight loss. Although their use for weight control was once very common, it is now quite rare. Now these drugs are recommended only for short-term management of obesity, as an adjunct to more effective methods. OTC nonamphetamine stimulants are now widely used as weight-loss aids (e.g., Dexatrim, Acutrim); they are equally ineffective. (See **Figure 5.2**.)

In the past, amphetamines were used to treat attention deficit hyperactivity disorder (ADHD). Children with this syndrome have short attention spans and are hyperactive, impulsive, easily distracted, and emotionally volatile. It is hard to understand how a stimulant is of value for the characteristic symptoms of ADHD. However, it is thought that concentration ability and attention span are enhanced, thus reducing problem behavior. Amphetamines have been largely replaced by methylphenidate (Ritalin), a drug with similar properties but with less potential for addiction. However, federal drug laws put Ritalin and amphetamines in the same category for control purposes.

The Monitoring the Future survey shows that in 2001, 16.2% of high school seniors reported any lifetime use of amphetamines, while 10.9% had used them in the 12 months prior to the survey. Use by other age groups is illustrated in Table 5.1

and Figure 5.1. Like cocaine, amphetamine use has not changed much over the last 10 years.

In the late 1980s, a smokable form of amphetamines arrived on the scene, moving from the Orient to Hawaii and then east across the United States. Crystal methamphetamine, called Ice, raised great concern because evidence suggested that smoking it was very addictive. Some predicted that Ice would become the drug epidemic of the 1990s.[1] It wasn't until 1999 that the national drug surveys began to gather data on methamphetamine use, so it is impossible to draw any conclusions regarding use of the drug prior to that time. However, arrests for drug law violations involving methamphetamines, as well as methamphetamine-related deaths and emergency room visits, were increasing during the 1990s.

Both amphetamines and cocaine reinforce repetitive drug-taking behavior, and this propensity becomes even greater with smokable forms (e.g., Ice and crack) and IV drugs because the effects are more pronounced and immediate. Both drugs rapidly provide a striking euphoria (sometimes described as orgasmic), but these effects wear off quickly (in as little as 10 minutes with crack). Because the euphoria is so enjoyable, many users feel compelled to take another dose. For some people, this need becomes obsessive, to the exclusion of everything else in their life. In addition, as the drug effect wears off, especially in a chronic user, the person experiences significant depression (dysphoria), so he or she is driven to take more drugs just to get out of a funk. Furthermore, family members and coworkers may respond positively to the user's increased energy, enthusiasm, productivity, and elevated moods, thereby inadvertently encouraging continued drug use. Continued use may cause psychological and physical dependency.

Hazards

While the addiction potential of amphetamines and cocaine is a real hazard, it has been overstated. Many people try these drugs or use them infrequently, but do not do so habitually. As Table 5.2 shows, less than 5% of those older than 26 years who have ever used these drugs have done so recently.

Amphetamines and Cocaine: Similarities and Differences[2,3]

Similar Effects*

Alertness	Magnification of pleasure
Insomnia	Talkativeness
Sense of well-being	Euphoria
Lower anxiety	Decreased social inhibitions
Increased energy	Increased self-esteem
Increased sexuality	Enhanced confidence
Dilated pupils	Sweating
Hypertension	Hyperthermia
Rapid heart rate	Increased respiration

Differences

Amphetamine effects typically last much longer (4 to 8 times). Cocaine must be taken much more frequently.

Cocaine is almost always illegally produced; dosage and purity are uncertain. Amphetamines often are made by pharmaceutical firms, where dosage and purity are standardized.

Amphetamines seem more closely related to hostile and violent reactions.

*Effects vary depending on the specific type of drug, the dosage, the way the drug is taken, the unique biochemical response of the user, and the setting.

[Table 5.2]

Lifetime, Past-Year, and Past-Month Use of Cocaine and Other Stimulants by Age Group, 2001

Age Groups	Lifetime	Past Year	Past Month
Cocaine			
12–17	2.3%	1.5%	0.4%
18–25	13.0	5.7	1.9
26+	13.6	1.2	0.6
12+	12.3	1.9	0.7
Stimulants			
12–17	3.7	2.2	0.7
18–25	9.5	3.4	1.3
26+	7.1	0.6	0.3
12+	7.1	1.1	0.5

Source: National Household Survey on Drug Abuse, 2001.

flight response. In addition, the drugs cause a variety of mood changes. As shown in the FYI box, the two drugs are very similar in effect; differences occur due to the degree of the user's prior experience with the drug, the dosage and purity of the drug, the way the drug is taken, and the circumstances surrounding its use. Equivalent doses taken in the same way (e.g., injected) have virtually identical effects. (See **Figure 5.3**.)

There are some differences between these two drugs. Amphetamines are usually taken by mouth, whereas cocaine is more often snorted, injected, or smoked. When used in these ways, cocaine is more likely to cause dependence, because the effects come and go rapidly. Furthermore, amphetamines last longer in the blood and nervous system before they are metabolized, which also tends to decrease the addiction potential of amphetamines relative to cocaine. Although the evidence is not unified, indications are that amphetamines cause people to react violently, particularly when large doses are taken in binges (e.g., "speed runs").[4] Violence occurs as paranoid delusions set in. This reaction may be exacerbated by sleep and food deprivation, characteristic of excessive use of the drug. Cocaine also may cause paranoia and confusion, but in clinical experience amphetamines are associated more frequently with violence.

A similarly small proportion of participants in the Monitoring the Future survey who have ever used these drugs are now using them daily. An important caveat is the possibility that the most habituated users, and those who have become the most dysfunctional and disabled, were not available to survey. Nevertheless, it should be understood that addiction is not a uniform phenomenon turning only on the pharmacological properties of a drug. Psychosocial characteristics and environmental circumstances are also involved.

Both amphetamines and cocaine are stimulants that act on the **central nervous system**. They cause physiological effects, such as increased heart rate and dilated pupils, that are similar to the fight-or-

Alertness

Insomnia

Sense of Well-being

Lower Anxiety

Increased Energy

Increased Sexuality

Dilated Pupils

Hypertension

Rapid Heart Rate

Magnification of Pleasure

Talkativeness

Euphoria

Decreased Social Inhibitions

Increased Self-esteem

Enhanced Confidence

Sweating

Hyperthermia

Increased Respiration

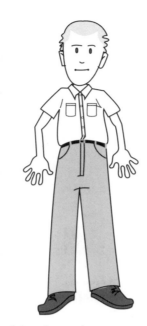

Figure 5.3 Common Effects of Cocaine and Amphetamines Stimulant drugs have numerous physical and emotional effects.

The health consequences of amphetamine and cocaine use are outlined in the FYI box, which compares the hazards of the two drugs. In some cases the hazards are the same. The unique health effects of the two drugs are also shown. Paradoxically, although both drugs tend to stimulate sexual drive and performance, chronic abuse often leads to sexual dysfunction and disinterest.[5] The legal sanctions for use of or trafficking in the drugs are identical. Addiction to the two manifests in similar behavior and lifestyle patterns.

It is important to understand that not every user will experience all of the effects or all of the hazards outlined in the accompanying boxes. Rather than predict the unique experience of an individual user, these boxes present cumulative clinical and epidemiological findings. Tobacco can be used as an example. Lung cancer is a frequent consequence of smoking; however, not all smokers get lung cancer. Disease risk is a matter of probability: The more cocaine or amphetamines used, and the longer use continues, the greater the risk that undesirable consequences will occur.

These drugs, particularly cocaine, not only are potentially hazardous to an unborn child, but some reports also show that infants can suffer harm from inhaling secondhand cocaine smoke.[14] (See **Figure 5.4**.) It could be hypothesized that smoking crystal methamphetamine (Ice) has a similar effect.

Media attention to a growing epidemic of crack babies and the consequences to school systems unprepared to serve their needs has been overblown. Evidence indicates that with adequate environmental supports, most of the early developmental deficits can be overcome.[15] Considering that most mothers who abuse cocaine and amphetamines during pregnancy are disadvantaged and dysfunctional, society is challenged in responding to the needs of these children.

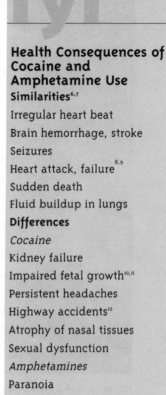

Health Consequences of Cocaine and Amphetamine Use

Similarities[6,7]

Irregular heart beat

Brain hemorrhage, stroke

Seizures

Heart attack, failure[8,9]

Sudden death

Fluid buildup in lungs

Differences

Cocaine

Kidney failure

Impaired fetal growth[10,11]

Persistent headaches

Highway accidents[12]

Atrophy of nasal tissues

Sexual dysfunction

Amphetamines

Paranoia

Violence[13]

Finally, beginning in the late 1980s the connection between cocaine use and the acquired immunodeficiency syndrome (AIDS) grew stronger. Cocaine is a short-term aphrodisiac that enhances sexual feelings. The sexual revolution did not need any help; unsafe sex was already far too common. However, in the inner cities, the exchange of sex for crack cocaine became prevalent among prostitutes and their customers.[16,17] Prostitutes and other female or male addicts provide sexual services in return for cocaine, which accounts for part of the increase in HIV infection in the heterosexual population.

In summary, both amphetamines and cocaine are addictive and can result in serious medical problems for users and unborn children. While millions of people have used these drugs, only a small proportion do so in an abusive and hazardous way.

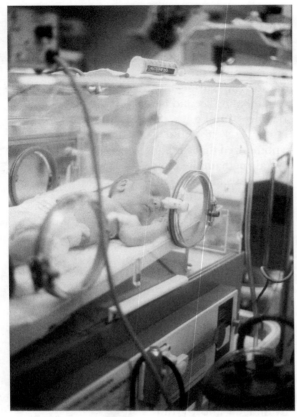

Figure 5.4 **A Crack Baby** Crack babies are born every day in major U.S. cities. (© Betts Anderson/Unicorn Stock Photos)

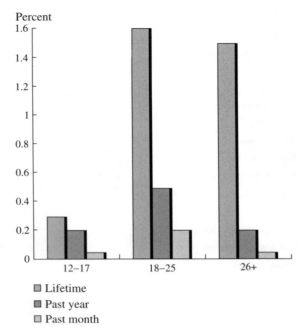

Percent

Figure 5.5 **Lifetime, Past-Year, and Past-Month Use of Heroin by Age Group, 2001**

Source: National Household Survey on Drug Abuse, 2001.

There has not been much change in the percentage of people currently using these drugs; in the case of cocaine, the current users seem to be using greater quantities than were typically used in the late 1980s.

Narcotics

Background

Prior to the 1980s, narcotics use, particularly IV heroin, was viewed as the quintessential drug abuse problem of the big cities. Although narcotics are still on the scene, they have been overshadowed by cocaine. As illustrated in **Figure 5.5**, heroin use is found in only a small segment of the population. When Monitoring the Future was initiated in 1975, 2.2% of high school seniors reported ever using heroin; from 1980 to 1994, the number hovered

around 1%, but increased in the late 1990s, reaching a peak of 2.4% in 2000. These figures represent a small proportion of the population, but even small percentages of the large U.S. population amount to a lot of people and big problems, especially when they are concentrated in certain areas, such as the central sections of New York, Chicago, Los Angeles, and Miami. The National Household Survey found that 456,000 people reported heroin use in 2001; this compares with 4.1 million who used cocaine. It must be reiterated that chronic drug abusers are less likely to be included in surveys, so the available statistics are undoubtedly conservative figures.

In spite of the relatively small number of people involved with heroin and other narcotics, these drugs still warrant some attention. First, narcotics use may be a significant problem in some communities. Second, the consequences of narcotics abuse are potentially severe. Finally, IV narcotics abuse, like all IV drug abuse, is directly related to the AIDS epidemic, a public health concern for all.

The original narcotic was opium, which historically was swallowed or smoked. During the 1800s, opium was purified to produce the more potent substances codeine and morphine. Heroin is the first and most infamous of a long line of synthetic narcotics, some more potent than morphine, whose introduction began in the 1890s. **Intravenous injection** technology also developed during the 19th century. These events greatly increased the potential dependency and hazard of the narcotics. Common examples of narcotics are shown in the FYI box.

The primary effect of narcotic drugs is relief of pain; pharmacologists call them *narcotic analgesics*. These drugs relieve pain without producing loss of consciousness. They cause sedation (i.e., a pronounced relaxation) and diminish the brain's interpretation of a sensation as painful (i.e., they raise the pain threshold). Narcotics also cause euphoria—feelings of lightheadedness and warmth. Other physical effects are shown in the FYI box entitled "Physical Side Effects of Narcotics."

Although all narcotics relieve pain and cause sedation and the side effects listed in the FYI box, there are differences among the drugs: Some are more potent, and some minimize certain effects and maximize others. Narcotics in general can be taken orally, smoked, snorted, or injected, either intravenously, **subcutaneously,** or **intramuscularly.** Morphine probably is used most widely in medical practice; heroin is entirely illegal, even in medical care, but it is the opiate most commonly taken by illicit drug users.

The other narcotic worth singling out is methadone, a synthetic drug developed in Germany in the 1940s. Methadone's effects are similar to morphine's, but they last much longer. Because methadone is very potent when taken orally and its effects last a long time, it has some efficacy in detoxifying heroin addicts. In treatment, an addict's use of heroin is abruptly ended. Because of cross-tolerance, methadone can immediately take the place of the heroin. Thus, the more severe symptoms of heroin withdrawal are blocked by methadone, and the client is then slowly weaned from methadone. Methadone's lasting effect means that only one dose in 24 hours is required, compared with three or four for heroin. Furthermore, because methadone is taken orally, needle use is immediately terminated, which has some behavioral implications in drug treatment. Methadone has not proved to be a panacea in treating narcotic addiction; some street trafficking in methadone occurs as well. Methadone maintenance is described further in Chapter 12.

Narcotics are used as an additive in some cough medicines (e.g., Robitussin A-C with codeine), in the relief of some forms of diarrhea, as premedication for surgery, and in treating acute pulmonary edema (i.e., water in the lungs). However, they serve their most important function in analgesia. Narcotics are the most potent pain relievers, particularly for dull, constant pain. They are used widely in treating heart attack pain and the intractable pain associated with cancer, and their sedation ability relieves the characteristic anxiety that exacerbates heart attacks. Because of narcotics' potential for dependency, physicians typically choose nonnarcotic analgesics as a drug of first choice; if pain still is not sufficiently controlled, a narcotic is the next choice.

Physicians must balance the pain-relieving capacity of a narcotic with its risk for causing dependency; conventional medical practice

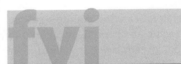

has guidelines for appropriate use. Because prescribing narcotics is a matter of professional judgment, some physicians may be too lax, facilitating a patient's dependency, while others are too conservative, tolerating a patient's continued suffering. Patients who chronically use narcotics in legitimate medical care still develop tolerance and physical dependency. However, the reversal of such a dependency is quite simple and usually successful. This expectation is in contrast to a street addict, whose addiction is complicated by extensive personal and social dysfunction.

Hazards

Illicit narcotics use has many hazards. The first is the significant risk of physical and psychological dependency. This potential has been exaggerated in the past—addiction does not occur after just one dose. In fact, there is a subset of users who

fyi

IV Drug Use and AIDS

After purchase, drugs in powdered form are commonly placed in a bottle cap "cooker." The powder is then diluted in tap water, heated to go into solution, and withdrawn into a needle and syringe. A suitable vein is identified and punctured, blood is withdrawn into the needle and syringe, and the solution is injected. Often, small quantities of drug are injected repeatedly, with intervening blood withdrawals. Thus, the injection apparatus, or "works," is easily contaminated with blood. Needles, syringes, and "cookers" are all shared. It is common practice to rent a used needle in a "shooting gallery," where intravenous drug users gather to administer drugs. After use, the contaminated "works" are rented to another user. The needle and syringe may be rented repeatedly until they are no longer usable. Thus, sequential anonymous sharing of blood-contaminated needles and syringes occurs among large numbers of persons. It would be difficult to design a system better suited to promote the transmission of blood-borne infection.

Source: G. H. Friedland and S. R. Klein, "Transmission of the Human Immunodeficiency Virus," *New England Journal of Medicine* 317, 18 (1987): 1125–1135.

seem to be relatively free from severe personal and social consequences. Nevertheless, dependency is real and often precludes a normal lifestyle. Because most street narcotics are expensive, users usually resort to stealing or prostitution to support their habit. In rare cases, a user may have free access to narcotics or adequate means to buy them and be able to live a normal and functional life.[18] These users are the exception. For most addicts, narcotic use becomes the central organizer of their lives. They get up in the morning and go to work: securing the money to buy drugs and locating a dealer with a supply for sale. This is followed by a few hours of relative tranquility, which may be spent sleeping or in more purposeful activities. After a short respite, they begin the cycle all over again.

In addition to having their lives controlled by an endless pursuit for the next high and being largely devoid of the things that provide genuine meaning in life, addicts continually face significant hazards and threats. Data from the national Drug Abuse Warning Network (DAWN) indicate that narcotics are one of the leading causes of drug-related deaths, after alcohol and tobacco.[19] One reason is that the drugs addicts buy do not come with quality assurances. The exact dose and ingredients are unknown. Although the dose is usually small,[20] it may be potent enough to kill before the needle is out of the arm.[21] Overdose is characterized by acute respiratory depression (i.e., the person stops breathing). The drugs often are mixed with other substances that may by themselves be hazardous. In the deaths reported to DAWN, 86% are from combinations, rather than single drugs.[22] Pure narcotics usually do no damage to the brain or other internal organs, but adulterants may damage blood vessel walls, lungs, liver, and kidneys. (See **Figure 5.6**.)

Besides these risks, addicts who use dirty needles almost certainly will get a variety of infections, including hepatitis B and AIDS. Intravenous drug use accounts for about 25% of male AIDS cases and about 39% of female AIDS cases.[23] IV drug use is a principal, though not the only, bridge by which AIDS reaches the heterosexual population. (See the FYI box.)

Users of illegal narcotics experience a world of social chaos and predation. Addicts are victims of

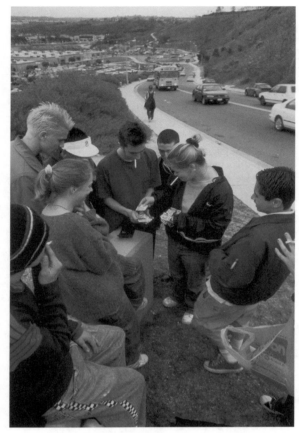

Figure 5.6 A Street Drug Buy People who buy drugs on the street face substantial risks. (© Spencer Grant/PhotoEdit)

violence at the hands of dealers and other junkies and are, of course, the targets of sometimes violent police action. Unlike alcohol, narcotics usually don't promote violent behavior. On the contrary, euphoria typically puts a user at peace with the world. However, an addict may resort to violence if money is required to get the next fix. This act is more a result of desperation than of anger or hostility.

Although legalization of narcotics might have serious pitfalls, many experts believe that the current legal framework for controlling these drugs makes life even more dangerous and depraved for the user and increases the toll borne by society. The issue of legalization is discussed in Chapter 14. It is sufficient to note here that the three principal dangers of narcotic abuse are overdose, infection, and violence. These dangers are not consequences

of the pharmacologic properties of the drugs, but rather of the illegal status of narcotics and needles. (See the FYI box entitled "Pros and Cons of Needle Exchange.") Indeed, some individuals who take narcotics for decades under ideal conditions have no noticeable ill effects.[24]

Nevertheless, narcotics abuse is a very grim reality for most users, and many, perhaps most,

fyi

Pros and Cons of Needle Exchange

Pros

Needle exchange is an effective bridge to treatment.

Clean needles save lives.

Many programs provide easier access to treatment.

Health professionals should offer clean needles as a viable alternative to using unclean needles.

Needle exchange programs serve as a contact point for hard-core drug abusers to bring them into public health and social services.

Active users can make behavior changes. But if we wait for all drug abusers to stop, the AIDS epidemic will continue to grow, threatening everyone.

We should put our energies into life-saving activities rather than giving verbal excuses for doing nothing.

Cons

Needle exchange subsidizes the drug culture.

Programs are designed to provide treatment, not needles.

Programs condone drug use and prolong addiction.

Distributing needles allows more people to begin using drugs.

Needle exchanges are genocidal to people of color.

Needle exchange programs send a mixed message: Drugs are illegal, but here is the paraphernalia.

Money for public services is in short supply; needle exchange shouldn't replace more important programs.

More data are needed to show that needle exchange programs are effective.

Distributing clean needles does not guarantee that they won't be shared.

never recover. In the meantime, they are a blight on the communities they haunt. While the narcotics problem may be relatively small, it is not decreasing. We are faced with a great challenge to prevent all we can and treat all we can. It remains to be seen if public policy in the first decade of the 21st century will be any more successful than it has been in the past. (See the Viewpoints box.)

Depressants

Background

Earlier in the chapter we noted that stimulants are resonant with the rapid pace of modern life. The flip side is that many people feel bludgeoned by life in the fast lane and seek a temporary release through drugs. Alcohol is the most popular choice, but there are others, such as barbiturate and nonbarbiturate sedatives and antianxiety drugs. Examples of these drugs are identified in the FYI box.

Alcohol, whose effects are very similar to these drugs' effects, is probably the most widely used drug in the self-management of stress. However, alcohol generally is not used in medical practice, and its role in society is very different in most ways.

Figure 5.7 shows statistics on the use of depressants in the general population. In 2001, the U.S. government estimated that about 806,000 persons had used depressants illicitly (i.e., not under the supervision of a physician) in the past 12 months. In 1975, 18.2% of high school seniors reported any lifetime use of depressants; by 2001 the figure was 8.7%, up from 5.5% in 1992. Only 0.1% of high school seniors reported using these drugs on a daily basis in 2001.

Examples of Depressant Drugs

Barbiturates (Nembutal, Seconal, phenobarbital)

Nonbarbiturates

  methaqualone (Quaalude, Sopor)

  meprobamate (Miltown)

  glutethimide (Doriden)

  chloral hydrate

  paraldehyde

Benzodiazepines (Libium, Valium, Dalmane, Restoril, Xanax)

A Perspective on Opium

Plants can live without animals but not animals without plants. We animals appear set upon destroying ourselves by nuclear or germ warfare and by drugs in war and peace. Some day by some such means—unless informed interest and public opinion gets busy—we shall possibly succeed. Then the symbol of eternal sleep [opium] will bloom on year by year, more appropriate than ever, and utterly indifferent.

Source: J. M. Scott, *The White Poppy: A History of Opium* (New York: Funk & Wagnalls, 1969).

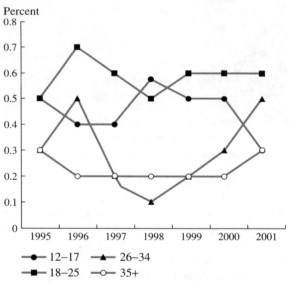

Figure 5.7 Use of Depressant Drugs, by Age, 1995–2001

Source: National Household Survey on Drug Abuse

Besides alcohol, barbiturates are the oldest drugs in the depressant category. They have been used for decades to treat insomnia, anxiety, and epilepsy and other seizure disorders and as anesthetics.

While barbiturates are very effective for these medical purposes, they also have a high risk for physical and psychological dependency. For this reason, they are used infrequently now for sedation or as sleeping pills. In addition, there is concern about accidental or intentional overdose, because in large enough doses, barbiturates depress respiration to the point of suffocation and death; this risk is exacerbated when they are used in combination with alcohol. A further concern is that people who take barbiturates may forget the earlier dose and later take more in a drug-induced stupor, leading to unintentional overdose.

A variety of drugs called *nonbarbiturate sedatives* have similar properties but differ chemically. Examples include chloral hydrate, paraldehyde, meprobamate, and methaqualone. The first two are rarely used now because of their objectionable smell and taste. Meprobamate (Miltown) was once prescribed enough that comedians and cartoonists joked about it in full expectation that audiences could relate and respond. (See **Figure 5.8**.) It has now been largely replaced by the benzodiazepines. Methaqualone is now entirely illegal, even in medical practice, because it has a very high dependency potential and has no benefits different from other available, safer drugs.

As mentioned previously, barbiturates and nonbarbiturates are similar in eliciting sedation or sleep; differing effects are a result of dosage. Benzodiazepines also cause sedation or sleep, depending on the dosage. However, they also have a direct effect on anxiety, which sets them apart from barbiturates and nonbarbiturates. One way to appreciate this distinction is to consider tolerance.

Barbiturates or nonbarbiturates may be used to relieve anxiety. They accomplish this by causing sedation, mildly depressing the central nervous system, and diminishing concentration and mental acuity. After continuous use for a period of time, a person usually develops physical dependency and tolerance, and larger, unsafe doses are needed to create the desired effects. Benzodiazepines used for sedation over a continuous period also show the development of tolerance, but the anxiety-reducing effects seem to be resistant to tolerance;[25] therefore, anxiety treatment effects continue without the need to increase dosage. Benzodiazepines may cause dependency, but this is a lesser concern than it is with barbiturates. They also cause less depression of the respiratory system. For these reasons, benzodiazepines are usually the first choice in drug therapy for anxiety. (See **Figure 5.9**.)

Hazards

Several undesirable consequences occur with the abuse of depressant drugs. Barbiturates and nonbarbiturates may cause respiratory failure and death. It is unlikely, though not unknown, for benzodiazepines to cause overdose unless they are combined with other drugs such as alcohol. Data on deaths and medical emergencies due to drugs are illustrated in Table 5.3 and **Figure 5.10**. These statistics demonstrate that depressant drugs are relatively rare causes of death or emergency room visits.

Another important hazard of depressant drug abuse is accidental injury. Just as with alcohol, the sedation caused by these drugs increases the risks of driving or operating machinery.

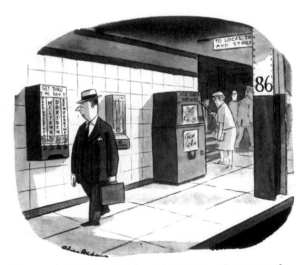

Figure 5.8 Charles Addams Cartoon The name of a depressant drug, Miltown, was once a household word.

(Drawing by Chas. Addams; © 1956–1984. The New Yorker Magazine, Inc.)

Table 5.3

Drug-Related Deaths, Selected Drugs and Selected Cities, 2000

	Chicago	Los Angeles	New York	Seattle
Heroin/morphine	499	473	194	118
Cocaine	464	471	492	104
Marijuana	23	32	37	1
Other narcotics	171	407	590	75
Benzodiazepines	43	142	25	33
Club drugs	9	27	5	3
Methamphetamines	2	155	3	15

Source: Drug Abuse Warning Network, 2001.

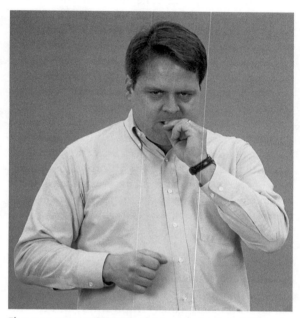

Figure 5.9 How Can We Cope with Anxiety Without Drugs?

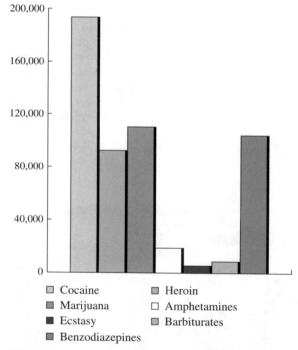

- ☐ Cocaine
- ☐ Heroin
- ■ Marijuana
- ☐ Amphetamines
- ■ Ecstasy
- ■ Barbiturates
- ■ Benzodiazepines

Figure 5.10 Emergency Room Visits for Selected Drugs, 2001

Source: Drug Abuse Warning Network, 2001.

Stimulant drugs temporarily improve a person's ability to function in the various tasks of life. Depressant drugs do not do this, except perhaps by relieving a disabling anxiety. Nevertheless, depressants are more likely to interfere with effective living. Impaired productivity at school or work occurs in much the same way as seen with alcohol abuse.

The final concern with depressants is physical and psychological dependency. Among the depressant drugs, barbiturates are the worst offenders in this regard, but abuse of benzodiazepines also leads to dependency. The statistics on the prevalence of benzodiazepine dependency are limited. Some people

| Table 5.4 |
| Past-Year Use of Marijuana, by Age Group and Grade Level, 1995–2001 | | | | | | |

Age Group	1995	1996	1997	1998	1999	2000	2001
12–17	14.2%	13.0%	15.8%	14.0%	14.2%	13.4%	15.2%
18–25	21.8	23.8	22.3	24.1	24.5	23.6	26.7
26–34	11.8	11.3	11.2	9.7	10.3	10.3	11.9
35+	3.4	3.8	4.4	4.1	4.0	3.8	4.1
Grade							
8	15.8	18.3	17.7	16.9	16.5	15.6	15.4
10	28.7	33.6	34.8	31.1	32.1	32.2	32.7
12	34.7	35.8	38.5	37.5	37.8	36.5	37.0

Source: Age group — National Household Survey on Drug Abuse; grade level — Monitoring the Future.

assume that dependency is common simply because of the widespread use of these drugs. In the 1970s and 1980s, about 15% of the U.S. population used one of the benzodiazepines at least once a year;[26] in 1985 these drugs accounted for more than 50% of all psychotropic drug prescriptions.[27] In recent years they have been surpassed by antidepressant drugs as the most commonly prescribed psychiatric drugs. Currently there is debate in the medical community about the relative advantages of **short-acting** benzodiazepines (e.g., Xanax) versus **long-acting** ones (e.g., Valium). Short-acting drugs in the group are less likely to produce residual sedation or grogginess, which might be important for elderly patients. However, long-acting benzodiazepines seem to have less pronounced withdrawal symptoms, less **rebound anxiety**, and less potential for dependency.[28]

The withdrawal syndrome associated with barbiturate addiction is considered one of the most dangerous and should be medically supervised over a period of two to three weeks. Abrupt discontinuance of benzodiazepines also will cause withdrawal symptoms, but the symptoms are usually less severe.

Marijuana

Background

Marijuana's claim to fame is that it is this country's most widely used illegal drug. It is also the illegal drug about which there is the most ambivalence. In the early 1990s, candidate Bill Clinton

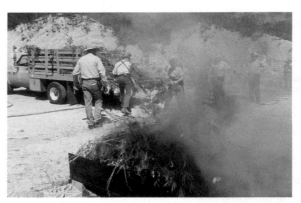

Figure 5.11 Destruction of Marijuana Plants by Police In spite of aggressive police tactics, the public is somewhat ambivalent about marijuana.

(© Alon Reininger/Unicorn Stock Photos)

was asked if he ever had used marijuana. When he said "I didn't inhale," some people doubted his honesty, but for most people, it was a nonissue. (See **Figure 5.11**.)

While marijuana use declined significantly through the 1980s, there has been almost no change from 1995 to 2001. Table 5.4 shows data for marijuana use in the population at large. In 2001, an estimated 83 million Americans had used marijuana sometime during their lifetime; about 12 million had used the drug in the past month.

Marijuana has been used for centuries in many regions, including the Middle East, Africa, Latin America, Asia, and the Caribbean. In the early 1990s,

Effects of Marijuana

Psychological

Relaxation

Euphoria

Sociability

Focus on the now

Drowsiness

Giddiness

Hunger

Anxiety

Lapses of attention

Impaired concentration

Impaired short-term memory

Perception that time is passing slowly

Physical

Red eyes (conjunctival reddening)

Increased heart rate (plus 20 to 50 beats per minute)

Dilation of bronchial tubes

Slowed reflexes

Decreased muscle coordination

Staggering and postural imbalance

Disruption of complex task performance

Effects are variable and dose dependent.

a tomb dating from the fourth century was uncovered near Jerusalem. It contained a woman and child who died in childbirth, and also marijuana ashes. Evidence suggests that the marijuana was used as medication during the birth.[29] While some other cultures have used marijuana primarily as a medicine or to ease the burden of heavy work, Western culture has used marijuana primarily as recreation. The principal effects of marijuana are shown in the FYI box.

Marijuana actually contains hundreds of chemicals, including about 60 known as cannabinoids. Cannabinoids as a group cause the effects for which marijuana is most known; delta-9-tetrahydrocannabinol (THC) is the most important substance in the group.[30] The other cannabinoids are present either in much smaller quantities or are much less potent. The average marijuana cigarette has about 3% THC. Sometimes the concentration is as much as 14%,[31] particularly with the marijuana called sinsemilla. Other forms of marijuana, such as hashish, have a THC content higher than joints (conventional marijuana cigarettes). Recently in the United States, youth have been hollowing out tobacco cigars and filling them with marijuana. These tobacco marijuana cigars are called *blunts*.

Marijuana may be taken orally, which gives a milder but longer effect than smoking it does.

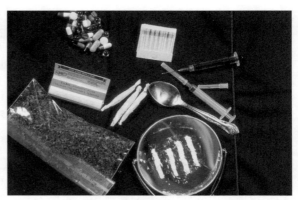

Figure 5.12 Drugs and Paraphernalia Marijuana use has created an industry that produces related items.

(© Dennis MacDonald/PhotoEdit)

Evidence suggests that the average THC content of cigarettes sold on the street increased from 1% to 3% throughout the 1970s and 1980s. Because both the acute effects and potential hazards are dose dependent, this increased potency caused concern among health officials.[32] (See **Figure 5.12**.) However, the dosage of any marijuana cigarette is unpredictable and variable, so it is impossible to make any assumptions that always apply.

As noted in the FYI box, marijuana has a variety of psychological and physical effects but does not cause violent, aggressive, or antisocial behavior. Contrary to what government officials stated in the 1920s and 1930s,[33] marijuana does not produce violent reactions, as other drugs do. Instead, marijuana usually makes users less violent than when they are not intoxicated with the drug. Even those users who develop a dependency for marijuana do not experience desperation, unlike heroin and cocaine addicts, who often commit crimes to get more drug. This behavior is not found among marijuana users because their dependency is not as compelling.

Research has been conducted to determine if marijuana has some useful therapeutic effects. A chemically synthesized form of THC (Marinol) has been produced by an American drug company. The most promising applications are as an antinausea drug used by people undergoing cancer chemotherapy and in the treatment of glaucoma. Some scientists maintain that marijuana has no medical applications that cannot be duplicated by other drugs with less troublesome side effects and less potential for addiction,[34] a view shared by the U.S. Public Health Service. However, others feel the government's opposition is politically motivated, and note that one survey showed that almost half of **oncologists** would prescribe THC if it were legal.[35] Regardless of the outcome of this debate, the association of marijuana with cancer treatment (see **Figure 5.13**) has led to the myth that marijuana can treat or somehow prevent cancer. Educators must counteract this myth.

Hazards

The consequences of marijuana use are real, though not extensive. As shown in Table 5.3, deaths attributed to marijuana are rare compared with heroin and

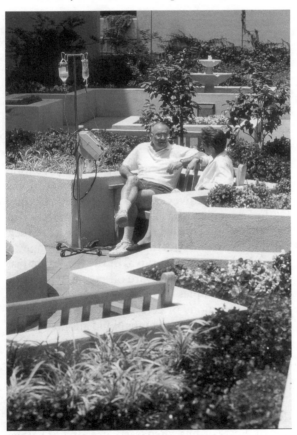

Figure 5.13 **A Patient Receiving Cancer Chemotherapy** Should people have access to marijuana as part of their therapy? (© Gary A. Conner/PhotoEdit)

cocaine, and certainly compared with tobacco and alcohol. Compared with cocaine, marijuana has been used by 5 times more people in the past year and almost 7 times more people in the past month. Compared with heroin, marijuana has been used by 42 times more people in the past year and 97 times more people in the past month. Given those facts, the lethal effects of marijuana appear to be minimal.

Research on marijuana and driving performance shows that driving is unsafe because of marijuana's physical and psychological effects. However, data to document the incidence of marijuana-related accidents are limited because the signs of marijuana intoxication are less obvious and less known than the signs of alcohol intoxication. Also, police agencies don't routinely test for marijuana, as they do for alcohol. However, safety experts agree that people should not drive under the influence of marijuana.

Another hazard of marijuana is lung damage. Heavy use of marijuana impairs breathing capacity. Marijuana smoke contains more tar and is more carcinogenic than tobacco smoke. This is certainly not good for health, but concern is tempered by the fact that marijuana is not used in the same way as tobacco cigarettes. The typical tobacco smoker smokes throughout the day to maintain a constant blood nicotine level. Marijuana smokers typically smoke only socially; even daily smokers rarely exceed three to four cigarettes.

For about three decades there has been a concern that marijuana leads to the "amotivational syndrome," which is characterized by lack of interest in goal-oriented activity, such as schoolwork, and apathy about managing the growing pains of adolescence to become a productive member of society. While the psychological effects of marijuana don't promote a "taking life by the throat" philosophy, there is scant definitive evidence of a chronic residual syndrome that continues even when the user is not under the influence. However, mainstream Western and Judeo-Christian values maintain that marijuana use is an unhealthy diversion from normal adolescent development and the pursuit of excellence. Whether there is an actual syndrome that draws users into unfocused, mediocre living is a moot point. Those who chronically abuse marijuana probably will not make maximum use of their personal gifts.

Marijuana use may cause physical and psychological dependency, and abrupt discontinuance of heavy use causes an **abstinence syndrome**. However, these withdrawal symptoms are mild, and a user would not go to great lengths to avoid them. Furthermore, the picture of dependency is not as squalid, or usually as violent, as is typical of cocaine or heroin addiction, perhaps because marijuana is more readily available and cheaper. Also, the effects of marijuana dependency are not as debilitating as other drug dependencies. Finally, the number of users who are marijuana dependent constitutes a relatively small proportion of those who have ever used the drug.

Other marijuana-related health concerns include an impaired immune system with decreased levels of **T lymphocytes**. Marijuana use also causes a reduction in reproductive hormones: In males, sperm count and motility are decreased; in females, ovulation and menstruation may become irregular. The clinical significance of these changes is not specific—no defined morbidity or mortality has been identified. On the other hand, adequate evidence suggests that marijuana use during pregnancy causes low birth weight and developmental anomalies, so prenatal use should be avoided.

In summary, marijuana has social and medical hazards, particularly when consumption is heavy and chronic. Educators must strive to prevent its

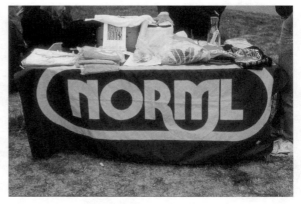

Figure 5.14 **Norml Materials** The National Organization for the Reform of Marijuana Laws (NORML) has promoted the decriminalization of the drug for many years. (© Aneal Vohra/Unicorn Stock Photos)

use. However, in the shadow of alcohol, tobacco, cocaine, and heroin, marijuana does not deserve the excessive concern or the big investment of public dollars it has garnered. (See Figure 5.14.)

Hallucinogens

Background

The curtain rose on drugs that mimic psychotic **hallucinations** during the baby boom generation's adolescence. However, this was not act one. Hallucinogenic drugs have a long tradition in human history. Throughout the natural world, such substances are found that provide advantage in natural selection and survival of the fittest; that is, hallucinogenic toxicities ward off potential enemies. Disparate examples include morning glory seeds, the skin secretions of certain toads, nutmeg, and mushrooms. In the past, humankind adopted plants with hallucinogenic properties not for pleasure or to relieve the grind of daily living, but instead to enhance religious experience, to heal, and to practice witchcraft.

In this era, the most familiar hallucinogen is LSD (lysergic acid diethylamide), though in recent years use of Ecstasy has surpassed use of LSD. (See Figure 5.15.) Accidentally discovered by a chemist in the 1930s, LSD has become the prototype of this drug group. The FYI box identifies various examples

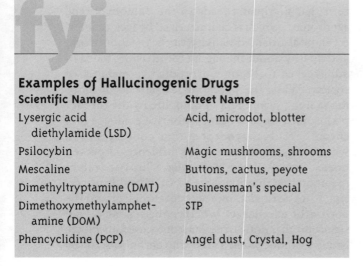

fyi

Examples of Hallucinogenic Drugs

Scientific Names	Street Names
Lysergic acid diethylamide (LSD)	Acid, microdot, blotter
Psilocybin	Magic mushrooms, shrooms
Mescaline	Buttons, cactus, peyote
Dimethyltryptamine (DMT)	Businessman's special
Dimethoxymethylamphetamine (DOM)	STP
Phencyclidine (PCP)	Angel dust, Crystal, Hog

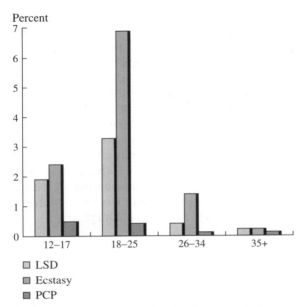

Figure 5.15 Use of Selected Hallucinogens, by Age Group, 2001

Source: National Household Survey on Drug Abuse.

Legend:
☐ LSD
☐ Ecstasy
■ PCP

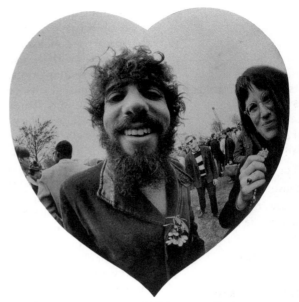

Figure 5.16 1960s Flower Children Hallucinogens were a prominent part of the 1960s counterculture.

(© John Brown–Chicago)

of hallucinogens. All hallucinogens have similar effects, but vary by potency, duration of action, and side effects. The setting in which the drug is used and the emotional condition and past experiences of the user also influence the drug experience.

During the 1960s, hallucinogenic drugs burst into headlines and broadcast media everywhere. For many, hippies and flower children languishing at an LSD-induced "love-in" was the memorable image of the drug scene. (See **Figure 5.16.**) The attention was caused by the novelty of the drugs and relief from the more familiar college beer bashes. In any case, hallucinogenic drugs have never attracted many drug users, perhaps because they do not meet the needs of the average teen or young adult.

In 2001, 12.8% of high school seniors reported any lifetime use of hallucinogens, and only 3.2% had used within one month of the survey. Lifetime use by seniors dropped slightly from 1997 to the present, after increasing from 1991 to 1997. The "alarming" increase in hallucinogen use that was proclaimed in the mass media in the early 1990s has dissipated.[36] Use of Ecstasy, however, has increased since 1996.

The sensory effect of a hallucinogenic drug experience may be similar to that of a large dose of marijuana, but otherwise it is unique from that of all other drugs of abuse. In fact, people who have used hallucinogens have difficulty articulating the experience to the uninitiated. Because most people have neither had a real nor a drug-induced hallucination, they can't relate. Furthermore, these sensory effects are very much an internal experience not apparent to an observer, unlike the mania of cocaine or amphetamines or the stupor of alcohol. The FYI box outlines the effects of LSD and other hallucinogens.

While many adolescents try hallucinogens out of curiosity, other people purposefully use these drugs. They seek an alternative to the technological, rational, and **materialistic** (in a scientific sense) aspects of life. They want to experience rather than think, and feel rather than know. Their goal may be to achieve enhanced creativity, a unique sensory experience, or a mystical **transcendence**, characterized by a sense of unity with the universe, feelings of peaceful bliss, and insights into self and

Effects of Hallucinogenic Drugs

Physical

Central nervous system stimulation

Dilated or unequal pupils

Hypersensitive reflexes

Involuntary contraction and relaxation of skeletal muscles

Gooseflesh

Tingling, numbness

Fever

Hypersalivation, nausea, vomiting

Rapid heart rate

Increased blood pressure

Sensory/Psychological

Visual distortions, illusions

Vivid, kaleidoscopic images

Distortions of space, size, distance

Distortions of body image, integrity, proportion

Distorted proprioception (sense of body position, alignment)

Synesthesia (confused sensory perception, such as seeing sound)

Anxiety, panic

Intense introspection

Effects are variable and dose dependent.

Hazards

The hazards of hallucinogens appear to be limited. Altered sensory perceptions create accident hazards; misperception of depth, distance, speed, and proportions might lead to many dangerous circumstances, the meaning of life. There is no objective evidence that creativity measurably improves with the use of LSD or similar drugs. However, unusual sensory experiences and transcendence occur in varying degrees whether they are sought after or not. For most users, this altered state comes and goes as the drug is absorbed and metabolized; there are no residual physical or emotional effects, or changes in personal views of self or life. However, some users under some circumstances experience fear, dread, and panic (a *bad trip*), which creates an undesirable emotional state that persists for days or weeks after the drug use. This experience may be more likely to occur in users who are emotionally unstable to begin with. For some other users, the transcendence may lead to an improved adjustment to life, particularly if this "psychedelic therapy" is in the context of disciplined character development.[37] However, this benefit is unpredictable and probably very rare.

some life threatening. There are no known cases of overdose due to LSD alone, and most hallucinogens are similarly benign. PCP is an exception and is discussed further in the next section.

Hallucinogens also can cause recurring flashbacks: Weeks or months after the drug is used, its sensory effects are repeated. This effect is unpredictable in terms of who will have flashbacks and when they will occur. The safety hazards of using hallucinogens then become more formidable.

Finally, hallucinogens may be hazardous to an unborn child. Although documentation on specific cases is limited, expectant mothers are encouraged to avoid all drugs during pregnancy.

Phencyclidine: A Special Case

Phencyclidine (PCP) is classified with the hallucinogenic drugs, but it is worthy of significantly more concern than other drugs in the group. PCP was introduced in 1957 as a human anesthetic agent. Undesirable side effects led to its relegation to only veterinary use as an animal tranquilizer. Because it is legally manufactured by drug companies and is easy to synthesize in clandestine laboratories, a significant amount of street trafficking and illicit use of PCP have occurred. The drug may be smoked, swallowed, snorted, or injected.

Monitoring the Future began collecting data on PCP in 1979. At that time, 12.8% of high school seniors reported any lifetime use of the drug; in 2001 that statistic had declined to 3.5%. Data from the National Household Survey and Monitoring the Future indicate that use of PCP is less than that of LSD or Ecstasy. However, the DAWN survey indicated in 2001 that there were more emergency room visits associated with PCP than with LSD or Ecstasy.

PCP causes the stimulation and sensory changes common with other hallucinogens. In addition, phencyclidine causes profound confusion, involuntary eye movements, difficulty in walking and muscle control, hypertension, agitation, disorientation, auditory hallucinations, and **paranoid delusions**. The cognitive alteration predisposes the user to violent behavior, although this propensity to violence has been overstated and is apparently rare. PCP use can also lead to psychological dependency.

PCP has been recklessly called the "killer drug," and media depictions of the drug's hazards have been hyperbolized. Nevertheless, PCP is more dangerous than the other hallucinogens and deserves concerted effort to discourage its use.

Club Drugs

The term **club drug** refers to a group of drugs that are categorized together, not necessarily because of similar chemical effects but because they are commonly used in dance clubs, bars, and dance parties called raves.[38] Examples include Ecstasy, GHB, ketamine, and Rohypnol. Use of these drugs by school-aged youth is shown in **Figure 5.17**. Ecstasy began to enjoy considerable popularity among college students in the late 1980s.[39] The other drugs have come on the scene more recently.

Ecstasy is the street name for methylenedioxymethamphetamine (MDMA). It combines the stimulant effects of methamphetamine with hallucinogenic properties. It is also known as "the party drug," X-TC, Adam, Clarity, and Lover's Speed.

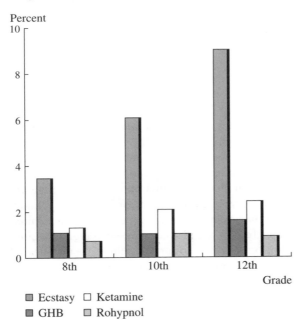

Figure 5.17 **Use of Selected Club Drugs by Grade, 2001**

Source: Monitoring the Future, 2001.

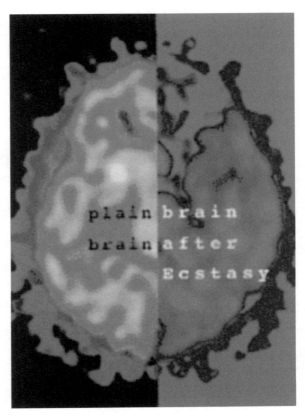

Figure 5.18 **Brain After Ecstasy**   These brain scans show the sharp difference in human brain function between an individual who has never used drugs (left) and one who has used the club drug Ecstasy many times (right).

Source: National Institute on Drug Abuse.

It is available in tablet, capsule, or powder form. For up to 24 hours after the drug is taken, the user can experience euphoria, enhanced mental and emotional clarity, and sensations of lightness and floating, but also confusion, depression, sleep problems, anxiety, depression, and paranoia. Acute pysical effects can include muscle tension, teeth clenching, nausea, blurred vision, faintness, chills, sweating, dehydration, hypertension, and tremors. There is great concern that use of Ecstasy can lead to permanent brain damage. (See **Figure 5.18.**)

Gamma hydroxybutyrate (GHB) is an anabolic steroid that has euphoric, sedative, and body-building effects. It was available over the counter until 1990, when the U.S. Food and Drug Administration made it strictly a prescription drug. It can come as a clear liquid, a white powder, or a tablet. It can cause high blood pressure, mood swings, and violent behavior. The immediate physical effects include sweating, headache, slowed heart rate, nausea, vomiting, impaired breathing, loss of reflexes, and tremors.

Ketamine is a nonbarbiturate anesthetic, sometimes called K, Ket, Special K, Vitamin K, and many other names. It can come as an injectable liquid, or in powder form for smoking or snorting. Its appearance causes it to be mistaken for cocaine or crystal methamphetamine. Ketamine produces a dissociative state in users—a feeling of disconnection from one's body and the objective, material world. Other effects are similar to those of PCP. Ketamine can cause fatal overdose by serious depression of breathing.

The last club drug is Rohypnol, a brand name for flunitazepam, a member of the benzodiazepam family. On the street it is known as roofies, rophies, and the "date rape" drug. Rohypnol is illegal in the United States even as a prescription drug; it is used in many other countries. The drug comes as a tablet, but can be crushed and dissolved in liquid. In this way it has been given to people surreptitiously to prevent them from resisting sexual assault. The immediate effects of Rohypnol are intoxication, muscle relaxation, drowsiness, slurred speech, and difficulty walking. Users are often unable to remember what happened while they were under the influence of Rohypnol. The drug can cause respiratory distress. In combination with alcohol, this can be fatal.

Like all street drugs, club drugs don't come with a warranty. Often buyers don't get what they think they are buying. (See **Figure 5.19**.) Furthermore, while the drugs may have effects that users find appealing, many of them damage the nervous system and other organs. Some are so potent that they cause death from overdose very readily.

If there is such a thing as responsible drug use, it is when a consumer knows what the effects of a specific dose of a specific drug are, and uses only enough to derive benefit without exceeding that dosage and increasing the risk of harm. The nature of club drugs as they are sold on the street precludes

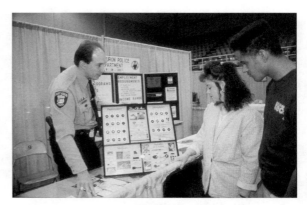

Figure 5.19 Illegal Drugs: What Is the Real Content of These Drugs? (© Dennis MacDonald/Unicorn Stock Photos)

this responsible behavior, and their use can only be considered a form of Russian roulette.

Summary

This chapter recounted a long list of drugs, what they do, and why they should be avoided. Readers will be interested primarily in the technology of prevention: What works? However, all of us might ponder the broader question: Why do we have so many drug problems (and other serious social problems), and how can they be solved?

Much of the world is drawn to the personal freedom and high standard of living found in the United States. Perhaps the bedrock of our founding philosophy is found in the words "We hold these truths to be self-evident, that all men are created equal, that they are endowed by their creator with certain unalienable rights and amongst these are life, liberty and the pursuit of happiness," taken from the Declaration of Independence. The United States finds itself in a curious, even embarrassing, position. In many countries, people are intoxicated by our slogans about equality and freedom, "reaching for the ideas at America's core." And yet we who know the American reality have much to be ashamed of.[40]

Is it possible that there is not enough responsibility reining in our freedom? Is self-serving freedom out of hand in America? Perhaps there is a malignancy on the American soul. Finding solutions to this broader problem presents a formidable challenge.

Scenario | Analysis and Response

There is no question that countries and groups that are involved in terrorism are involved in the international illegal drug trade. It is true that buyers of illegal drugs are possibly channeling money to terrorists. However, this is also true of people who buy gasoline. Since many terrorist drug dealers are also being supported by money earned from the sale of petroleum, the case can be made that people who use petroleum products (or drive gas-guzzling cars) are supporting terrorism.

While it is a worthy goal to discourage people from using drugs, all prevention strategies must be honest. The public loses confidence in programs that lack credibility. This compromises the value of legitimate programs and prevention concepts.

Learning Activities

1. Obtain a copy of a middle school health textbook. Assess the amount of space devoted to each of the drugs addressed in this chapter and compare it with that devoted to alcohol and tobacco. Make a judgment about the appropriateness of the attention given to the various drugs based on the personal and societal harm done by each.

2. Visit a law enforcement agency and try to get statistics or anecdotal estimates concerning the extent of local trafficking in the drugs discussed in this chapter.

3. Visit an emergency room and try to get information about the frequency with which the drugs discussed in this chapter are involved in cases served in that facility.

4. Interview a pharmacist to learn about the controls placed on prescription use of depressants, stimulants, and narcotics. Determine whether the controls are too stringent or too lax and whether the pharmacist thinks the control mechanisms should be changed.

5. Visit a local hospice and find out about its policies regarding pain control in terminal patients. Is there any concern regarding excessive use of drugs? How does the hospice work with patients who are unwilling to use prescription narcotics or other mood-altering drugs?

Notes

1. M. Sager, "The Ice Age." *Rolling Stone,* February 8, 1990, 53–57, 110, 114, 116.

2. F. H. Gawin and E. H. Ellinwood, "Cocaine and Other Stimulants: Actions, Abuse, and Treatment," *New England Journal of Medicine* 318, 18 (May 5, 1988): 1173–1182.

3. J. R. DiPalma and G. J. DiGregorio, *Basic Pharmacology in Medicine,* 3d ed. (New York: McGraw-Hill, 1990), 107–108, 246–249.

4. K. A. Miczek and J. W. Tidey, "Amphetamines: Aggressive and Social Behavior," in *Pharmacology and Toxicology of Amphetamine and Related Designer Drugs,* K. Asghar and E. De Souza, eds., NIDA Research Monograph 94 (Rockville, MD: DHHS, 1989).

5. Gawin and Ellinwood, "Cocaine and Other Stimulants."

6. L. L. Cregler and H. Mark, "Medical Complications of Cocaine Abuse," *New England Journal of Medicine* 315, 23 (December 4, 1986): 1495–1500.

7. DiPalma and DiGregorio, *Basic Pharmacology in Medicine.*

8. R. L. Minor, B. D. Scott, D. D. Brown, and M. D. Winniford, "Cocaine-Induced Myocardial Infarction in Patients with Normal Coronary Arteries," *Annals of Internal Medicine* 115, 10 (November 15, 1991): 797–805.

9. R. Hong, E. Matsuyama, and K. Nur, "Cardiomyopathy Associated with the Smoking of Crystal Methamphetamine," *Journal of the American Medical Association* 265, 9 (March 6, 1991): 1152–1154.

10. J. J. Volpe, "Effect of Cocaine Use on the Fetus," *New England Journal of Medicine* 327, 6 (August 6, 1992): 399–407.

11. D. A. Bateman, S. K. C. Ng, C. A. Hanson, and M. C. Heagarty, "The Effects of Intrauterine Cocaine Exposure in Newborns," *American Journal of Public Health* 83, 2 (February 1993): 190–193.

12. P. M. Marzuk, K. Tardiff, A. C. Leon, M. Stajic, E. B. Morgan, and J. J. Mann, "Prevalence of Recent Cocaine Use Among Motor Vehicle Fatalities in New York City," *Journal of the American Medical Association* 263, 2 (January 12, 1990): 250–256.

13. Miczek and Tidey, "Amphetamines."

14. Bateman et al., "The Effects of Intrauterine Cocaine Exposure in Newborns."

15. H. G. Mirchandani, et al. "Passive Inhalation of Free-Base Cocaine (Crack) Smoke by Infants," *Archives of Pathology and Laboratory Medicine* 115 (1991): 494–498.

16. J. A. Inciardi, A. E. Pottieger, M. Forney, D. D.Chitwood, and D. C. McBride, "Prostitution, IV Drug Use, and Sex-for-Crack Exchanges Among Serious Delinquents: Risks for HIV Infection," *Criminology* 29, 2 (1991): 221–235.

17. M. Balshem, G. Oxman, D. Van Rooyen, and K. Girod, "Syphilis, Sex and Crack Cocaine: Images of Risk and Morality," *Social Science and Medicine* 35, 2 (1992): 147–160.

18. Andres Goth, *Medical Pharmacology* (St. Louis: C.V. Mosby, 1974), 302.

19. Substance Abuse and Mental Health Services Administration, Office of Applied Studies, *Mortality Data from the Drug Abuse Warning Network, 2000,* DAWN Series D-19, DHHS Publication No. (SMA) 02-3633 (Rockville, MD: DHHS, 2002).

20. J. A. Inciardi, *The War on Drugs II* (Mountain View, CA: Mayfield, 1992), 69.

21. Ibid., 76.

22. Substance Abuse and Mental Health Services Administration, *Mortality Data.*

23. Centers for Disease Control and Prevention, "Update: AIDS—United States, 2000." *MMWR Weekly* 51 (July 12, 2002): 592–595.

24. Goth, *Medical Pharmacology*, 301.

25. DiPalma and DiGregorio, *Basic Pharmacology*, 227.

26. Ibid., 337.

27. H. Koch, National Center for Health Statistics, *Highlights of Drug Utilization in Office Practice, National Ambulatory Medical Care Survey, 1985; Advanced Data Vital and Health Statistics,* DHHS Publication No. (PHS) 87-1250 (Rockville, MD: DHHS, 1987).

28. D. D. Hallfors and L. Saxe, "The Dependence Potential of Short Half-Life Benzodiazepines: A Meta-Analysis," *American Journal of Public Health* 83, 9 (September 1993): 1300–1304.

29. "Marijuana Medication," *New York Times,* June 1, 1993, C5.

30. Bateman et al., "The Effects of Intrauterine Cocaine Exposure in Newborns."

31. DiPalma and DiGregorio, *Basic Pharmacology*, 341.

32. National Institute on Drug Abuse, *Marijuana and Health: 9th Report to the U.S. Congress,* DHHS Publication No. (ADM) 82-1216 (Rockville, MD: DHHS, 1982), vi.

33. L. Sloman, *Reefer Madness: A History of Marijuana in America* (Indianapolis: Bobbs-Merrill, 1979), 30–63.

34. E. T. Herfindal, D. R. Gourley, and L. L. Hart, eds., *Clinical Pharmacy and Therapeutics* (Baltimore: Williams & Wilkins, 1988), 294.

35. P. Cotton, "Government Extinguishes Marijuana Access, Advocates Smell Politics," *Journal of the American Medical Association* 267, 19 (May 29, 1992): 2573.

36. E. Negin, "CBS' '48 Hours' Fails Acid Test," *American Journalism Review* 15, 2 (March 1993): 10.

37. S. Cohen, "The Chemical Transcendental State: An Experience in Search of an Explanation," in *The Psychopharmacology of Hallucinogens,* R. C. Stillman, and R. E. Willette, eds. (New York: Pergamon Press, 1978), 324–329.

38. A. M. Arria, G. S. Yacoubian, E. Fost, and E. D. Wish, "Ecstasy Use Among Club Rave Attendees," *Archives of Pediatrics and Adolescent Medicine* 156, 3(2002): 295–296.

39. S. J. Petrouka, "Incidence of Recreational Use of 3,4-Methylenedioxymethamphetamine (MDMA-Ecstasy) on an Undergraduate Campus," *New England Journal of Medicine* 317, 24 (December 10, 1987): 1542–1543.

40. S. A. Hewlett, *When the Bough Breaks: The Cost of Neglecting Our Children* (New York: Basic Books, 1991), 275–276.

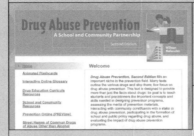

Chapter Learning Objectives

Upon completion of this chapter, students will be able to:

1. Explain the relationship between violence and drug abuse and between drug abuse prevention and violence prevention.

2. Describe the nature and extent of school and community violence.

3. Compare and contrast violence risk and protective factors with drug abuse risk and protective factors.

4. Outline a variety of factors thought to promote violence and identify possible prevention strategies for each.

5. Point out and explain the components of a school safety plan.

6. Identify several national resources for violence prevention programs.

Scenario

On April 20, 1999, America was shaken from within as a horrible event was reported in international news. Two high school students in Littleton, Colorado, had entered their school with firearms and bombs, killing 12 other students, one teacher, and finally themselves. Twenty-three other students were seriously wounded. Prior to that day, the boys had been in trouble with the police, charged with neighborhood vandalism and breaking into an automobile. One of the boys was taking antidepressant drugs prescribed by a psychiatrist.

The boys belonged to a recognized fringe social group in the school called the "Trench Coat Mafia." Ironically, the oversized coats they wore on April 20 facilitated the smuggling in of weapons without detection. Over the previous two years, the boys had turned in written and video assignments with extremely violent and hateful content. A counselor had talked to one of the boys and his father about this material. One of the boys had a Web site on which he posted content with extreme violence and hate. Because he

Chapter 6

School and Community Violence Prevention

Introduction

From the very beginning humans have perpetrated violence on one another. Folklore images of cavemen incorporate an easy acceptance of brutality, particularly toward women. In the Judeo-Christian tradition, the first recognized act of violence occurred at the dawn of recorded civilization: Cain's murder of Abel. While the means of inflicting violence have varied through time, the underlying motivations are largely constant. In a sense, violence is yesterday's news.

However, because the human species is endowed with the ability and inclination to make life better, every generation makes an effort to cope with violence and its consequences. This has been easier in some eras than others. While much has been

had threatened a neighborhood boy, that boy's parents made copies of the Web site's material and brought it to the local police.

At home, the boys were constructing pipe bombs and maintaining detailed journals outlining their plans for violence and retaliation against fellow students who they felt had ridiculed and ostracized them. The boys were absorbed in violent music and video games.

A girlfriend of one of the boys was old enough (18) in Colorado to buy three guns for him, and a 22-year-old man bought an assault weapon for them as well.

In hindsight, all of these factors came together on that fateful day. Many of the events just chronicled were observed or observable by other students, parents, teachers and school staff, neighbors, police, and mental health professionals. Many wonder why it happened. The most sobering question is "Why wasn't it prevented?"

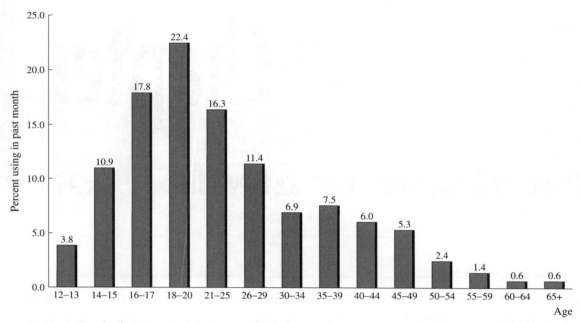

Figure 6.1 **Past-Month Illicit Drug Use by Age, 2001**

Source: National Household Survey on Drug Abuse.

learned about the nature and causes of violence during the previous 100 years, we are far from being able to dismiss it from the social agenda. Americans at the dawn of the 21st century have great anxiety about being victims of violence. This anxiety includes violence in schools and among youth.

Schools are constituent of the communities in which they are located. The strengths and weaknesses of families and children will be manifest in the school. Because both drug abuse and violence are common in communities, it is to be expected that these problems will be found in schools, experienced by students and adults in the school setting.

Parents and society have paradoxical attitudes about our schools. On the one hand, people are often cynical and dismayed by perceptions of poor school performance and media reports of student alcohol and drug abuse, violence, and sexuality. On the other hand, the knee-jerk response of society is to ask schools to help solve a wide range of social problems. At one and the same time, we blame the schools, yet look to them for solutions.

In spite of these mixed attitudes toward and expectations for schools, it is appropriate for schools to address school and community violence. Because drug abuse and violence are so intertwined and because the prevention and early intervention strategies for each problem are parallel, this text includes this chapter on violence and its prevention.

There are many similarities between drug abuse and violence. Both problems are significantly clustered among teens and young adults. **Figure 6.1** illustrates the prevalence of illicit drug use by age category; **Figure 6.2** shows homicide by age. These figures demonstrate the pattern of significant youth involvement in each.

It is worth noting that while young people are significantly involved in both drug abuse and violence, these behaviors are much more likely to occur outside of school hours and off school grounds than in schools. Because schools incorporate a high degree of structure, supervision, and continuous monitoring of students by adults, they are relatively drug and violence free. **Figure 6.3** compares the prevalence of homicide and suicide among young people at schools and in community locations.

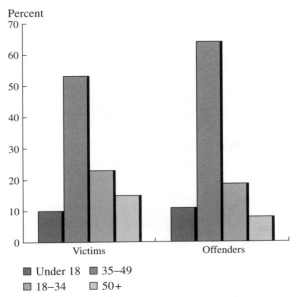

Figure 6.2 **Homicide Victims and Offenders by Age, 1976–1999**

Source: U.S. Department of Justice, 2000.

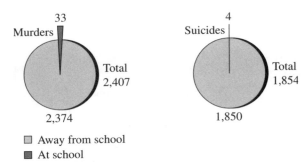

Figure 6.3 **Youth Homicide and Suicide at School and Away from School, 1998–1999**

Source: U.S. Department of Justice.

The figure clearly shows that youth are much more vulnerable in family, neighborhood, and other community settings than at school.

Another association between drug abuse and violence is the concept of risk and protective factors. Factors that put youth at risk for drug abuse largely intersect with risk factors for violence. Those factors that might decrease the risk of youth involvement in drug abuse also tend to decrease their risk for violence. These factors are shown in Table 6.1.

The range of pharmacological effects of alcohol, tobacco, and other drugs is broad and varied. Violence is one category of those effects. In theory, drug abuse can lead to violence through two pathways. Drugs that create extreme stimulation, such as amphetamines and cocaine, induce the fight-or-flight mechanism. The user is physiologically stirred to fight. In the right circumstances, a person so stimulated responds to provocation in ways more violent than in a nondrugged state.

The other pathway is through drugs that cause depression of the central nervous system, such as alcohol. When the senses and consciousness are impaired by drugs that depress the brain, the person is less aware of danger and is less cognizant of ordinary rules of social interaction. Without the normal inhibitions that serve as social barriers, people under the influence of a depressant drug will sometimes act on hostile or violent impulses.

Finally, many of the prevention programs designed for school settings address both drug abuse and violence. The movement for science-based programs and best-practice principles incorporates curriculum and program activities for both drug abuse and violence prevention strategies. For this reason and all the reasons cited previously, this chapter is included to help students understand violence as well as drug abuse and to facilitate the inclusion of violence prevention with school and community drug abuse prevention programs.

Nature and Extent of School and Community Violence

Monitoring and assessing the proportions of our violence problem require reference to statistics. Data on violence are gathered by a variety of agencies at the local, state, national, and international level. However, there is an important caveat when drawing conclusions from such data. In the medical and public health field, we have excellent and generally very reliable data on births and deaths because they are distinct events and there is a standardized procedure for keeping track of them: birth and death certificates. Less available and reliable are statistics on the incidence and prevalence of diseases, per se. Reporting of these is much more cumbersome

Table 6.1

Risk and Protective Factors for Violence

Domain	Risk Factors		Protective Factors
	Early Onset (Age 6–11)	**Late Onset (Age 12–14)**	
Individual	General offenses	General offenses	Intolerance to deviance
	Drug abuse	Restlessness	High IQ
	Being male	Difficulty concentrating	Being female
	Aggression	Risk taking	Positive social orientation
	Hyperactivity	Aggression	Perceived sanctions for
	Antisocial behavior	Being male	bad behavior
	TV violence exposure	Physical violence	
	Medical/physical problems	Antisocial attitudes	
	Low IQ	Crimes against persons	
	Dishonesty	Low IQ	
		Drug abuse	
Family	Poverty	Harsh, lax, or inconsistent	Supportive relationship with
	Antisocial parents	discipline	parents/other adults
	Harsh, lax, or inconsistent	Poor supervision	Parent's positive evaluation
	discipline	Low parental involvement	of peers
	Separation from parents	Antisocial parents	Parental monitoring
	Neglect	Broken home	
		Poverty	
		Abusive parents	
		Family conflict	
School	Poor attitude	Poor attitude	Commitment to school
	Poor performance	Poor performance	Recognition for involvement
		Academic failure	in school activities
Peer group	Weak social ties	Weak social ties	Friends who engage
	Antisocial peers	Antisocial peers	in conventional activities
		Gang membership	
Community		Neighborhood crime	
		Neighborhood drugs	
		Neighborhood	
		disorganization	

Source: *Youth Violence: A Report of the Surgeon General* (Washington, DC: U.S. Public Health Service, 2001).

Available: http://www.mentalhealth.org/youthviolence/surgeongeneral/SG_Site/chapter4/sec1.asp#RiskFactors.

and uncertain. Even though there are some reporting systems in place (e.g., the Centers for Disease Control Reportable Disease System, state cancer registries), reporting is less than perfect.

This problem is paralleled in the violence field. Violence that ends in death or arrest is well documented. However, about half of all violent crime goes unreported.[1] Sometimes domestic violence and sexual violence between intimates are not recognized as criminal or socially unacceptable behavior, even by the victims. Therefore, the general assumption guiding the use of statistics on violence is that the numbers usually underrepresent the frequency of violent incidents. Child abuse is an exception to this assumption. While a lot of child abuse is not reported, a significant proportion of reports is not verified.

International Data

International violence statistics are compiled by Interpol (International Criminal Police Organization) and the World Health Organization (WHO) from reports of individual countries. These data are useful in guiding national policy and expenditure debates and in making comparisons between nations, but have little value for programs in local communities. For more information, Interpol's Web site can be found at http://www.interpol.com, and the WHO Web site can be found at http://www.who.int/home-page/. At the WHO site, interested readers should look for the World Report on Violence and Health.

National Data

At the national level, there are several different sources of violence data: the National Crime Victimization Survey (NCVS), the FBI's Uniform Crime Reports (UCR), and the Centers for Disease Control and Prevention. The NCVS is a national household survey to gather data on the victims of crime and violence, including personal information on the victims, the relationship of victims to offenders, when and where crimes take place, whether self-protective measures were used, whether incidents were reported to the police, and what victims were doing when victimized. The survey has been conducted every year since 1973 and includes both reported (to the police) and unreported crime. The survey design circumvents the bias of variations in police efficiency and record keeping. Persons 12 years old or older are interviewed in sample households; about 50,000 households were included in the survey in 2001. The self-reports gathered provide a quantitative description of the extent and nature of being a victim of crime. This source provides no direct information about perpetrators or the causes of crime. Homicide is not included in the NCVS since victims cannot be interviewed.

The UCR is maintained by the FBI and is based on records of local police departments concerning reported crimes and arrests made. The UCR does not include unreported crimes, but it does include crimes against children younger than 12 (who are not interviewed in the NCVS) and crimes against commercial establishments, and provides information about offenders. The UCR also provides information about homicides and permits comparisons between local communities and states.[2] For more information about the Uniform Crime Reports and the National Crime Victimization Survey, see http://www.ojp.usdoj.gov/bjs/abstract/ntmc.htm.

Within the U.S. Centers for Disease Control and Prevention, there are two agencies involved in violence surveillance: the National Center for Injury Prevention and Control, Division of Violence Prevention; and the Youth Risk Behavior Survey. The data gathered by the Division of Violence Prevention include statistics on homicides and suicides, as derived from death certificates recorded by states, with additional data provided by the National Center for Health Statistics and the U.S. Bureau of the Census. In addition, the division maintains data on intimate partner violence, child abuse, and firearm-related violence. For more information about the National Center for Injury Prevention and Control, see http://www.cdc.gov/ncipc/ncipchm.htm.

The CDC's Youth Risk Behavior Survey (YRBS) provides data on the health risk behavior of high school students. The national sample of schools and students in grades 9 to 12 is representative of the U.S. high school population. In addition, state departments of education are encouraged to use the survey with a random sample of each state's high schools. Local school districts also may use the survey, independent of the state education agencies. Examples of behaviors inventoried include alcohol and drug use, seatbelt wearing, and unprotected sex. The survey includes several items of direct interest in violence prevention: physical fighting, carrying a weapon, fear of being victimized by violence at school, and suicidal thoughts and behavior. In 1999, the survey found that 35.7% of adolescents had fought at least once in the 12 months preceding the survey, while 17.3% had carried a weapon at least one day in the 30 days preceding the survey.[3] For more information on YRBS, see http://www.cdc.gov/nccdphp/dash/yrbs/index.htm.

Other Data Sources

In addition to the national sources of violence statistics, state police agencies make violent crime reports available to the public, while state health agencies provide statistics on homicide. Local police agencies can provide statistics on local violent crime, but they may be less organized to readily disseminate these data to citizens.

As an important supplement to government sources of violence statistics, specific studies of various aspects of violence can be found in published periodical literature. Many agencies in the private sector also provide statistical information on violence. Examples include the Children's Defense Fund, the Center to Prevent Handgun Violence, the National Crime Prevention Council, the National Center on Child Abuse and Neglect, and local child abuse and spouse abuse service agencies. These resources are easy to find by searching the Internet.

Even though there are many agencies that gather and disseminate violence statistics, there are many data needs that challenge the violence prevention field. In some cases, the deficiencies are simply a matter of funding: No one is gathering data because of limited funding. An example is the lack of national data on violence among certain racial and ethnic groups. In other cases, there are problems of methodology and technology. An example is getting an accurate figure for the prevalence of rape. Rape is frequently unreported, and the estimates obtained by various survey designs are widely discrepant.

Categories of Violence

Violence is behavior that purposefully seeks to inflict physical injury on one's self or another individual. Although words can be described as violent, this chapter is concerned with deeds. The motives for violence are numerous; most of those motives are viewed as illegitimate (e.g., racial hatred, greed, rage). In contrast, some violence has varying degrees of social acceptance (e.g., corporal and capital punishment, war); whether these types of violence are legitimate is often debated. What follows is a brief overview of various forms of violence.

Domestic Violence

Domestic violence may be defined as violence between intimates: current or former spouses or other sexual partners. Another definition is violence that occurs between family members: the abuse of children, violence between spouses, and violence by adult children against parents (usually elderly) or other vulnerable adults. It can also include violence between current or former dating partners. Definitional confusion is not the only uncertainty about domestic violence.

There is only a vague consensus as to what constitutes child abuse. Most people would agree that children who require medical treatment as a result of purposeful adult actions have been abused. However, the line between punishment and abuse is not clearly distinguished by society. For example, some people consider spanking to be child abuse, whereas others believe that it is appropriate under certain circumstances.

About 12% of American adults report that they were abused as children; 75% of adults believe the child abuse problem is worse today than when they were growing up.[4] In 1999 there were just over 800,000 cases of child abuse substantiated by investigation; 58% were in the form of neglect or emotional abuse, 21% physical abuse, and 11% sexual abuse.[5] Child abuse is hidden within spouse abuse when it occurs during pregnancy: Estimates are that about 4% to 17% of pregnant women are battered by their partners.[6] Furthermore, children who observe spouse abuse are emotional victims, predisposed to becoming batterers when they reach adulthood.

Child abuse has decreased consistently since about 1994. In 1998, there were about 3 million victims of child abuse reported; about 900,000 of those reports were substantiated.[7] Because society deems child abuse victims to be innocent and helpless, precautions have been put in place to encourage individuals and various professionals to report any suspected child abuse. This pressure and other factors have resulted in many reports of child abuse that are never substantiated. The substantiation rate is about 33%.[8] Some of the unsubstantiated reports are honest mistakes, while an unknown percentage of others are genuine but unproven.

Americans, indeed people worldwide, have not forgotten the O. J. Simpson case, which riveted the attention of so many people on wife battering. Violence between husbands and wives is another common form of domestic violence. This commonality is paradoxical in a culture that has traditional mores of nurturing and sheltering women. Nevertheless, wife battering occurs because these very closest of relationships by their very nature may include the most irksome and continuous points of conflict. In addition, society grants an informal license for a degree of violence in marriage relationships that would immediately be rejected in other settings with other people.

Although domestic violence between adults is perpetrated by both males and females, the most virulent violence is usually done by males against female partners. This type of violence may be between spouses, but also includes violence between former spouses and between boyfriends and girlfriends. In 1998, about 700,000 U.S. women were physically assaulted by their male partners; about 150,000 men were assaulted by their female partners.[9] In a study of murders in which the victim and assailant were from the same family, 41% of the cases involved a husband or wife killing his or her spouse.[10] However, violence perpetrated against women by a male intimate partner is 10 times more likely than violence against men by a female intimate partner.[11]

The statistics on domestic violence are not precise: This crime is notorious for underreporting. About 72% of family violence is committed by a boyfriend or girlfriend, or a current or ex-spouse. The ratio of female to male domestic violence victimization is about 5:1. The rate of domestic violence slowly decreased during the 1990s. However, in 1998 there were about 876,000 female victims of spouse abuse.[12] National surveys have shown that each year, women are physically abused in about 10% of couples.[13]

Elder abuse is also not new, but it has become more recognized because of the development of the discipline of gerontology. Like child abuse or spouse abuse, elder abuse is not always violent, but may be verbal or financial (e.g., taking money from an elderly family member without his or her consent).

It appears to have become more common simply because people are living longer, increasing the chances for significant generational overlap and prolonging the time when adults are called to be caretakers for weakened parents. The economic and emotional stress generated by the caretaker role is, in part, the cause of elder abuse. Sometimes adult children who are struggling financially or who are socially dysfunctional resent the economic and social accomplishments of their parents and act out their resentments against them. Many other factors may be involved, such as alcohol abuse. Data on elder abuse are limited and not unequivocal, but studies indicate that 1% to 10% of the elderly population have been abused.[14] In a study conducted by the U.S. Administration on Aging in 1996, about one-half million older persons in domestic settings were found to be abused or neglected, or experienced self-neglect; the study also found that for every reported incident of elder abuse, neglect, or self-neglect, approximately five go unreported.[15]

Sexual Assault

Domestic violence often is sexual in nature. However, much sexual violence also occurs outside of marriage and family relationships. This may include date rape, rape and sexual assault between acquaintances, and rape and sexual assault between strangers. The National Crime Victimization Survey indicates that less than half of rapes are reported to the police. In 2000, that survey reported 261,000 rapes, both attempted and completed, and sexual assaults. Only 90,000 rapes and sexual assaults were reported to the police. About 1% of women over the age of 11 were raped or sexually assaulted in 2000, a rate 52% lower than it was in 1993.[16] An additional number (not documented) of women experience other types of forced sexual activity. Some women are at much greater risk of rape and sexual assault: those aged 16 to 24, and those living in the central city portions of large metropolitan areas.[17]

Disagreement exists about what rape is, who is a rape victim, and how many rapes actually occur. Police records only reflect those incidents that are reported. Estimates on the reporting rate vary widely.

However, some in the ranks of feminism maintain that many women don't recognize when they have been raped because they don't regard as rape nonconsensual sex with a spouse or boyfriend, or they may disregard certain types of activities that others would consider rape (e.g., unwanted finger penetration). These advocates claim that cases of rape actually number in the range of 1 to 2 million each year. How rape is defined has a tremendous impact on the rate that is determined.

Abortion

In 1997 there were about 1.33 million abortions, about 340 for every 1,000 babies born.[18] This will not be a focus of this book. However, the act of abortion is considered by some to be a form of violence. Those who believe that an embryo and fetus have essential human traits and a living soul consider abortion to be homicide. Those who believe that personhood does not occur until birth or at least late in pregnancy reject the association of the term *murder* with abortion. Considering all the alternatives for dealing with contraception and unwanted pregnancy, abortion does have an element of brutality about it that resonates with society's propensity to solve conflicts with violence. Ironically, there has been significant violence generated between the opposing camps in the abortion debate, most often perpetrated by extremists among pro-life advocates.

Workplace Violence

Over six hundred homicides occur at work each year, the third leading cause of occupational fatalities. The job is frequently a site of violent behavior, though rates of workplace violence declined during the 1990s. Each year in the United States, about 1.7 million violent incidents take place at work,[19] including 7% of all rapes.[20] Nationally, the annual rate of workplace homicide is about 1 per 100,000 workers. Worksite violence may be between workers in conflict or may be perpetrated by a disgruntled worker against management personnel. However, about 83% of worksite homicides are perpetrated not by employees but by outsiders attempting robbery or other crimes against the employment establishment.

Violence in Labor Disputes

According to one author, "The United States has had the bloodiest and most violent labor history of any industrial nation in the world."[21] This has been seen in labor disputes in agriculture, mining, the auto industry, trucking, and other areas of work. There have been many instances of violence perpetrated by striking workers against management or strike breakers. For example, during a Greyhound Bus strike in 1991, strikers fired on a bus driven by a replacement driver, wounding seven passengers; over the next few months of the strike, shootings of buses occurred 52 times.[22] The issue has even been discussed in the U.S. Congress, leading to the introduction of the Freedom from Union Violence Act of 1997. However, labor unrest today more often leads to peaceful demonstrations, court battles, and consumer boycotts than to violence.[23]

Terrorism

Although the idea of terrorism is not new, the term has been seared into the popular consciousness by the events of September 11, 2001. (See **Figure 6.4.**) The means of terrorism are far more menacing now than in past decades because of modern technology, such as chemical and biological weapons. Terrorism is violence committed for political rather than economic or interpersonal reasons. Prior to the 1990s, the United States had been relatively unscathed by terrorism compared with Europe and the Middle East. However, the first bombing of New York's World Trade Center in 1994 and the final destruction of those buildings in 2001 have demonstrated for all time that Americans are not immune to international terrorism; we are reminded each time we must pass through metal detectors at the airport. The activity of the Ku Klux Klan in the 20th century is a notable example of indigenous American terrorism; more recent examples include activities by extremists in the antiabortion movement and by environmental terrorists and, in April, 1995, the bombing of the federal building in Oklahoma City. Currently, many Americans feel

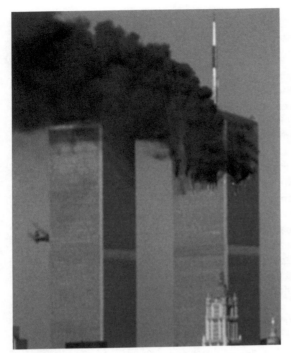

Figure 6.4 The U.S. feels more vulnerable to international terrorism than ever before.

(© Moshe Bursuker AP Wide World Photos)

endangered by the activities of underground militia movements and hate groups (see the FYI box.)

At first glance it seems that although Americans are among the most violent of Earth's inhabitants, they have not been frequent perpetrators of terrorism. Nevertheless, this is a form of violence that threatens people in every major city and airport, and around military and government installations, and now seems to be a permanent feature of life in the 21st century.

Legal Intervention

Violence carried out by government officials must be included in any inventory of the forms of community violence. This includes capital punishment, of which there have been about 700 instances since 1977.[24] In 1998, police officers committed 367 acts of justifiable homicide, killing in the line of duty a person in the act of committing a felony.[25] Recently there have been serious proposals by state legislatures to enact provisions for corporal punishment

(e.g., caning) of offenders, a practice common in other countries.[26] In the pluralism of our society, some found the actions of the Singapore government in caning American youth Michael Faye a human rights abuse, while others found it to be an inspiring model of public policy.

In addition to the violence that is part of criminal sentencing, there is an undetermined amount of violence that occurs among prisoners, not sponsored by officials, but often without their consistent intervention.[27] For example, some researchers maintain that male-on-male rape in prisons is actually a more frequent event than male-on-female rape in the community.[28]

Finally, an undetermined amount of police brutality or excessive force is committed by officers against suspects or arrestees, outside the bounds of criminal law. The Rodney King and Abner Louima incidents are noted examples of police brutality. Given the unique stresses of police work, the character of some segments of society, and the personalities of many attracted to the police profession, there is probably a continuing but unmeasured amount of police misconduct. Minorities tend to feel that they are the victims of police brutality more often than whites.[29] Many commentators attributed the outcome of the O. J. Simpson trial at least in part to the differences between whites and blacks in their attitudes toward the integrity of the police and the criminal justice system.

In spite of public perceptions, limited documentation indicates that excessive use of force by police officers is relatively rare, and pales in the face of the high level of community violence that officers must address.[30] Just as an aside, 1,159 police officers were killed (accidentally or intentionally) in the line of duty between 1990 and 1999.[31] Although we are one of the world's most violent societies, there is some consolation that illicit governmental violence against persons is relatively rare in the United States.[32]

Incidence and Trends of Violence in America

America's violence problem is made up of all the components outlined previously. It is important for researchers and policy analysts to be able to monitor the population patterns and changes that

Domestic Terrorism

During the 1990s, paramilitary organizations began to crop up around the United States. Some of the organizations had roots that go back decades, but there was a dramatic proliferation in militias and their membership during the early part of the decade. That growth was generally spurred by local economic hardships and resentment toward immigrant and nonwhite groups, but also specifically by the violent 1992 attack by federal agents on the Idaho farm of white separatist Randy Weaver and the 1993 attack on the Branch Davidians in Waco, Texas.

The militias are not affiliated with government or the official military. Rather, they are contemptuous and suspicious of government and believe the government is trying to take away their rights, especially the right to possess firearms. They assemble themselves for the purpose of military-type training in preparation for the confrontation with government officials that they believe is coming.

Members are predominantly poor, uneducated white men who feel isolated and disenfranchised from government and mainstream social institutions. About 30% of the militias are unified around a theme of racism, but other groups are more concerned about environmentalism encroaching on land rights, perceived abuses of taxation and the IRS, the belief that U.S. political and economic "elites" are plotting with the United Nations to create a "new world order" that will take away freedoms, opposition to abortion, and, of course, gun ownership.

Many of the leaders are educated, technologically sophisticated, and media savvy; they disseminate their propaganda over the Internet and with fax networks. Because the militia groups are covert, there is no exact way to count their numbers. Leaders in the militia movement claimed a membership that was large and growing. Outside experts have estimated membership ranging from 10,000 to 40,000. Since the Oklahoma City bombing, militia membership has declined, though hate groups still number in the hundreds in the United States.

While the primary threat of militias involves violent confrontations with law enforcement and other government officials, there is also serious concern about their propagation of terrorist acts that present a hazard to all.

In addition to militias, hundreds of so-called hate groups are active in the United States. These organizations sponsor written and spoken words, public demonstrations, and acts of violence against various minority groups. Typical targets include African Americans, Hispanics, Jews, and immigrants of all kinds. Examples of hate groups include several branches of the Ku Klux Klan, the World Church of the Creator, Aryan Action, Posse Comitatus, and the League of the South (see Figure 6.5). For more information about hate groups, visit the Web site for the Southern Poverty Law Center at http://www.splcenter.org/.

Domestic terrorism is an issue about which school personnel and others interested in violence prevention should be informed. Youth, or their parents, may be involved in these groups, and may express involvement in related activities and events or share ideas from militias and hate groups that conflict with multicultural tolerance and respect. It is also a grim reality that acts of terrorism or other antisocial behavior are committed by hate groups, environmental activists, and antiabortion advocates in U.S. communities. School personnel and other professionals may be asked to assist students with the emotional trauma that results from such activities.

occur in those individual components. However, for the present purpose, it is only important to look at the big picture. How much violence occurs every year, and is it getting better or worse? How much violence takes place at school or involves school-aged youth, and is it getting better or worse? It will be sufficient to have a general sense of these broad measures of violence as a background for planning and implementing school-based prevention programs.

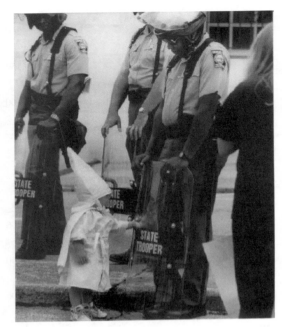

Figure 6.5 There are many hate groups that promote intolerance and violence. (© Todd Robertson)

How Much Violent Crime Is There and What Is the Trend?

According to the FBI, there is a murder in the United States every 33.9 minutes, a forcible rape every 5.8 minutes, a robbery every 1.3 minutes, and an aggravated assault every 35 seconds.[33] This type of crime is significantly more common in the United States than in most other developed countries.[34] Law enforcement agencies compile a standardized statistic called "violent crime," which includes murder, forcible rape, robbery, and aggravated assault. This statistical measure increases or decreases year by year, but the recent trend is that it decreased by 33% from 1991 to 2000.[35] Over that same period, the murder rate fell 37%.[36]

The causes for this decline in homicide are not clear. However, some experts predict that homicide and violent crime will increase over the next decade because the segment of the population that is most violent—adolescent and young adult males—will increase.

School Violence

Violence at schools tends to be most frequent and lethal at the middle school and high school level, but it also occurs in elementary school and on college campuses. It includes student fighting, possession and use of weapons, and sometimes large group melees. Some schools report violence over racial tensions.[37] Other schools have reported incidents of violent hazing within organized sports.[38] It is important to recognize that school violence is not only between students, but can also be directed by students against school personnel.[39]

It is well known that schools reflect the surrounding community conditions. When violence is a harsh norm in homes, playing fields, and streets, it will come to school as a perverse show-and-tell. During the 1998–1999 school year there were 33 homicides and 4 suicides at U.S. schools.[40] In the 1993–1994 school year, 12% of all elementary and secondary school teachers (341,000) were threatened with injury by a student from their school, and 4% (119,000) were physically attacked by a student.[41] There are about 14,000 serious violent crimes perpetrated against teachers each year.[42]

In 1999, students aged 12 to 18 experienced about 186,000 nonfatal serious violent crimes (rape, sexual assault, robbery, and aggravated assault) when they were at school. The victimization rate for serious violent crime at school and away from school generally declined from 1992 to 1999.[43] Rates were higher in urban schools, higher for African Americans and males, higher for secondary school students, and higher in public than in private schools.[44] Weapon carrying and physical fighting are less common at school than in other community settings. (See **Figures 6.6 – 6.10.**) As shown in Figures 6.6 to 6.8, while school violence is disturbing, it is less common than youth violence in other places.

School violence is very alarming for many, and the figures are disturbing. However, this can be a situation of the glass being either half full or half empty. According to the CDC's 1999 Youth Risk Behavior Survey, 33% of students were involved in a fight in a 12-month period, but only 4% were injured. Only 12.5% of high school students fought

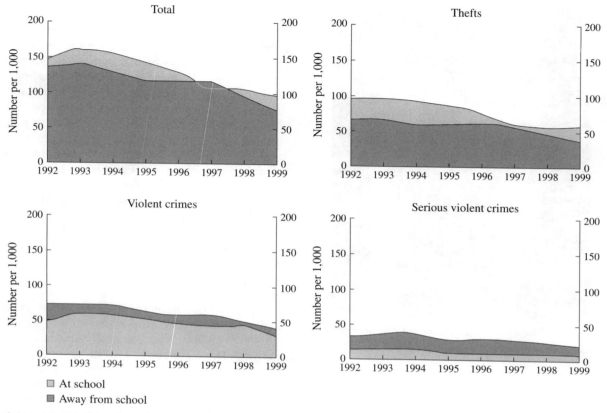

Figure 6.6 **Number of Nonfatal Crimes Against Students Aged 12 to 18 per 1,000 Students, by Type of Crime and Location, 1992–1999**

Source: U.S. Department of Education.

on school property. Only 6.6% of students felt too unsafe to go to school on at least one day during the previous 30.[45]

In February 1992, the U.S. Department of Education published a report of a survey of 830 public school principals, representative of the United States as a whole. The report indicated that 77% of principals considered fighting by students to be only a minor problem or no problem at all. Weapons possession by students was considered by 98% of the principals to be a minor or no problem.[46] There is no question that there is a school violence problem, but it is possible to overreact and exaggerate the extent of school violence. It must be remembered that the youth violence problem is much greater when youth are not in school.

As described earlier, the data that track the actual incidence of violence in American schools show a serious problem, but one that is often overblown. However, data that describe violence in which school-aged youth are perpetrators or victims are a bit more alarming. From 1970 to 1980 the homicide victimization rate for youth aged 15 to 24 increased by 33%; the increase from 1980 to 1991 was 44%. It is encouraging to note that there has been continuous progress since about 1994. (See Figure 6.9 and Table 6.2.) These trends are even more dramatic for males, particularly African American and Hispanic males. While the homicide rate for all adolescents aged 14 to 24 in 1999 was 10.7 per 100,000, the comparable rate for African American males in that age range was 66.9, more than six times greater. (See Figure 6.10.)

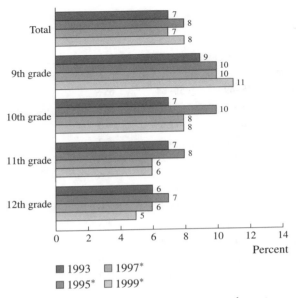

Figure 6.7 Percentages of Students in Grades 9 to 12 Reporting Being Threatened or Injured with a Weapon on School Property During the Last 12 Months, by Grade, Selected Years

Source: U.S. Department of Education.

Why Violence Must Be Addressed

It would appear self-evident that violence in schools and communities should be eliminated, or at least reduced and controlled. While violence among other animals is accepted as part of the natural order, all human societies have had sanctions against violence, although the criteria and standards have varied widely. Nevertheless, in the modern world, the value of violence control is always balanced against other values in which society can invest. (See Table 6.3.) Legislatures debate the relative merit of building prisons and hiring police officers versus investing in schools, highways, and art museums. Schools must make choices concerning how the minutes of the school day are allocated and budgets apportioned.

Consequently, policymakers must be able to justify the implementation of violence control programs at the cost of other possible uses of the money. Ideally, the case will be made on the basis of objective data and careful needs assessment. Unfortunately, many times school and public policy is unduly influenced by misinformation and misperceptions. Some deny that there is a local

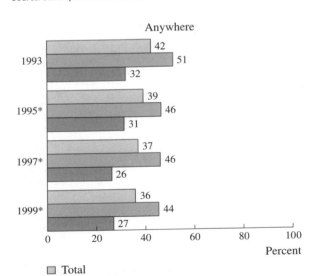

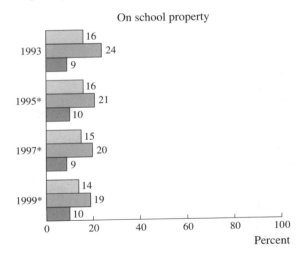

Figure 6.8 Percentages of Students in Grades 9 to 12 Reporting Having Been in a Physical Fight in the Last 12 Months, by Gender, Selected Years

Source: U.S. Department of Education.

Table 6.2

Violent Crime Victimization Rate per 1,000 Persons in Each Age Group, 1990–2000

	12–15	16–19	20–24	Age of Victim 25–34	35–49	50–64	65+
1990	101.1	99.1	86.1	55.2	34.4	9.9	3.7
1991	94.5	122.6	103.6	54.3	37.2	12.5	4.0
1992	111.0	103.7	95.2	56.8	38.1	13.2	5.2
1993	115.5	114.2	91.6	56.9	42.5	15.2	5.9
1994	118.6	123.9	100.4	59.1	41.3	17.6	4.6
1995	113.1	106.6	85.8	58.5	35.7	12.9	6.4
1996	95.0	102.8	74.5	51.2	32.9	15.7	4.9
1997	87.9	96.3	68.0	47.0	32.3	14.6	4.4
1998	82.5	91.3	67.5	41.6	29.9	15.4	2.9
1999	74.5	77.6	68.7	36.4	25.2	14.4	3.9
2000	60.1	64.4	49.5	34.9	21.8	13.7	3.7

Source: U.S. Department of Justice, Bureau of Justice Statistics.

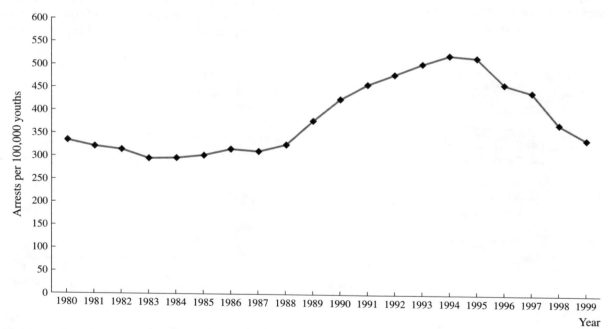

Figure 6.9 **Arrest Rates of Youths Aged 10 to 17 for Serious Violent Crime, 1980–1999**
Source: *Youth Violence: A Report of the Surgeon General* (Washington, DC: U.S. Public Health Service, 2001).

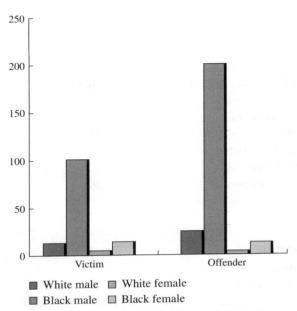

Figure 6.10 **Homicide Victimization and Offending Among 18- to 24-Year-Olds, per 100,000 Population, by Race and Gender**

Source: U.S. Department of Justice, Bureau of Justice Statistics.

Legend:
- White male
- White female
- Black male
- Black female

[**Table 6.3**]

The Risk of Violence Compared with Other Threats to Health

Event	Rate per 1,000 Adults per Year
Accidental injury	220
Any violent victimization	31
Assault	25
Injury in auto accident	22
Death from all causes	11
Violent injury	11
Serious assault	8
Heart disease death	5
Cancer death	3
Rape (women only)	1
Accidental death—all causes	0.4
Pneumonia/influenza death	0.4
Motor vehicle accident death	0.2
Suicide	0.2
HIV infection death	0.1
Homicide death	0.1

Source: U.S. Department of Justice.

violence problem, asserting that violence (like drugs) is only a concern in major cities; others overestimate the proportions of violent crime, believing assault and robbery are much more common than they really are. Local communities must assess the dimensions of their own violence problem and make appropriate plans.

In a general sense, violence is a problem that must be dealt with because it inflicts pain and suffering on victims; robs potential victims of quality of life as they limit their activities out of fear; and costs society billions of dollars in medical costs, expenses in the criminal justice system, lost productivity in the workplace, and increases in the cost of business. One study found that 23% of victims suffer some economic loss, such as medical expense or lost wages.[47] When schools experience violence, it disrupts the education process. Children attending school in fear are not going to perform at their highest potential. Teachers working in fear are not going to demonstrate excellence in the classroom. School violence, or

the threat of it, is a destructive influence with serious consequences for current students and future generations.

Factors That Promote Violence

Many factors have been associated with violence. Some are related to the physical, mental, and emotional characteristics of individuals. Other factors are related to the family environment and relationships between children and adults. Still another set of factors is related to a student's adjustment and orientation to the school atmosphere and schoolwork. Finally, a number of factors relate to peer group and community influences. (See Table 6.1.)

A couple of observations can be made about these factors. First, the factors are numerous and diverse. It is clear that there is no single overriding factor in youth violence. There is no one dominant

[**Table 6.4**]

Effect Sizes of Selected Risk Factors

Early Risk Factors (Age 6–11)	Effect Sizes (r)	Late Risk Factors (Age 12–14)	Effect Sizes (r)
		Large Effect Size	
General offenses	.38	Weak social ties	.39
Drug abuse	.30	Antisocial peers	.37
		Gang membership	.31
		Moderate Effect Size	
Being male	.26	General offenses	.26
Poverty	.24		
Antisocial parents	.23		
Aggression	.21		
		Small Effect Size	
Hyperactivity	.13	Restlessness	.20
Poor parent–child relations	.15	Difficulty concentrating	.18
Harsh, lax, inconsistent discipline	.13	Risk taking	.09
Weak social ties	.15	Harsh, lax discipline	.08
Antisocial behavior	.13	Low parental involvement	.11
TV violence exposure	.13	Aggression	.19
Poor attitude to school	.13	Being male	.19
Low IQ	.12	Poor attitude to school	.19
Broken home	.09	Academic failure	.14
Dishonesty	.12	Physical violence	.18
Neglect	.07	Neighborhood crime/drugs	.17
Antisocial peers	.04	Antisocial parents	.16
		Low IQ	.11
		Broken home	.10
		Poverty	.10
		Abusive parents	.09
		Family conflict	.13

Source: *Youth Violence: A Report of the Surgeon General* (Washington, DC: U.S. Public Health Service, 2001).

influence that if addressed properly could eliminate or greatly reduce violence problems. Instead, a holistic approach is required, one that considers a variety of factors. A corollary to this, in thinking about the list of factors, is that many of the factors are beyond the ordinary influence and responsibility of schools. An effective response to violence requires not just school programs, but also involvement by parents, social service agencies, churches, and a variety of other institutions and agencies. This situation is identical to that of effective drug abuse prevention, which also requires a holistic approach.

A second observation is that some of the factors related to violence are more important than others. In other words, some of the identified factors have a more pronounced effect on the development of violent behavior. (See Table 6.4.) For example, being involved in drug abuse at a young age is much more predictive of future violence than is exposure to TV violence. As shown in Table 6.4, some factors are much more deserving of a school

Table 6.5

Strategies to Decrease Community Violence

School	Community
Community collaboration	Community policing
Conflict mediation	Diminishing poverty
Curriculum	Drug addiction treatment
Discipline and school rules	Gun control
Dropout prevention	Health care system referrals
Family resource centers	of violent injuries
Parent education	Recreation programs
Security	Reducing media violence
Student assistance programs	
Teacher training and support	

Source: *Youth Violence: A Report of the Surgeon General* (Washington, DC: U.S. Public Health Service, 2001).

and community's attention than others as we try to use prevention resources most effectively. This is tempered by the fact that some factors, though they may be less important, are more easily altered. For example, it might be easier to make TV programming more socially responsible than to reduce or eliminate the antisocial attitudes of some parents.

In general, the number of factors should be a source of optimism, because there are apparently many ways in which we can influence more peaceful and prosocial development and behavior. There is unrealized potential for many segments of the community to play a constructive role in this important enterprise.

Violence Prevention Strategies

This text is unable to provide extensive details on the array of specific strategies that could be used to address violence prevention and intervention. Because there are so many underlying factors that influence the development of violence, there are many possible strategies. Table 6.5 outlines real and potential prevention strategies. The reader should recognize that the list is very general, in that each item will be more or less relevant in different circumstances. Also, the strategies vary with respect to their proven value in violence prevention. Some items have well-established effectiveness, whereas others are only experimental.

The solution to violence, like most social problems, is not unilateral and will not come by school-based efforts alone. A comprehensive approach, as espoused by the public health model, will be required. Though school personnel will not be centrally involved in community interventions, their understanding will help them to see their efforts from a team perspective and enable them to work together more effectively within a holistic approach to violence prevention. The FYI box lists resources to help in this effort.

Components of a School Safety Plan

The following five points serve as a general outline of the components of a school safety plan. Each specific plan will be different because of the unique characteristics of communities, students, school personnel, needs identified, and resources available.

1. *Convene a safe school planning team.* Because the solution of school violence problems requires the participation of many segments of the school and community, it is important to establish a planning team that is inclusive. Having broad representation of students, parents, teachers, administrators, Board of Education members, government representatives, business representatives, religious leaders, law enforcement officials, health care professionals, and others will better ensure success.
2. *Conduct a school site assessment.* Each year the planning committee should gather data on actual school and community violence trends and take stock of the programs and resources in place. This assessment should provide a basis for future planning.

Some National Resources in Violence Prevention

Blueprints for Violence Prevention

http://www.colorado.edu/cspv/blueprints/Default.htm

This site is maintained by the Center for the Study and Prevention of Violence (CSPV) at the University of Colorado at Boulder. CSPV designed and launched a national violence prevention initiative to identify and replicate violence prevention programs that are effective. The project, called Blueprints for Violence Prevention, has identified 11 prevention and intervention programs that meet a strict scientific standard of program effectiveness. The 11 model programs, called Blueprints, have been effective in reducing adolescent violent crime, aggression, delinquency, and substance abuse. Another 19 programs have been identified as promising programs. To date, more than 500 programs have been reviewed, and the Center continues to look for programs that meet the selection criteria. The Blueprints Initiative is a comprehensive effort to provide communities with a set of demonstrated effective programs and the technical assistance and monitoring necessary to plan for and develop an effective violence intervention.

Early Warning, Timely Response: A Guide to Safe Schools

http://www.ed.gov/offices/OSERS/OSEP/Products/earlywrn.html

This publication of the U.S. Department of Education offers research-based practices designed to assist school communities with identifying warning signs of violence early and develop prevention, intervention, and crisis response plans. The guide includes sections on the characteristics of a school that is safe and responsive to all children, early warning signs, getting help for troubled children, developing a prevention and response plan, responding to crisis, and resources.

Healthy People 2010 Injury and Violence Prevention

http://www.health.gov/healthypeople/document/HTML/Volume2/15Injury.htm

The national Healthy People project includes a focus on intentional, violent injuries. This link leads to the chapter in the *Healthy People 2010* document that addresses both intentional and unintentional (accidental) injuries. There are many statistics and prevention concepts regarding violent injuries.

Indicators of School Crime and Safety

http://nces.ed.gov/pubs2002/crime2001/

This site, maintained by the U.S. Department of Education, provides an ongoing database of statistics on the various dimensions of school violence. It can serve as a useful benchmark for comparing local school violence assessments.

Minnesota Center Against Violence and Abuse

http://www.mincava.umn.edu/

This site is a clearinghouse for information, statistics, and resources on all dimensions of the violence problem.

National Violence Prevention Resource Center

http://www.safeusa.org/

Sponsored by the Centers for Disease Control and Prevention and the Federal Working Group on Youth Violence, this site has extensive statistics and information on various forms of violence.

Safe and Drug-Free Schools Program

http://www.ed.gov/offices/OESE/SDFS/

The Safe and Drug-Free Schools program is the federal government's primary vehicle for reducing drug, alcohol, and tobacco use and violence through education and prevention activities in our nation's schools. This program is designed to prevent violence in and around schools and to strengthen programs that prevent the illegal use of alcohol, tobacco, and drugs; involve parents; and coordinate with related federal, state, and community efforts and resources.

Youth Violence: A Report of the Surgeon General

http://www.surgeongeneral.gov/library/youthviolence/toc.html

This report, produced in 2001 by the Office of the U.S. Surgeon General, outlines the nature and extent of youth violence in the United States, reviews the literature on the underlying causative factors, and sets out a plan of action to address this pressing national problem.

3. *Develop strategies and implement violence prevention programs to address school safety concerns*. Typical strategies include the following:
   - Including all students in school events and activities.
   - Establishing clear rules about bullying, violent behavior, and conflict.
   - Implementing school security as appropriate (limiting access, using ID badges, hiring security officers, etc.).
   - Establishing a hotline for reporting suspicions or concerns about violent students.
   - Training teachers for identification and referral of high-risk students.
   - Using specific violence prevention and conflict resolution curricula. Examples include the Seattle Social Development Project, Life Skills Training, and Midwestern Prevention Project. Many curricula claim to address violence prevention. Unfortunately, many of them have uncertain effectiveness because they have never been adequately evaluated. Because this has been a pervasive problem, there is increasing pressure on schools to adopt curricula that have met criteria of effectiveness. The criteria are stated in different ways, but the important elements are as follows: being evaluated with a rigorous experimental design, showing evidence of significant deterrent effects, and replicating those effects at multiple sites or various studies. Chapters 7 to 10 of this text contain information about the criteria of effectiveness that relate to drug education curricula, but the criteria are equally relevant in violence prevention. For further information, students are encouraged to contact their state department of education or the U.S. Department of Education's Safe and Drug-Free Communities Program.
   - Referring high-risk students and families to community services and resources.

4. *Establish a social support team*. The purpose of this team is to identify students who are in trouble, and to marshal appropriate support and assistance. The team could include teachers, parents, students, counselors, and law enforcement officers. The specific objective is to intervene with high-risk students before the most severe consequences occur.

5. *Develop a crisis response plan*. In spite of the best intentions and earnest efforts by school and community, there is a chance that a violence-related crisis will occur. When such a crisis occurs, the response will be much more effective if there is a contingency plan already in place. It should be decided in advance what steps should be taken, and by whom. Of course, schools hope to never have to use the crisis plan, and most will not. However, if the need arises, everyone involved will be grateful that guidelines were in place and that people knew what to do. For more specific information about a crisis plan, see the U.S. Department of Education's *Early Warning, Timely Response: A Guide to Safe Schools* (http://www.ed.gov/offices/OSERS/OSEP/Products/earlywrn.html).

Summary

Violence in the United States is a significant problem, one more severe than in most other countries. It is a very diverse problem, consisting of many different forms. People's perceptions of the violence problem are, in part, molded by the media, which tends to portray violence as more excessive and unremitting than it actually is. Consequently, school violence is seen by the public as a huge problem. The truth is that although violence among young people is frequent, especially among African American males, it usually takes place outside of schools. Nevertheless, schools have a central role in addressing the problem of community violence.

Scenario | Analysis and Response

The events that took place in the spring of 1999 in the Littleton, Colorado, high school could not have been anticipated explicitly. It is difficult for most people to foresee that anyone is capable of such evil acts. Nevertheless, it is abundantly clear in retrospect that those boys were seriously troubled, and intervention prior to the day of the shootings should have occurred.

The two student perpetrators had many characteristics of high-risk youth: history of trouble with the police, antisocial attitudes, exposure to TV violence, and poor parental supervision, just to name a few. These risk characteristics were not apparent to everyone; various individuals had bits and pieces of the puzzle, so no single responsible person had the complete perspective on the risk posed by the students. Nevertheless, the hard lessons are that the warning signs of youth violence must not be ignored, and that schools must have in place a mechanism for collecting disparate observations of troubled behavior in a way that leads to meaningful intervention.

Learning Activities

1. Gather statistics that assess violence in your community. Examples are police records on homicide, assault, rape, and domestic violence, and records on incidents of school violence.

2. Search the Internet and the government documents section of your library to determine what agencies gather and disseminate violence statistics on a state or national basis.

3. Interview teachers or other school personnel to get a subjective assessment of the extent of violence in the local school system. Also discover what the schools are doing to respond to violence problems.

4. Interview someone over the age of 70. Ask that individual how he or she feels about community violence, and how he or she thinks the extent and nature of violence have changed over his or her lifetime.

5. Select five countries, including the United States. Do library research to compare the five countries on measures of violent crime.

6. Interview someone who is not a native-born American. Discuss the nature and frequency of violence in the United States compared with his or her birthplace. Explore his or her perceptions of why there are differences.

Notes

1. M. W. Zawitz, P. A. Klaus, R. Bachman, et al., *Highlights from 20 Years of Surveying Crime Victims: The National Crime Victimization Survey, 1973–1992* (Washington, DC: U.S. Department of Justice, Bureau of Justice Statistics, 1993).

2. U.S. Department of Justice, Federal Bureau of Investigation, "Uniform Crime Reporting Summary System, Frequently Asked Questions." Available: http://www.fbi.gov/search?NS-search-page=document&NS-rel-doc-name=/ucr/ucrquest.htm&NS-uery=unreported+crime&NS-search-type=NS-boolean-query&NS-collection=FBI_Web_Site&NS-docs-found=1&NS-doc-number=1.

3. L. Kann, S. A. Kinchen, et al., "Youth Risk Behavior Surveillance—United States, 1999," *Morbidity and Mortality Weekly Report, Surveillance Summaries* 49, SS05 (2000): 1–96.

4. K. Maguire and A. Pastore, eds., *Sourcebook of Criminal Justice Statistics* (Washington, DC: U.S. Department of Justice, Bureau of Justice Statistics, 1994), 278, 216.

5. U.S. Bureau of the Census, *Statistical Abstract of the United States* (Washington, DC: Government Printing Office, 2001), 199.

6. Centers for Disease Control and Prevention, "Physical Violence During the 12 Months Preceding Childbirth, 1990–1991," *Morbidity and Mortality Weekly Report* 43, 8 (1994): 132–137.

7. U.S. Bureau of the Census, *Statistical Abstract*.

8. Ibid.

9. Ibid.

10. M. A. Straus and R. J. Gelles, "How Violent Are American Families?" in *Physical Violence in American Families: Risk Factors and Adaptations to Violence in 8,145 Families*, M. A. Straus and R. J. Gelles, eds. (New Brunswick, NJ: Transaction Publishers, 1990), 95–112.

11. U.S. Department of Justice, "Two-Thirds of Women Violence Victims Are Attacked by Relatives or Acquaintances," Bureau of Justice Statistics press release, January 30, 1994.

12. U.S. Bureau of the Census, *Statistical Abstract*.

13. S. Plichta, "The Effects of Woman Abuse on Health Care Utilization and Health Status: A Literature Review," *Women's Health Issues* 2, 3 (Fall 1992): 154–163; C. M. Rennison and S. Welchans, "Intimate Partner Violence," U.S. Department of Justice, Bureau of Justice Statistics,

May 2000. Available: http://www.ojp.usdoj.gov/bjs/pub/pdf/ipv.pdf.

14. Administration on Aging, U.S. Department of Health and Human Services, *The National Elder Abuse Incidence Study: Final Report*, September 1998. Available: http://www.aoa.gov/abuse/report/default.htm.

15. Ibid.

16. C. M. Rennison, "Criminal Victimization 2000: Changes 1999–2000 with Trends 1993–2000," U.S. Department of Justice, Bureau of Justice Statistics, June 2001.

17. R. Bachman, *Violence Against Women: A National Crime Victimization Survey Report* (Washington, DC: U.S. Department of Justice, Bureau of Justice Statistics, 1994), 6.

18. U.S. Bureau of the Census, *Statistical Abstract,* 71.

19. D. T. Duhart, "Violence in the Workplace, 1993–99," U.S. Department of Justice, Bureau of Justice Statistics, December 2001. Available: http://www.ojp.usdoj.gov/bjs/pub/pdf/vw99.pdf.

20. U.S. Department of Justice, "Workplace Violence," Bureau of Justice Statistics press release, July 24, 1994.

21. P. Taft and P. Ross, "American Labor Violence: Its Causes, Character, and Outcome," in *Violence: Patterns, Causes, Public Policy*, N. Weiner, M. Zahn, and R. Sagi, eds. (San Diego: Harcourt Brace Jovanovich, 1990).

22. J. Bovard, "A Federal License to Maim," *National Review,* March 21, 1994, 53–55.

23. Neil Alan Weiner, Margaret A. Zahn, and Rita J. Sagi, *Violence: Patterns, Causes, Public Policy* (San Diego: Harcourt Brace Jovanovich, 1990).

24. U.S. Bureau of the Census, *Statistical Abstract,* 203.

25. Ibid., 195.

26. P. Henkels, "A Good Beating Might Not Be So Bad," *Wall Street Journal,* July 7, 1994, A13; E. Bailey, "Paddling Bill Defeated in Assembly Panel," *Los Angeles Times,* June 23, 1994, A1.

27. D. Roberts, "Imprisoning Violent Youths Exposes Them to Physical and Sexual Abuse," in *Youth Violence*, M. Biskup and C. Cozic, eds. (San Diego: Greenhaven Press, 1992), 234–242.

28. S. Donaldson, "The Rape Crisis Behind Bars," *New York Times,* December 29, 1993, A11.

29. R. Bray, "What Blacks Think of White Cops," *New York Times,* July 11, 1994, 33–35.

30. W. Tucker, "Is Police Brutality the Problem?" *Commentary,* January 1993, 23–28. See also J. Katz, "Is Police Brutality a Myth?" *New York Times,* July 11, 1994, 38–40.

31. U.S. Bureau of the Census, *Statistical Abstract.*

32. Amnesty International Annual Report 2001. London, United Kingdom. Available: http://web.amnesty.org/web/ar2001.nsf/home/home?OpenDocument.

33. U.S. Department of Justice, *Uniform Crime Reports for the United States* (Washington, DC: Federal Bureau of Investigation, U.S. Department of Justice, 2000), 4. Available: http://www.fbi.gov/ucr/cius_00/contents.pdf.

34. A. Reiss and J. Roth, *Understanding and Preventing Violence* (Washington, DC: National Academy Press, 1993).

35. U.S. Department of Justice, *Uniform Crime Reports,* Section II, 12. Available: http://www.fbi.gov/ucr/cius_00/00crime2_2.pdf.

36. Ibid., Section II, 15. Available: http://www.fbi.gov/ucr/cius_00/00crime2_3.pdf.

37. A. Tuck, "Fulton Drafts Anti-Bigotry School Policy," *Atlanta Constitution,* January 8, 1991, D1, D4.

38. K. Dupont, "You Don't Forget It," *Boston Globe,* October 1, 1990, 37, 46.

39. P. Kaufman, X. Chen, et al., "Indicators of School Crime and Safety: 2001," National Center for Education Statistics, U.S. Department of Education, 2001. Available: http://nces.ed.gov/pubsearch/pubsinfo.asp?pubid=2002113.

40. Ibid.

41. Ibid.

42. Ibid.

43. Ibid.

44. Ibid.

45. Centers for Disease Control and Prevention, "Youth Risk Behavior Surveillance—United States, 2001," *Morbidity and Mortality Weekly Reports, Surveillance Summaries* 51, SS04 (2002): 1–64.

46. National Center for Education Statistics, *Public School Principal Survey on Safe, Disciplined, and Drug-Free Schools* (Washington, DC: U.S. Department of Education, 1992).

47. P. Klaus, *The Costs of Crime to Victims* (Washington, DC: U.S. Department of Justice, Bureau of Justice Statistics, 1994).

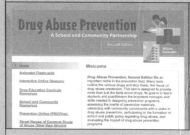

web resources

The Web site for this book offers many useful resources for educators, students, and professional counselors and is a great source for additional information. Visit the site at **http://healtheducation.jbpub.com/drugabuse/**.

Chapter Learning Objectives

Upon completion of this chapter, students will be able to:

1. Summarize the multiple dimensions of prevention.

2. Compare primary prevention to secondary and tertiary prevention.

3. Discuss the continuum of primary prevention efforts and the new classification system.

4. Relate the three components of the public health model to ATOD prevention.

5. Compare and contrast past prevention efforts.

6. Examine the concept of universal values.

7. Describe parents' prevention roles.

8. Summarize the underlying assumptions of unsuccessful community prevention programs.

Scenario

Kim, a health teacher at Franklin Middle School, is head of the site-based team at the school. The principal has just informed the site-based team that the school has received a $10,000 grant from Nellie, Inc., to address ATOD issues. The CEO of Nellie wants to bring in a well-known recovering addict to talk to a full-school assembly. In addition, the local sheriff will come to the assembly with a "drug kit" showing all the paraphernalia and examples of drugs confiscated during the past year. Kim appreciates the grant funds, but has some other suggestions for how the money can benefit the school's ATOD prevention efforts. She wants to expand the health education curriculum to include life skills and form a school/community committee to coordinate the school's efforts. What recommendations would you make if you were Kim? How would you handle this situation?

Chapter 7

Single-Focus Approaches to Prevention

Introduction

Illegal alcohol, tobacco, and other drug consumption and abuse are costly. Illegal drug and alcohol consumption alone costs our society nearly $277 billion a year.[1] (See **Figure 7.1.**) The overall contribution of illicit drug abuse to productivity losses, health care costs, and other costs rose steadily throughout the 1990s.[2] **Figure 7.2** shows the proportional increases in each of the various categories from 1992 to 1998. For productivity losses, an annual increase of 6.0% was estimated, with costs for drug-abuse-related illness and incarceration increasing the fastest. Health care costs increased at a rate of 2.9% annually but were moderated by a decrease in costs for HIV/AIDS patients. The cost of other effects includes costs of the criminal justice system, costs for reducing the supply of drugs, and social welfare costs. This rate rose at approximately 6.6% annually, with the largest increases resulting from police protection and legal adjudication costs.

In another study conducted for the Office of National Drug Control Policy (ONDCP), researchers concluded that trade in illicit drugs was approximately $70 billion a year during the later 1990s; however, as recognized from the previous statistics, the indirect costs to society far exceed the direct expenditures. "Drug use fosters crime; facilitates the spread of catastrophic health problems, such as hepatitis, endocarditis, and AIDS; and disrupts personal, familial, and legitimate economic relationships. The public bears much of the burden of these indirect costs because it finances the criminal justice response to drug-related crime, a public drug-treatment system, and anti-drug prevention programs."[3]

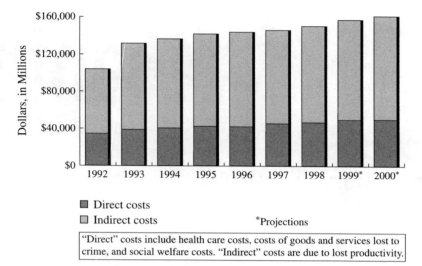

"Direct" costs include health care costs, costs of goods and services lost to crime, and social welfare costs. "Indirect" costs are due to lost productivity.

Figure 7.1 **The Economic Costs of Drug Abuse in Constant 2000 Dollars (Direct vs. Indirect)**
Source: Office of National Drug Control Policy.

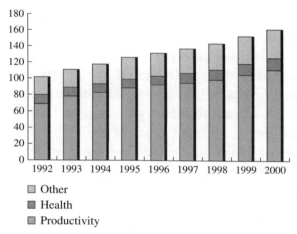

Figure 7.2 **Trends in the Components of the Cost of Illegal Drugs, 1992–2000, in Billions of Dollars (1999–2000 Projected)**
Source: Office of National Drug Control Policy.

Every day we see, read, or hear about adolescents or adults who have compromised their quality of life by abusing ATOD. They can no longer contribute positively to our schools, communities, or world because of the debilitating effects of ATOD. The authors, like many educators in the prevention field, regret when anyone suffers the consequences of abuse. We believe that "demand-side" strategies of prevention must continue to be strengthened to reduce the occurrence of these life tragedies. Table 7.1 shows that the expenditures for illicit drugs have steadily decreased since 1988, but Figures 7.1 and 7.2 show that the costs to society have continued to rise. These statistics are convincing evidence that the number of chronic and occasional users of illicit drugs, tobacco, and alcohol remains unacceptably high. So, what can we do about it? What does the history of expenditures for prevention efforts teach us?

During the 1970s and 1980s, government officials and community leaders seemed skeptical of prevention's potential to reduce ATOD use. The majority of appropriated funds went to treatment facilities to address addiction problems and to law enforcement to reduce the supply of drugs on the streets. Primary prevention received very little of the ATOD budget. In the 1990s, prevention specialists were optimistic that a larger portion of the funds appropriated for ATOD would be placed in primary prevention because government administrators were often quoted as supporting primary prevention.

[Table 7.1]						
Total U.S. Expenditures on Illicit Drugs, 1988–1998						
	1988	**1990**	**1992**	**1994**	**1996**	**1998**
Cocaine	$76.9	$61.3	$49.4	$42.2	$41.3	$39.0
Heroin	21.8	17.6	10.9	10.5	11.7	11.6
Methamphetamine	3.2	2.6	2.3	3.3	2.4	2.2
Marijuana	11.3	13.5	12.5	11.4	9.0	10.7
Other Drugs	3.3	2.2	1.5	2.6	2.7	2.3
Total	**$116.5**	**$97.2**	**$76.6**	**$70.0**	**$67.1**	**$65.8**

Figures are in billions; 1998 dollar equivalents. Columns may not add due to rounding.

Source: Office of National Drug Control Policy, *What America's Users Spend on Illegal Drugs, 1988–2000* [Executive Summary]. (Cambridge, MA: Abt Associates, 2001).

viewpoints

Quotes

I want to change the way we think about health—by putting prevention first. We will never have a large enough budget to address all the health care needs of our citizens if we do not start thinking about prevention and taking personal responsibility for our health.

—Former Surgeon General Jocelyn Elders, Senate confirmation hearings, July 1993

The more you invest in the front end, the less you're going to have to pay down … the line.

—Former Attorney General Janet Reno, *USA Today,* July 27, 1993

(See the Viewpoints box.) However, the trend remained constant: The largest portion of funding was spent on supply-reduction efforts and treatment. Officials paid lip service to the need for more funding of educational efforts, but gave the majority of funds to agencies connected with supply-reduction efforts such as law enforcement and interdiction.

Upon entering the new millennium, prevention specialists and educators once again are optimistic that national, statewide, and local attention will focus on reducing the demand for ATOD and that more dollars will be appropriated for curbing ATOD use. Key supporters of this approach must continue to take an active role in educating legislators and community leaders. The Physician Leadership on National Drug Policy, a group of 37 leading physicians, assisted in this effort when it issued a statement supporting the need for demand reduction.[4] As part of its policy recommendations, the group called for the reprioritization of funding so that at least half of the federal drug-control budget would address demand reduction. Will the American Medical Association continue to provide leadership in supporting this recommendation? Top government officials now speak favorably of and publicly endorse demand reduction. Will federal government officials continue to provide the leadership to shift the focus from supply reduction to demand reduction? Why are prevention specialists and educators continuing to advocate for more funding for primary prevention, including comprehensive strategies for addressing young children who live in high-risk environments? The answer to this last question is simply that prevention is the best way to reduce illegal ATOD use. Although not inexpensive, demand-reduction efforts remain more cost-effective than either treatment or supply reduction. (See the FYI box.)

Community leaders, parents, and educators can effectively participate in demand-reduction efforts by gaining a better understanding of primary prevention. They need to study (1) what has been tried in the past, (2) where ATOD prevention fits in the larger picture of prevention efforts, (3) the common characteristics of successful prevention programs, and (4) the strategies best suited for their schools and community. This chapter defines prevention and addresses past prevention approaches. Some of the components from past efforts are still valuable today, whereas others should be discarded or replaced.

A Public Health Approach to ATOD Prevention

Prevention has been described as a dynamic, assertive process of promoting wellness in individuals, families, and communities through creating the appropriate conditions (environmental factors) and developing personal attributes and skills (individual factors).[5] The public health field provides an epidemiological model of health that includes a third dimension: the agent. Agents can be etiological agents (e.g., drugs) or change agents (e.g., community health workers, teachers, and others who transform knowledge into new ideas and innovations). The public health field also provides a well-known model for defining the three levels of prevention efforts: primary, secondary, and tertiary.

Primary prevention refers to efforts usually directed at a time before an unwanted behavior begins. These efforts can be directed at individuals (the host), the substance itself or change agents (the agent), or community conditions (the environment). For example, fifth-grade students (the host) can practice refusal skills that may deter ATOD use in adolescence. Policymakers can monitor the tobacco and alcohol industries to ensure that the addictive properties of these agents are not strengthened, such as by increasing the nicotine in cigarettes (the agent). Community health educators and teachers can serve as change agents in the community. Environmental factors include negative conditions such as poverty or overcrowding and positive conditions such as neighborhood watch groups or activities for youth. The FYI box on page 125 provides some additional examples of factors to consider.

Secondary prevention efforts occur at a stage where ATOD use is first manifested or has just begun. ATOD use starts at younger ages today, with estimated onset now between the ages of 10 and 14.[6] Secondary prevention uses intervention techniques and strategies directed at individuals who are still believed capable of stopping ATOD use. For example, intensive skill-building sessions are conducted for students caught using ATOD on school property. In these sessions, students learn signs and symptoms of ATOD abuse and become knowledgeable about referral procedures and available resources to get further help. Zero-tolerance programs are designed to intervene with students who are caught using or possessing ATOD on school grounds. Student assistance programs prevent adolescents from becoming further involved in ATOD use by providing early intervention before treatment is necessary.

Tertiary prevention efforts occur when ATOD use behaviors are already fixed, so these efforts are aimed at reducing the consequences of use, even if ATOD use isn't stopped. Again, children and adolescents are targeted because ATOD patterns established in early adolescence can persist throughout life. Research shows that ATOD dependency and abuse patterns are more likely to develop in youth who begin ATOD use early.[7] As an example of tertiary prevention, a heroin addict may be given methadone through a local treatment program with the stipulation that he or she must submit to routine drug tests. The program is designed to reduce the user's illegal drug consumption and purchases, not to cure him or her.

Classifying ATOD Primary Prevention Efforts

A recent important change in primary prevention is the development of a classification system for preventive intervention research, suggested by the Institute of Medicine (IOM). This system is now being used in discussions of ATOD prevention, particularly when addressing science-based principles, practices, and methods. Programs are classified on a continuum according to the population and intended purpose of the intervention. Three classifications of prevention approaches have been delineated: universal, indicated, and selective.[8] **Universal prevention strategies** are designed to address large populations, such as all the students in a school or district. **Selective prevention strategies** are designed to address target groups or subgroups of the population, such as children of alcoholics or underachievers. **Indicated prevention strategies** are designed to address subpopulations who are already using ATOD or are displaying risk factors such as behavioral problems in school.[9] These classifications are addressed later, in the discussion of school, parent, and community programs that focus on salient risk and protective factors.

Another schematic for intervention strategies can be found in the guidelines set by the Center for Substance Abuse Prevention (CSAP) for state incentive grant recipients. The six categories are (1) information dissemination, (2) prevention education, (3) alternative drug-free activities, (4) problem identification and referral programs, (5) community-based processes, and (6) environmental approaches.[10] These categories are also highlighted in the discussion of current findings related to what works in prevention.

The Public Health Role in Prevention

Throughout history, public health agencies held major responsibility for primary prevention. Concurrently, health service agencies had major responsibility for secondary and tertiary prevention and for remediation (reactive and corrective efforts). Public health agencies worked closely with health care agencies because their missions were distinct and separate. Coincidentally, most appropriated funds were dedicated to health service agencies for health-related disorders and diseases, not to public health agencies for preventive efforts.

After 1980, funding appropriations for health issues, including ATOD, changed. Soaring health care costs necessitated that primary prevention receive more attention. With the change in funding, health service agencies began expanding their mission by redefining many secondary, tertiary, and remedial efforts as primary prevention (using the term *primary care*). More recently, we have witnessed the change in terminology from *prevention* to *prevention interventions*. With this broadened focus, turf battles among health service agencies and public health agencies accelerated, causing each to define their missions more clearly and protect their programs more vigorously.

The blurring of roles and a limited, competitive funding pool make coalition building difficult. Prevention specialists support the concept of collaboration and resource sharing among agencies, but politics often prevents efficient use of funds.

Prevention specialists struggle to keep agencies and organizations working together despite the apparent overlap in their roles, missions, and services. Today, public health agencies have both benefited and been thwarted by the expanding role of prevention.

Dimensions of Prevention

Prevention encompasses multiple processes, a comprehensive and directed approach, and collaborative effort. Efforts are directed at reducing risk factors, and enhancing protective factors and developmental assets. Although prevention specialists may not agree on a common definition of prevention, most specialists agree that the overall goal of prevention is to foster a climate in which the following are true.[11]

- Alcohol use is acceptable only for those of legal age and only when the risk of adverse consequences is minimal.
- Prescription and over-the-counter drugs are used only for their intended purposes.
- Other abusable substances (e.g., gasoline or aerosols) are used only for their intended purposes (see **Figure 7.3**).
- Illegal drugs and tobacco are not used at all.

The following descriptions of key components of prevention are adapted from a California

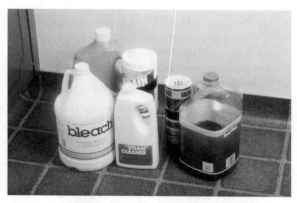

Figure 7.3 Gasoline, Paint, and Household Chemicals Are Abusable Substances Prevention efforts also are directed at the abuse of common household substances.
(© Tony Freeman/PhotoEdit)

Department of Education document.[12] Additional components have been included to create a broader understanding of the dimensions of prevention.

Multiple Processes

Prevention includes multiple processes that involve people proactively protecting, enhancing, and restoring the health and well-being of individuals and their communities. Health is viewed as something positive, a joyful attitude toward life; it is not just the absence of disease.[13]

Protective Factors

Primary prevention may involve activities, programs, and practices that can alter an individual's opportunities, risks, and expectations.[14] For example, opportunities may include new jobs, increased availability of literacy programs, and access to GED programs. Risk reduction may include increased visibility of local police, a Neighborhood Watch program, and better gun control. Expectations may include increased community pride, hope for children's futures, and increased support from those who live with privilege.

Comprehensive Approach

Prevention must be comprehensive, involving many systems, such as educational, medical, law enforcement, religious, and business communities. Prevention efforts are focused on programs and strategies that deal with individual risks, protective factors, developmental assets, and environmental conditions.[15]

Directed Efforts

For prevention to be successful, efforts must address the reciprocal relationships and interactions among the host, environment, and agent (reciprocal determinism). They can be directed toward the potential or active users (the host), toward the sources, supplies, and availability of drugs (the agent), and toward the social climate that encourages, supports, reinforces, or sustains the problematic use of alcohol or other drugs (the environment).[16]

Proactive Process

Prevention is an initiative-taking, **proactive** process intended to promote and protect health and reduce or eliminate the need for remedial treatment of the physical, social, and emotional problems associated with the consumption of drugs and alcohol.[17]

Developmental Assets

Developmental assets, building blocks of healthy development, can help children and adolescents develop into caring and responsible adults. Internal and external developmental assets allow for a proactive approach to preventing ATOD abuse.[18]

Collaborative Effort

Prevention is a collaborative school, family, and community process of planning and implementing multiple strategies that (1) reduce specific risk factors contributing to tobacco, alcohol, and drug use and related behavioral problems among youth and (2) strengthen protective factors to ensure young people's good health and well-being. Collaboration occurs when agencies truly work together on a common problem rather than work independently to pursue their own agendas.[19]

Learning from the Past

Past prevention efforts often focused on a single component of the epidemiological model of health, not on the reciprocal relationships and interactions of the components. The underlying assumption of each singularly focused effort differed depending on the target. Prevention efforts that targeted the host were characterized by the assumption that individuals control their own behavior and choose abstinence, moderation, or abuse. In these efforts, professionals provided adequate information for informed decision making and then relied on the individual's sound judgment.

Prevention efforts focused on the agent were characterized by attempts to control the substance being ingested, inhaled, injected, or applied. The substance, not the individual, was viewed as the culprit. Controlling or removing the substance, it was

reasoned, eliminated the abuse. Theoretically, this method could work, but, in reality, the demand for drugs continues and, consequently, the supply remains.

Prevention efforts dealing with the environment were characterized by a focus on societal attitudes toward alcohol and drug use, living conditions, and resources. Advocates surmised that a society with a lower tolerance for drunkenness and drug abuse had fewer problems, and that poor living conditions and inadequate resources contributed heavily to alcohol and other drug abuse.

This section addresses past prevention strategies within the United States. The singular approach of each effort is highlighted according to the epidemiological model for prevention.

The Information Model

The first prevention efforts in the United States, which focused on the host, began in the 1890s. At that time, the Women's Christian Temperance Union (WCTU) successfully convinced all states to require public school instruction in tobacco, alcohol, and other drugs. The WCTU believed that educating youth about the evils of alcohol was the way to eliminate its use. The temperance movement later shifted its focus from the immorality of drinking to the elimination of the temptation, thus supporting prohibition.

Prohibition attempted to prevent the abuse of ATOD by eliminating the agent. Although prohibition was not successful in eliminating alcohol, the country did experience a decline in overall alcohol use. Complete elimination of alcohol was never achieved.

In the 1960s, the second wave (or resurgence) of educational efforts focusing on the host (young people) began. Parents and community leaders believed that young people lacked accurate information about the harmful effects and consequences of drugs and that young people would refrain from drug use if they knew the dangers. As a result, teachers used scare tactics to convey information about drugs.

Former addicts visited classrooms or general school assemblies to give personal accounts of their horrible struggles with drugs. They talked about

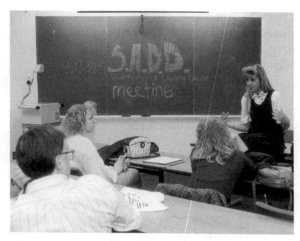

Figure 7.4 A Former Drug Addict Speaks to a Class
Using former addicts and drug dealers as school assembly speakers is an ineffective, albeit well-intentioned, prevention strategy. (© Aneal Vohra/Unicorn Stock Photos)

health problems, ruined family relations, skirmishes with law enforcement, and the gruesome details of life as a drug addict. Their message was clear: "If you don't watch out, you'll turn out just like me. You'll be the next addict. I'm here so you won't have to go through what I did." (See **Figure 7.4**.)

Scare tactics often involved inaccurate, overblown information or outright lies. Classroom teachers told stories of deformed infants with grotesque features or missing limbs who were born to mothers who used marijuana or LSD. Teachers further warned students about chromosomal damage to unborn fetuses. They talked about bad trips and bizarre behavior in LSD users, and about dealers who adulterated drugs so that even one-time users risked death.

This information model relied on the individual (host) to choose abstinence. The message was "Don't use drugs. The consequences are too unpredictable. The risk is too great."

Scare tactics sometimes backfired, resulting in increased experimentation. For example, students thought that if teachers had lied about marijuana, perhaps they had lied about cocaine, too. Some students decided to try the drugs and find out for themselves. Research clearly showed that neither scare tactics nor information alone was an effective way to change health behaviors, including ATOD use.[20-22]

Two variants of the information model, fear arousal and moral suasion, were found in the tobacco literature of this period. First, researchers found that by strengthening young people's beliefs in their susceptibility to the negative effects of ATOD, the potential for their use decreased.[23] Second, researchers found that strengthening young people's beliefs that ATOD use was morally wrong inoculated them against potential use.

Information dissemination can be effective when used with other strategies. The working draft of *Science-Based Practices in Substance Abuse Prevention: A Guide* provides several statements regarding the positive effectiveness of the information model:

- Educational programming regarding ATOD can increase knowledge regarding the hazards of substance use and aid in the development of negative attitudes toward ATOD use.
- Information dissemination campaigns should be viewed as complementary to more intensive and interactive prevention approaches.
- Traditional education about harms and risks associated with substance use and abuse cannot, by itself, produce measurable and long-lasting changes in substance abuse-related behavior and attitudes. Educational approaches that combine the conveyance of information about the harms of substance abuse with the fostering of skills (problem solving, communication) and promoting protective factors have been shown to be more effective.
- Didactic approaches are among the least effective educational strategies. Research suggests that interactive approaches engaging the target audience are more effective. The approaches include cooperative learning, role plays, and group exercises."[24]

The Responsible-Use Model

The responsible-use model, which focuses on the host, began in the 1960s and continues to be advocated by some prevention specialists. These advocates believe that government-imposed abstinence is not fair or effective and that individuals should be allowed to make decisions for themselves based on accurate information.

They also believe that students need accurate information about all drugs, including positive as well as negative consequences, to make informed decisions. They believe people use drugs because they innately seek an altered state of consciousness, and experimental and recreational drug use is a quick way to achieve this altered state.

Supporters of this model contend that drugs are not inherently good or bad; the problem is how they are used or abused. For instance, cocaine alone doesn't create problems, but when greedy dealers cut adulterants into the cocaine, risk is increased. Also, the government puts responsible users at risk by keeping drugs illegal and heavily regulated. Supporters of responsible use believe that keeping certain drugs illegal inflates their price and thus contributes to crimes and burglaries because abusers turn to crime to support their expensive habit. When drugs were legal in this country, they were inexpensive and not associated with crime. (A recent argument for this viewpoint is that stiffer penalties for illegal steroid use have been followed by an increase in their black-market prices and a decrease in quality.)

Advocates today appeal to the common sense and good judgment of persons who choose to try drugs. (See **Figure 7.5.**) They believe that many drugs are regulated because of fear of the unknown, illogical reasoning, and cultural bias. These proponents feel that an individual's freedom of choice regarding drugs is being denied through ignorance rather than sound, scientific judgment.

Opponents of the responsible-use model argue that the psychological effects of psychoactive drugs prevent users from making reasoned, logical choices. They say that some drugs have such powerful chemical effects that consumers cannot be allowed to make decisions about their use. In the 1970s and early 1980s, proponents of the responsible-use model thought cocaine was a relatively safe drug when it was used recreationally. During that time, cocaine was believed to be nonaddicting, that is, physical dependence did not occur and psychological dependence was unlikely for occasional users.

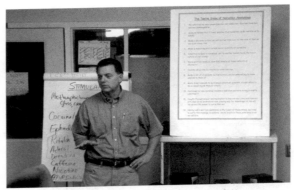

Figure 7.5 A Teacher Discusses Responsible Use
(© Spencer Grant/PhotoEdit)

Today, however, statistics on cocaine and its derivative, crack, do not support this contention. Furthermore, opponents view this position as irresponsible support of recreational drug use. Opponents also point to alarmingly high rates of alcohol-related problems by students, suggesting that responsible use is not possible for adolescents.

Research related to this prevention model is unavailable because legal regulations preclude its viability. Proponents and opponents continue to debate the merits of this controversial model. At this writing, governmental agencies fund only those projects that advocate abstinence, not responsible use. Although alcohol is not an illicit drug, its use by adolescents is illegal. Therefore, governmental agencies advocate the same strong message: "There is no responsible use of alcohol or illicit drugs by adolescents."

The Affective Education Model

Proponents of affective education, a model of the 1970s, believed that young people's attitudes toward ATOD determined whether they would use them (again, the focus was on the host). Practitioners and researchers suggested that young people's **values** were not thoroughly grounded and that they were unable to express their feelings adequately. Research showed that people who used drugs often had difficulty identifying and expressing feelings and exhibited a poorly developed sense of values and life goals. Affective education efforts focused on

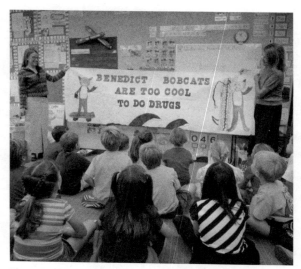

Figure 7.6 A Forced-Choice Classroom Exercise
(© Spencer Grant/PhotoEdit)

clarifying values, exploring feelings, and enhancing self-esteem. Through educational strategies and techniques, students received opportunities to clarify their values about ATOD. Teachers served as catalysts to help students determine their values, but the teachers themselves remained "value free." Proponents believed that students with high self-esteem chose abstinence; therefore, improving a student's self-esteem would result in reduced ATOD use. (See Figure 7.6.)

Opponents of this model believed that teachers needed to instill society's values rather than allow students to undertake the **valuing process** themselves. They argued that society valued abstaining from drug use and that students were too young to know right from wrong.

Thus erupted the battle over who should teach values. Some parents wanted values taught only in the home and religious institutions, not in the school. Other parents wanted school personnel involved in teaching values because most parents communicate inadequately with their children.

Teaching values remains controversial. In 1977, Reo Christenson provided a list of 20 values he felt everyone could accept as universal. (See the Viewpoints box.) How many of these values do you accept? Do your classmates agree with you? Are these values still relevant today?

Research found that some affective education efforts were successful in changing values, but evidence did not suggest that changes in values could be linked to changes in behavior.[25,26] Thus, these efforts alone were not effective in preventing ATOD use.

Today, character education based on character development and values education has been endorsed by a number of prevention proponents. Character education, like other affective approaches, does not suggest a direct and simple correlation between values and behavior. Situations in the real world are complex, requiring problem-solving and critical-thinking skills. Most situations are not either/or; rather, they exist within the both/and arena. Some scholars suggest that students learn more lessons through social interactions in the school than through formal education. Most prevention specialists wrestle with explaining to children and adolescents the incongruence between the values expressed by parents and role models and the behaviors they exhibit (the vicarious factor). Character education helps students address the complex nature of the decision-making process, the weighing of values and beliefs to make value-laden decisions.[27]

The Character Education Partnership suggests 11 principles that can serve as the criteria for schools and other groups when planning character education.[28]

1. Character education promotes core ethical values as the basis of good character.
2. *Character* must be comprehensively defined to include thinking, feeling, and behavior.
3. Effective character education requires an intentional, proactive, comprehensive approach that promotes the core values in all phases of school life.
4. The school must be a caring community.
5. To develop character, students need opportunities for moral action.
6. Effective character education includes a meaningful and academic curriculum that respects all learners and helps them succeed.

Values We Can All Accept

1. The most important thing in life is the kind of persons we are becoming, the qualities of character and moral behavior we are developing.
2. Self-discipline, defined as the strength to do what we know we ought to do even when we would rather not, is important in our lives.
3. Being trustworthy, so that when we say we will or will not do something we can be believed, is important.
4. Telling the truth, especially when it hurts to do so, is essential to trust, to self-respect, and to social health. Unless we can tell the truth when it is painful to us and seemingly injurious to our short-run interests, we are not truthful persons.
5. Being honest in all aspects of life, including our business practices and our relations with government, is important.
6. Doing work well, whatever it may be, and the satisfactions that come from this attitude, are important.
7. Personal courage and personal responsibility are important in the face of group pressures to do what, deep down, one disbelieves in.
8. While respecting the rights of others, it is important to use honorable means in seeking our individual and collective ends.
9. "Can it survive the sunlight?" is one of the most reliable tests of dubious conduct in private as well as in public life.
10. It is important to have the courage to say, "I'm sorry, I was wrong."

11. Recognizing inconspicuous, unsung people who have admirable qualities and live worthwhile lives is important.
12. Good sportsmanship should be understood and celebrated. Winning is not all-important.
13. It is necessary to get facts straight and to hear both sides before drawing conclusions adverse to a person, group, or institution.
14. It is important to listen, really listen, to persons with whom we are having disputes or difficulties.
15. Treating others as we would wish to be treated is one of the best guides to human conduct. This principle applies to persons of every class, race, nationality, and religion.
16. Another good guide is this: If everyone in comparable circumstances acted as you propose to act, would it be for the best?
17. No person is an island; behavior that may seem to be of purely private concern often affects those around us and society itself.
18. Adversity is the best test of our maturity and mettle.
19. Respect for law is essential to a healthy society, but responsible, nonviolent civil disobedience can be compatible with our ethical heritage.
20. It is important to acquire respect for the democratic values of free speech, a free press, freedom of assembly, freedom of religion, and due process of law. We should recognize that this principle applies to speech we abhor, groups we dislike, persons we despise.

Source: Reo M. Christenson, "McGuffey's Ghost and Moral Education Today," *Phi Delta Kappan,* June 1977, 738.

7. Character education should strive to develop students' intrinsic motivation.
8. The school staff must become a learning and moral community in which all share responsibility for character education and attempt to adhere to the same core values that guide the education of students.
9. Character education requires moral leadership from both staff and students.

10. The school must recruit parents and community members as full partners in the character-building effort.
11. Evaluation of character education should assess the character of the school, the school staff's functioning as character educators, and the extent to which students manifest good character.

Alternative Programs

Alternative programs proliferated with the advent of "natural highs" in the late 1970s. Natural highs were programs designed to create a safe environment for risk taking, such as river rafting, ropes courses, and wilderness experiences. The concept was that involving high-risk youth in these activities would occupy their leisure time and fulfill their need for thrill seeking. Because these activities tend to cost more than classroom activities, most alternative programs focus on high-risk youth. In fact, so many programs began that a halt was called for until evaluations could be made to support their effectiveness.

Research regarding alternative programs shows mixed results. Some universal programs appeared to show small positive effect. Kumpfer cited the positive results of alternative activities such as African and jazz dance, storytelling, karate, and creative arts through the Targeted Primary Prevention Housing Project Demonstration Program.[29] Some alternative programs may be more effective when used selectively or as indicated programs. Tobler found that alternative activities such as river rafting worked well with high-risk children, particularly those who missed adequate adult supervision, had limited access to a variety of activities, or lacked opportunities to develop social skills.[30] (See **Figure 7.7.**) Some alternative programs may demonstrate iatrogenic effects, such as attending rock concerts or sports events with older peers or adults.[31] Despite the limitations of alternative programs, they still occur. Activities range from volunteering in local soup kitchens and participating in neighborhood cleanups to vocational counseling and job placement services. Alternative programs, particularly those involving high-risk students, are classified as selective or indicated prevention approaches.

The working draft of *Science-Based Practices in Substance Abuse Prevention: A Guide* provides several statements regarding alternative programs.

- Alternatives should be part of a comprehensive prevention plan that includes other strategies with proven effectiveness. Environmental strate-

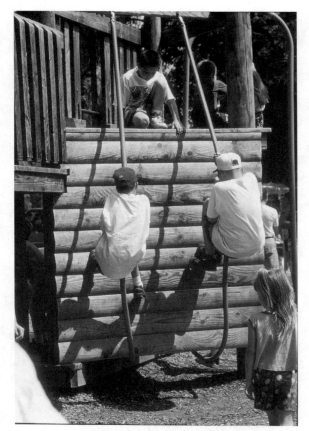

Figure 7.7 Young People in an Outward Bound Activity Exposing youth to physically and mentally challenging tasks is a common prevention strategy.

(© Chuck Schmeiser/Unicorn Stock Photos)

gies that reduce the availability of ATOD appear to be among the more effective strategies.

- The appropriateness and effectiveness of alternatives depend in part on the target group.
- Community service has been related to increased sense of well-being and more positive attitudes toward people, the future, and the community and allows youth to "give back" to their community.
- Mentoring programs provide youth with structured time with adults and are related to reductions in substance use and increases

in positivity toward others, the future, and school. Also, participation in these programs is related to increased school attendance.

- The more highly involved the mentor, the greater the positive results.
- Provision of organized recreation/cultural activities by community agencies can decrease substance use and delinquency by providing both drug-free alternatives and monitoring and supervision of children.
- Alternatives provide a natural and effective way of providing prevention services to high-risk youth.
- Alternatives can be part of a comprehensive prevention effort in the community, establishing strong community norms against misuse of alcohol and use of illicit drugs. Although a one-shot community event may not change the behavior of participants, such an event can serve as strong community statement that supports and celebrates a no-use norm.[32]

Parent Programs

Parental influence is often cited as the primary reason that youth do not use drugs. The National Center on Addictions and Substance Abuse found that 42% of teens who don't use marijuana cite their parents for their decision. The Partnership for a Drug-Free America (PDFA) suggests that adolescents are up to 50% less likely to use drugs if they learn about risks at home.[33] A recently released national study by PDFA found that more parents are talking with their children more often about ATOD, and the parents appear to be having an impact.[34] The PDFA notes the following about who is talking and what parental concerns are:

- 81% of mothers said they frequently talked with their children about how drugs can mess up their lives, compared with 63% of fathers.
- 77% of mothers said they frequently talked with their children about how drugs can mess

up their education, compared with 57% of fathers.

- One of every three parents (32%) believes "what I say will have little influence on whether my child tries marijuana." The numbers are even higher for African American and Hispanic parents (40% and 43%, respectively).
- Nearly six in ten (57%) parents have tried marijuana at some point in their lives.

As prevention specialists and educators, we have always intuitively known that parents were a key component of successful prevention efforts. Today research has compellingly documented the effectiveness of supportive, skillful parents in helping children and adolescents avoid ATOD use. Research also has documented effective parenting interventions designed to facilitate building healthy families. CSAP's family-based Prevention Enhancement Protocols Systems (PEPS), entitled *Family-Based Approaches to Prevention*, identified 10 different approaches: parent education, parent support, behavioral parent training, affective parent training, family support, in-home family support, family education, family skills training, and several types of family therapy. Three types of parenting interventions had the highest level of effectiveness: (1) behavioral parent training, primarily targeting parents with young children, (2) family skills training, for parents of elementary school-aged children, and (3) family therapy for adolescents and parents.

Behavioral parent training programs appear to be effective in reducing youth risk factors such as conduct disorders, aggression, and school problems and strengthening resiliency factors and social competencies. This parent training typically occurs over 12 to 20 weeks. Examples include Webster-Stratton's Child and Parent video series, Patterson's Parent Training, and Alvy's Effective Black Parents and Los Ninos Bien Educados.

Family skills training involves training for both parents and youth. Parents receive intensive skills training, and youth receive social and life skills training. Family practice sessions are also incorporated. Examples include Kumpfer's Strenthening Families Program, Aktan's SafeHaven Program,

1. Role model
2. Educator or information resource
3. Family policymaker and rule setter
4. Originator of and participant in enjoyable family activities
5. Consultant and educator about peer pressure

6. Monitor of children
7. Collaborator with other parents
8. Identifier and confronter
9. Intervener in children's ATOD use
10. Manager of their own feelings

Miller-Hyde's Dare to Be You, and Catalano's Focus on Families.

Family therapy is conducted by highly trained therapists who work with families and youth who are at high risk for substance abuse (e.g., initiation of drug use, juvenile delinquency, or conduct disorders). Examples include Alexander and Parson's Functional Family Therapy, Szapocznik's Structural Family Therapy, and Liddle's Family Therapy. The National Clearinghouse for Alcohol and Drug Information (NCADI) provides more information about effective parent programs for those who are interested.

Parents often assume a number of different roles and responsibilities in guiding their children's development. The CSAP publication *Parent Training Is Prevention* identified 10 prevention roles for parents. (See the Hints & Tips box.)

- *Parents as role models:* Parents influence children by the way they model health-promoting and health-compromising behaviors. Parents' attitudes toward and use of mind-altering drugs, such as tobacco, alcohol, caffeine, and OTC and prescription drugs, affect their children. Parents serve as models for how feelings are expressed and how values are processed.[35] (See Figure 7.8.)

- *Parents as educators and consultants:* Parents influence their children by what they say as well as what they do. They are the primary educators about the risks of ATOD use, the

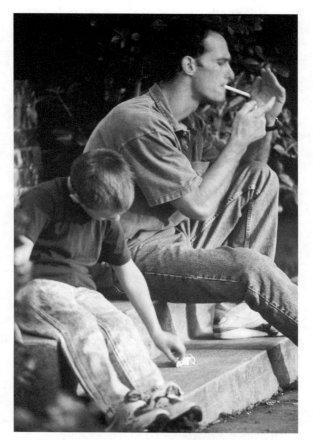

Figure 7.8 Children Look to Parents as Role Models
Drug and alcohol use by parents has a great influence on their children's drug use behavior.

(© Peter Poulides/Stone/Getty)

impact of peer pressure, and how to resist peer pressure.

- *Parents as policymakers:* As rule setters, parents must ensure that children and adolescents know three things: exactly what the rule is, exactly what the parent expects, and exactly what the consequences will be if the rule is broken.[36]
- *Parents as monitors:* As monitors and supervisors, parents make house rules, provide rewards and consequences, and evaluate existing plans.
- *Parents as identifiers:* As identifiers and confronters, parents detect ATOD use, confront the child or adolescent, and follow through on consequences. Parents need adequate training to assume this role.
- *Parents as family activity planners:* Parents can provide opportunities for children and adolescents to participate in family activities that range from household tasks to leisurely play. Children and adolescents benefit from performing meaningful tasks and gain skills they carry into adulthood. The recognition and rewards they receive provide a sense of empowerment.
- *Parents as collaborators:* Parents can work with other parents on social events and community prevention projects.
- *Parents as interveners:* As partners in prevention, parents need to be active in school and community coalitions. All families can benefit from parental involvement in school and community ATOD efforts. Unfortunately, many prevention specialists find that the parents who want to participate in programs are the ones who least need them; they are already providing guidance for their children. Nevertheless, all parents can learn necessary or additional skills for handling children and adolescents who use alcohol, tobacco, and other drugs, and they should be recognized and rewarded for their role in prevention efforts.

- *Parents as managers of their own feelings:* Parents with children or adolescents who are ATOD users need skills to manage their own feelings. Successful parenting requires learning to exit rather than explode, listening without feeling guilty or accepting excuses, standing firm, forgiving, and controlling their own actions while refraining from trying to control their child's or adolescent's actions.[37]

Working with parent groups can be extremely rewarding, but prevention specialists typically encounter the same frustrations as community health educators. They struggle to find ways to reach the parents who most need their services. CSAP's *Prevention Monograph 5* suggests strategies for broadening outreach efforts to parents. Because parents of at-risk children and adolescents are hard to reach, prevention specialists must use every possible opportunity to address ATOD issues within a broader effort. Suggested outreach efforts include the following:

1. Take advantage of milestone transitions. Examples: changing grade levels, moving from elementary to middle school, joining a club or band.
2. Communicate with parents during other life events. Examples: moving to a new location, family breakups.
3. Use minitransitions to communicate with parents. Example: family trips or vacations.
4. Increase parents' awareness and knowledge of potential risks. Examples: gateway drugs, heredity issues.
5. Increase parents' knowledge and understanding of parenting skills. Examples: communicating with children, discipline.
6. Develop materials for parents. Examples: audiocassettes, print material.
7. Create resource centers in libraries. Example: print and AV materials in public libraries.
8. Create resource packets for intermediaries to distribute. Examples: family resource centers, businesses.

9. Use intermediaries that have direct access to parents in transition. Examples: schools, employers, services.
10. Work with local media. Examples: radio, television.
11. Influence the mass media to help reach parents. Examples: storylines for shows, new aspects of ATOD research.
12. Conduct research on the knowledge, attitudes, and practices of parents. Examples: knowledge of gateway drugs, attitudes toward ATOD use.

Parent training programs have proliferated, so it becomes extremely important for prevention specialists to keep abreast of research regarding program effectiveness. Many effective parent resources are already available for community groups to implement. Pick one that meets your community's needs.

Common Elements of Unsuccessful Programs

The prevention models discussed in the preceding section were successful to some extent in effecting change in knowledge, values, communication, self-esteem, or attitudes. Yet, many of these programs were implemented as single-focus programs. They seldom demonstrated a lasting change in ATOD behavior because ATOD abuse cannot be solved with any single approach. ATOD abuse is caused by multiple factors and remains a community dilemma, not an individual, parent, school, or religious problem. Many communities have designed and implemented prevention efforts, but the expectation of quick fixes and magical solutions has led to frustration. Often prevention programs were based on unsubstantiated methods or approaches, usually ensuring their failure.

In a CSAP document, Goplerud summarized nine underlying assumptions found in many unsuccessful community prevention programs.[38] Communities that built programs on the following erroneous assumptions experienced frustration and failure.

1. One-shot interventions produce immediate success. Reality: One-shot interventions can demonstrate short-term success, but this doesn't necessarily translate into long-term benefits. Students may be temporarily awed by someone's devastating story of drug abuse or a demolished car on the school lawn, but the short-term impact doesn't create long-term healthy behaviors.

2. Programs designed by and for middle-class people should work for everyone. (Whatever works for low-risk students will work for all students.) Reality: While universal prevention programs have a critical role in ATOD prevention, some students will need selective or indicated prevention programs.

3. Prevention is inexpensive. Reality: Prevention must be comprehensive and sustained. This requires a long-term commitment to funding successful efforts. Professional staff, continuous education, staff development, and accessible office locations are expensive, but cost-effective.

4. Behavior change is possible through simple education programs. Reality: Behavior change is a complex process that requires maintenance and support. Changing individuals' levels of knowledge or improving attitudes is more easily accomplished than changing health behaviors.

5. All peer counselor programs have positive results. Reality: Peer counseling programs are only as effective as the training and skills of the peers who are chosen to conduct the programs. The research is mixed regarding the effectiveness of this strategy.

6. Parent programs, mass media campaigns, and "Just Say No" clubs alone can meet the needs of everyone. Reality: Each effort must be designed for the appropriate target group. Individual differences must be taken into account when designing a universal program.

7. Involving youth in nondrug recreational activities prevents ATOD use. Reality: Youth who spend three or more hours involved in sport, music, or artistic endeavors have developed

one beneficial asset. However, youth need more than one protective factor to make healthy lifestyle choices.

8. Using parts of an effective program will still give favorable results. Reality: All effective research-based programs must be replicated in their entirety to be valid and reliable. If a school or community chooses parts of an effective program, that new program must be reevaluated for its effectiveness. Often, successful programs have been conducted with considerable grant funding, making replication difficult if not impossible.

9. **Teacher-proof curricula** can be designed. Reality: The teacher who delivers and implements a curriculum must be trained and competent. No curriculum can be independent of the instructor.

A review of singularly focused programs and poorly designed community efforts reveals how our previous successes were limited. Communities cannot combat ATOD problems with quick, inexpensive fixes. They must design programs based on principles and practices that we now know increase the likelihood of success.

Past prevention efforts often focused on singular approaches that failed to produce the desired community outcomes. These efforts failed for a variety of reasons, but a common characteristic was the lack of connection to a broader, comprehensive health promotion program. The most promising, cost-effective way to reduce illegal ATOD use is prevention, not treatment or law enforcement. Community leaders, parents, and educators must collaborate to produce successful multifaceted prevention strategies.

Summary

Illegal ATOD consumption and abuse are costly. As primary prevention receives more funding, more agencies (including treatment-focused agencies) have become involved in ATOD prevention. Demand-side reduction efforts receive less money than supply-side strategies, showing that the country's

major focus is still on preventing drugs from reaching users.

Primary prevention intervention strategies fall into three classifications: universal, selective, and indicated. Within the three levels of prevention (primary, secondary, and tertiary), efforts focus on the environment, host, and agent (the public health model).

Parental influence is the primary reason young people do not use drugs. Parents have a number of roles to play within the prevention effort. Three types of parenting interventions have the highest level of effectiveness: behavioral parent training, family skills training, and family therapy for adolescents and parents.

Past prevention efforts often focused on a single component of the ATOD problem. Communities that modeled programs on erroneous assumptions and single dimensions of prevention experienced frustration and failure. One-shot programs have repeatedly failed in producing long-term change.

Scenario | Analysis and Response

As a health educator, Kim is aware of the need for a comprehensive school/community prevention effort. What does the research suggest regarding scare tactics? What does the research suggest regarding the showing of drugs and paraphernalia to students?

The coordinated school health program includes a comprehensive school-based curriculum. How might parents become involved in selecting an appropriate curriculum?

Grant funds can be either beneficial or detrimental to coalition building. The site-based team will have ultimate responsibility for the spending of the grant funds. How can the site-based team be strengthened through this decision-making process?

Learning Activities

1. Contact your local school district or a community agency to determine which parent training programs they are currently using. Are these programs supported by governmental agencies as effective? If not, what can you do to promote better programming efforts?

2. Gather information about the alternative programs available in your community. In a small group, brainstorm other alternative programs that could be initiated in your community.

3. Gather information about the one-shot programs currently being implemented in your school or community. What advocacy strategies can the class implement to increase awareness regarding the ineffectiveness of this approach?

Notes

1. "Changing Patterns of Drug Use in America," in *Reducing Drug Abuse in America* (Washington, DC: Office of National Drug Abuse Policy, 1999). Available: http://www.ondcppubs/publications/drugabuse/toc.html.

2. Office of National Drug Control Policy, *The Economic Costs of Drug Abuse in the United States, 1992–1998* (Washington, DC: Executive Office of the President, 2001). Available: www.whitehousedrugpolicy.gov/publications/.

3. Office of National Drug Control Policy, Office of Programs, Budget, Research, and Evaluation, *What America's Users Spend on Illegal Drugs, 1988–2000* (Cambridge, MA: Abt Associates, 2001). Available: www.whitehousedrugpolicy.gov/publications/.

4. "Top Docs Call for Refocusing Drug War on Prevention, Treatment," June 26, 2000. Available: www.jointogether.org/sa/wire/news/features/reader/0,1854,263595,00.html.

5. W. A. Loftquist, *Discovering the Meaning of Prevention: A Practical Approach to Positive Change* (Tucson, AZ: AYD Publications, 1983), 2.

6. P. Higgins, *The Prevention of Drug Abuse Among Teenagers: A Literature Review* (St. Paul, MN: Amherst H. Wilder Foundation, 1988).

7. J. D. Hawkins, D. Lishner, and R. F. Catalona, "Childhood Predictors and the Prevention of Adolescent Substance Abuse," in *Etiology of Drug Abuse: Implications for Prevention*, C. L. Jones and R. J. Battjes, eds., NIDA Research Monograph 56 (Rockville, MD: NIDA, 1985), 54–125.

8. Institute of Medicine, *Reducing Risk for Mental Disorders: Frontiers for Preventive Intervention Research* (Washington, DC: National Academy Press, 1994).

9. K. L. Kumpfer, *Identification of Drug Abuse Prevention Programs: Literature Review* (Washington, DC: NIDA Resource Center for Health Service Research; Rockville, MD: National Institute on Drug Abuse, 2000).

10. Center for Substance Abuse Prevention, *A Discussion Paper on Preventing Alcohol, Tobacco, and Other Drug Problems* (Rockville, MD: Substance Abuse and Mental Health Services Administration, U.S. Department of Health and Human Services, 1993).

11. *Prevention Primer: An Encylopedia of Alcohol, Tobacco, and Other Drug Prevention Terms* (Rockville, MD: National Clearinghouse for Alcohol and Drug Information, 1993), 98.

12. *Framework for Preventing Alcohol and Drug Problems* (Sacramento, CA: California Department of Education, 1991).

13. Central Valley Regional Prevention Forum, *Framework for Community Prevention* (Tulare, Kings, Fresno, Madera, Merced, and Mariposa Counties, CA, 1988).

14. *Prevention Plus II: Tools for Creating and Sustaining Drug-Free Communities* (Rockville, MD: Office of Substance Abuse Policy, 1989).

15. *The White House Conference for a Drug Free America* (Washington, DC: US Government Printing Office, 1988).

16. *Community Prevention System Framework for Alcohol and Other Drug Prevention* (Rockville, MD: Office of Substance Abuse Prevention, 1990).

17. L. Wallack, J. Ratcliffe, and F. Wittman, in *Comprehensive Alcohol and Drug Abuse Prevention Strategies* (California Health Research Foundation, 1984).

18. P. Benson, *All Kids Are Our Kids: What Communities Must Do to Raise Caring and Responsible Children and Adolescents* (San Francisco: Jossey-Bass, 1997).

19. *Not Schools Alone* (Sacramento, CA: California Department of Education, 1990).

20. R. L. Bangert-Drowns, "The Effects of School-Based Substance Abuse Education: A Meta-analysis," *Journal of Drug Education* 18 (1988): 243–264.

21. N. S. Tobler, "Meta-analysis of 143 Adolescent Drug Prevention Programs: Quantitative Outcome Results of Program Participants Compared to a Control or Comparison Group," *Journal of Drug Issues* 16, 4 (1986): 537–567.

22. E. Schaps, R. DiBartolo, J. Moskewitz, C. S. Palley, and S. Churgin, "A Review of 127 Drug Abuse Prevention Program Evaluations," *Journal of Drug Issues* 11 (1981): 17–43.

23. L. Johnston, P. O'Malley, and J. Bachman, *Use of Licit and Illicit Drugs by America's High School Students 1975–1988, Final Report* (Rockville, MD: National Institute on Drug Abuse, 1988).

24. P. G. Brounstein, J. M. Zweig, and S. E. Garnder, *Science-Based Practices in Substance Abuse: A Guide* (Washington, DC: Division of Knowledge Development and Evaluation, Center for Substance Abuse Prevention, 1998).

25. S. Kim, "A Short and Long-Term Evaluation of 'Here's Looking at You,'" *Journal of Drug Education* 18 (1988): 235–242.

26. E. Schaps, J. M. Moskowitz, J. H. Malvin, and G. H. Scheffer, "Evaluation of Seven School-Based Prevention

Programs: A Final Report on the Napa Project," *International Journal of Addiction* 21 (1986): 1081–1112.

27. R. S. Thomas, "Assessing Character Education: Paradigms, Problems, and Potentials." Available: www.quest.edu/content/whatsnew/archives/wnarticles2.html.

28. T. Lickona, E. Schaps, and C. Lewis, *Eleven Principles of Effective Character Education* (Washington, DC: The Character Education Partnership, 1997). Available: www.character/org/principles/index/cgi.

29. K. Kumpfer, E. Morehouse, B. Ross, C. Fleming, J. Emshoff, and L. DeMarco, *Prevention of Substance Abuse in COSA Programs* (Rockville, MD: ADAMHA/OSAP, 1988). Available from ADAMHA/OSAP, 5600 Fishers Lane (Rockwall II) Building, Rockville, MD, 20857.

30. Tobler, "Meta-analysis."

31. J. D. Swisher and T. W. Hu, "Alternatives to Drug Abuse: Some Are and Some Are Not," in *Preventing Adolescent Drug Abuse: Intervention Strategies,* T. J. Glynn, C. G. Leukefeld, and J. P. Ludfords, eds., NIDA Research Monograph 47 (Washington, DC: National Institute on Drug Abuse, 1983), 141–153.

32. P. G. Brounstein, J. M. Zweig, and S. E. Gardner, *Science-Based Practices in Substance Abuse: A Guide* (Washington, DC: Division of Knowledge Development and Evaluation, Center for Substance Abuse Prevention, 1998).

33. Partnership for a Drug-Free America, "Partnership Attitude Tracking Study 1999: New National Study Released: More Parents Talking About Drugs More Often, and Appear to Be Having an Impact," press release. Available: www.drugfreeamerica.org/research/pats99_parents/page4.html.

34. Ibid.

35. G. D. McKay, "Parents as Role Models," in *Parent Training Is Prevention: Preventing Alcohol and Other Drug Problems Among Youth in the Family,* DHHS Publication No. (ADM) 91-1715 (Rockville, MD: DHHS, 1991).

36. M. H. Popkin, "Parents as Family Policymakers and Rule Setters," in *Parent Training Is Prevention: Preventing Alcohol and Other Drug Problems Among Youth in the Family,* DHHS Publication No. (ADM) 91-1715 (Rockville, MD: DHHS, 1991).

37. B. A. Lundy and D. Smith, "Parents as Managers of Their Own Feelings," in *Parent Training Is Prevention: Preventing Alcohol and Other Drug Problems Among Youth in the Family,* DHHS Publication No. (ADM) 91-1715 (Rockville, MD: DHHS, 1991).

38. E. Goplerud, *Technical Assistance Guide for Prospective Demonstration Grant Applicants,* unpublished manuscript, Office of Substance Abuse Prevention, March 1989.

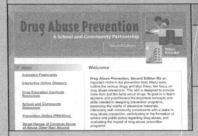

Chapter Learning Objectives

Upon completion of this chapter, students will be able to:

1. Define key terms such as *health, community health promotion,* and *community health education.*

2. Describe several health behavior and ATOD planning models.

3. Summarize the ATOD risk and protective factors found in the six life domains.

4. Summarize the developmental assets that protect the student against ATOD use and other negative health consequences.

5. Compare the basic tenets of community health promotion and ATOD prevention.

6. Compare and contrast the traditional community service model and the community empowerment service model.

7. Evaluate the lessons taught by successful community prevention programs for schools, parents, and communities.

8. Examine the implications of parents' acceptance or rejection of their children.

9. Examine the implications of parents' restrictiveness or permissiveness with their children.

Scenario

Lakeville is a small farming community (population 2,987). The community has one elementary school and a combined junior/senior high school. Several weeks ago, a number of events occurred that created consternation for local citizens. First, two parents of junior high school boys lodged complaints with the principal that their sons were being bullied and hav-ing lunch money stolen by older students. The parents of these older students were unwilling to inter-vene, believing that boys will be boys. Second, a high school junior was seriously injured in a car wreck. For the past three years, at least one student has been killed or seriously injured in a late-night accident after the Homecoming dance. Empty beer cans were found

Introduction

Adolescents today are faced with many health-related decisions, some of which are health promoting and some of which are health compromising. It is a mistake to believe that these decisions, including whether or not to use alcohol, tobacco, and other drugs, are made in a vacuum. Alcohol and drug problems are related to a myriad of other health and social problems, such as teen pregnancy, HIV infection, school discipline problems, and juvenile crime. The Web of Influence model provides a graphic representation of how ATOD abuse and other adolescent problems relate to risk and protective factors. (See **Figure 8.1.**) The model provides a strategy for classifying individual, family, and community risk and protective factors. These factors are the primary focus of community-wide health promotion efforts.

Because so many health-compromising behaviors are interrelated with ATOD abuse, this chapter includes background information on community health promotion, including definitions of health and health education and selected models for health behavior change. For readers knowledgeable in health education, this material can

in the vehicles. Third, some citizens complained that court judges were too lenient with alcohol and drug cases. It seemed as if most offenders were getting off with very light sentences or probation.

Lakeville is a close-knit community, and these events have many community members wondering what to do. Residents are aware that the resources available for dealing with ATOD problems are limited. They're forming a community task force, and they want you, a prevention specialist, to offer them suggestions for committee membership. Once the task force is formed, what steps should be taken to ensure success?

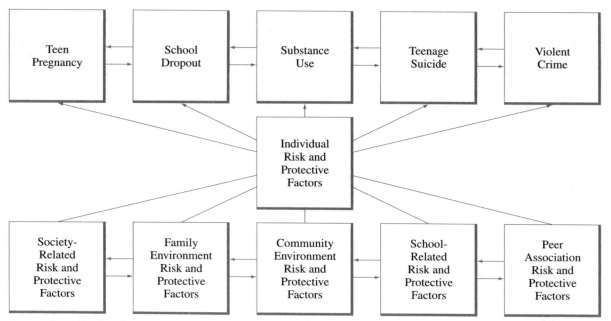

Figure 8.1 **Web of Influence**

Source: Centers for Substance Abuse Prevention, DHHS Publication No. (SMA) 99-3302.

serve as a review. For other readers, this material serves as an introduction for coordinating ATOD efforts with a comprehensive health promotion program.

In addition to community health promotion, successful ATOD prevention efforts for community partnerships are highlighted, with definitions and parameters of prevention from the ATOD literature, models for ATOD prevention, and components of successful ATOD community development.

Community Health Promotion

Some of the most promising prevention efforts have been directed at populations, rather than individuals, and are referred to as *community health promotion and disease prevention*. A *community* is defined in a variety of ways, including as a geographic area or as a collection of people (a population) who have a common cause or set of beliefs and values. Community health promotion and disease prevention efforts target "the educational, social, and environmental actions conducive to the health of a population."[1] These actions are numerous, complex, and interdependent. Educational

actions may include strategies for a broad range or a specific group of individuals, such as high-risk youth, families, special populations, and policymakers. Social actions may encompass changes in economic, political, legal, and organizational dimensions. Finally, environmental actions may address physical and biological factors, such as housing conditions or toxic exposure. (See **Figure 8.2.**) According to the Joint Committee on Health Education Terminology, health promotion and disease prevention, both individual and community, can be defined broadly as:

> The aggregate of all purposeful activities designed to improve personal and public health through a combination of strategies, including the competent implementation of behavioral change strategies, health education, health protection measures, risk factor detection, health enhancement, and health maintenance.

Community health promotion efforts, like ATOD prevention efforts, often lack adequate funding. According to the CDC, "In 1990, the medical-care

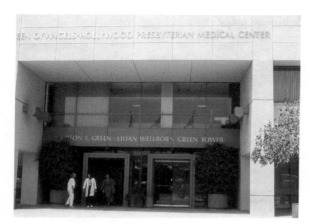

Figure 8.2 An Urban Health Care Facility Health promotion includes access to medical care resources.

(© Melanie Brown/PhotoEdit)

costs for persons with chronic diseases, which are in large part preventable, accounted for an estimated $425 billion…61%…of the nation's total medical-care costs. However, in 1994, the total reported expenditure for chronic disease-control activities in states was $1.21 per person. That amount represents only a modest increase in expenditures from the $0.99 per person in 1989."

Community health promotion, like ATOD prevention, emphasizes **collaboration** between the school and community. The community is responsibile for addressing social, political, and environmental issues; providing health education; and supporting school-based educational efforts. The school's role is to provide students with a coordinated school health program that includes ATOD prevention. Without question, the school is the key social system in the community, and its influence should not be underestimated. The Carnegie Council on Adolescent Development believes that the school has a preeminent role in the lives of children and adolescents. A report stated: "Schools could do more than perhaps any other single institution in society to help young people, and the adults they will become, to live healthier, longer, more satisfying, and more productive lives." Community health promotion focuses on empowering the school and community to (1) involve people in their own development, (2) recognize and

use their assets, (3) determine their needs and set priorities, and (4) gain control over their social and political environment. Through school and community collaboration, community health promotion seeks to maximize services, funds, and prevention efforts.

For thirty years, ATOD prevention efforts have paralleled community health promotion efforts. ATOD prevention efforts were focused specifically on mobilizing the community to fight ATOD use and abuse, whereas community health promotion efforts were focused on mobilizing communities to address a broad array of health issues, including chronic diseases such as heart disease and cancer. Many of the lessons learned by researchers conducting community health promotion efforts are invaluable for researchers conducting ATOD prevention efforts.

In *The Strategy of Preventive Medicine,* Rose summarized the basic tenets learned in community health promotion:[2]

- Risk factors for a large number of diseases and health problems are distributed in populations in a graded manner.
- There is often no obvious and clinically meaningful risk factor threshold that differentiates those at risk and those not at risk for a chronic disease.
- For many chronic diseases, there are many more people in a population at a relatively moderate level of risk than at the highest levels of risk.
- Addressing only the very high risk (clinically recognized) segment of a population misses the opportunity to improve the risk profile of the entire population.
- Modest risk lowering among many persons with moderate risk factor levels will shift the risk factor profile on the entire population in a favorable manner.
- A population-wide approach to intervention is thus called for, the objectives of which should be to reduce the average level of a population's risk through intervention for all and to intervene intensively for those few at the highest level of risk.

In another sphere of influence, researchers in HIV prevention have created a community development

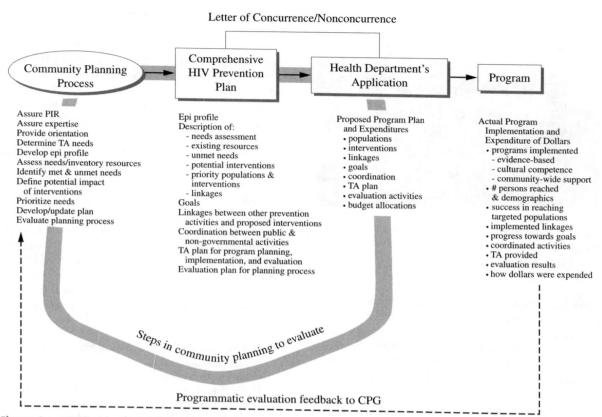

Figure 8.3 **HIV Prevention Community Planning** PIR, parity, inclusion, and representation; TA, technical assistance; epi, epidemiological; CPG, community planning group.

Source: Centers for Disease Control (http://www.cdc.gov/hiv/pubs/hiv-cp.pdf).

planning process in their efforts to reduce one of the six problem priority areas identified by the Centers for Disease Control and Prevention: sexual behaviors that result in HIV infection, other sexually transmitted diseases, and unintended pregnancy. (The other problem priority areas are tobacco use, poor eating habits, alcohol and other drug risks, behaviors that result in intentional and unintentional injuries, and physical inactivity.) The nine steps are elaborated in the following paragraphs. (See **Figure 8.3.**)

First, the community planning team must develop an epidemiologic profile. This step includes assessing and describing the extent, distribution, and impact of HIV/AIDS in the community. Second, the planning team must conduct a needs assessment of the prevention needs of the community.

Third, the planning team must assemble a resource inventory to determine the community's capability to respond to the epidemic. These resources include social networks, educational institutions, businesses, and other community-building activities. Fourth, the planning team conducts a gap analysis to determine the unmet needs of the community. This gap is determined by comparing the needs assessment to the resource inventory.

In step 5, potential strategies and interventions are determined. These strategies and interventions are based on the epidemiologic profile, needs assessment, and resource inventory. Step 6 is the prioritizing of HIV prevention needs based on the high-risk population needs and on identified interventions and strategies. Step 7 is the development of a comprehensive HIV prevention plan consistent with the priority needs and resources identified in previous steps. The plan should be reviewed, revised, and refined on a periodic basis. Step 8 is evaluation of the planning process. The effectiveness of the community planning process and the prevention plan should be evaluated throughout the entire planning process. Step 9 is the update of the comprehensive prevention plan. The periodic review may result in additional objectives and updating of the needs, resources, and comprehensive plan.

The steps for HIV prevention share many similarities with ATOD prevention planning, as you will read in the following section.

ATOD Community Development

In the ATOD field, the federal government has promoted efforts to transfer the knowledge learned by researchers into the hands of prevention providers at the local level. A major difficulty for researchers has been the dissemination of their findings to practitioners, those persons who are responsible for planning and implementing programs at the local level. A lack of adequate dissemination has led to many errors and mistakes in program development and implementation and to a squandering of local, state, and federal funds. Six regional Centers for the Application of Prevention Technologies (CAPTs) have been established to provide technical assistance to states, jurisdictions, and local communities in applying science-based prevention research. CAPTs are responsible for transferring science-based research to prevention providers from such federal agencies as the Center for Substance Abuse Prevention (CSAP), the Substance Abuse and Mental Health Services Administration (SAMHSA), the National Institute on Alcohol Abuse and Alcoholism (NIAAA), the National Institute on Drug Abuse (NIDA), the Office of Juvenile Justice and Delinquency Prevention (OJJDP), and the U.S. Department of Education (DOE). Science-based information "is that which has been identified and/or substantiated through an expert consensus or analytic process using commonly agreed upon criteria for rating research endeavors."[3] The process of technology transfer is illustrated in Figure 8.4.

Community partnerships to reduce ATOD abuse have received considerable federal funding. Over time,

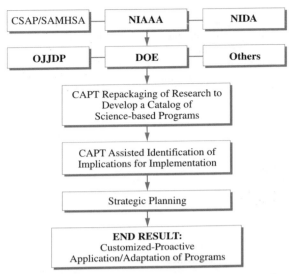

Figure 8.4 The Transfer of Science-Based Research

Source: Centers for the Application of Prevention Technologies, http://www.captus.org.

researchers have determined specific characteristics that make community partnerships more effective, including the following:[4]

- A comprehensive and widely shared vision agreed upon by group members
- A strong core of committed partners, including key policymakers
- An inclusive and broad-based membership
- Avoidance or quick resolution of severe conflict
- Decentralized units to address neighborhood issues
- Minimal staff turnover
- Extensive prevention activities and strong prevention policies
- Implementation of strategies that are tailored to specific needs within the community

These characteristics, identified by studying successful community partnerships for ATOD prevention, can support community health promotion specialists' efforts to build successful coalitions. How might these principles be applied to Lakeville's ATOD problems? How might they be applied to the target problem areas identified by the CDC?

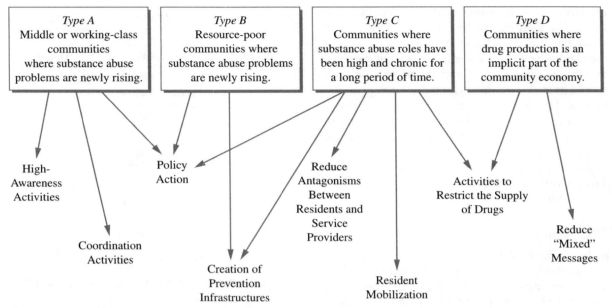

Figure 8.5 Matching Strategies to Community Type

Another factor for prevention specialists to consider is that "no one shoe fits all." The SAMHSA/CSAP's community partnership projects have led to the identification of a helpful fourfold typology that can help prevention specialists plan specific strategies to meet their community's needs. (See **Figure 8.5.**) What suggestions would you make to the citizens of Lakeville based on this information?

The Western CAPT has provided a framework for building a successful community prevention program targeting the risk and protective factors for ATOD. The seven steps are community readiness, needs assessment, prioritizing, resource assessment, targeting efforts, best practices, and evaluation. (See **Figure 8.6.**) An elaboration of each of these steps and tools for assessing the components of a successful prevention program can be found at the website of the Western CAPT (www.open.org/~westcapt/index.htm). Compare these seven steps to the community health promotion model discussed in the previous section.

Health and Wellness

Prevention specialists must appreciate the multidimensional nature of **health** if they are to promote community health efforts effectively. More often

than not, when people are asked to describe what it means to be healthy, they speak of what *not* to do. They say, "Don't drink, don't smoke, don't eat fatty foods, don't use too much salt, and don't drive without wearing seatbelts." They conclude that being healthy means not being sick. In some respects, this description reflects the concept of

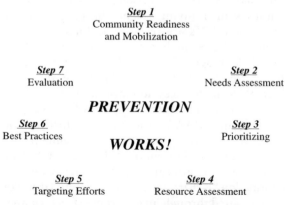

Figure 8.6 Building a Successful Prevention Program

Source: Center for Substance Abuse Prevention's Western Center for the Application of Prevention Technologies, http://www.open.org/~westcapt/index.htm.

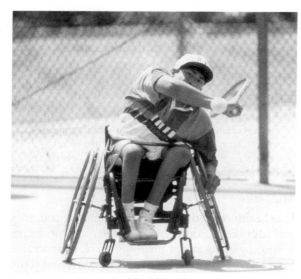

Figure 8.7 **A Disabled Person Can Be Considered Healthy** How healthy can this person be?

(© Phil McCarten/PhotoEdit)

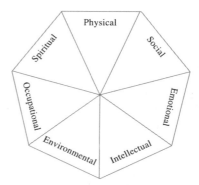

Figure 8.8 **Dimensions of Wellness**

prevention: to stop something from happening. Occasionally, when asked to define health, people focus on the positive aspects of health, describing health as feeling good, being physically fit, being the ideal weight, and getting enough sleep. Describing what to do instead of what not to do is more in line with **health promotion**: making something positive happen.

Although no universally accepted definition of health exists, the World Health Organization has provided the most frequently cited definition:

> Health is a state of complete physical, mental, and social well-being and not merely the absence of disease or infirmity.[5]

In this definition, health is more than the absence of disease; it is a multidimensional concept. (See Figure 8.7.)

Today, words such as *wellness* or *holistic health* are used interchangeably with the word *health* to signify a distinction from illness. The concept of high-level **wellness** was first defined in 1959 by Halbert Dunn as "an integrated method of functioning which is oriented toward maximizing the potential of which the individual is capable, within the environment where he is functioning."[6] Dunn recognized the recip-

rocal relationship between individual potential and environmental factors. This relationship is seen in current planning models and theories.

In 1980, Hettler defined wellness as "an active process through which the individual becomes aware of and makes choices toward a more successful existence."[7] His model of wellness has six dimensions: social, intellectual, spiritual, emotional, physical, and occupational. A significant distinction between the WHO definition and Hettler's view of wellness is the latter's inclusion of the spiritual domain. Some health educators also include an environmental dimension to wellness. (See Figure 8.8.)

Holistic health addresses the mind, body, and spirit as a whole, with the sum being greater than the parts. In 1983, Ardell, another strong advocate for wellness, defined it as "a conscious and deliberate approach to an advanced state of physical and psychological/spiritual health."[8] He divided wellness into five dimensions: self-responsibility, nutritional awareness, stress awareness and management, physical fitness, and environmental sensitivity. These definitions of health and wellness emphasize the multidimensional, positive focus of health.

ATOD prevention efforts and community health promotion efforts that focus on individuals would do well to remember the benefit of focusing program efforts and funding on healthy development, which is a proactive approach rather than a reactive one. For example, are the public schools in your area practicing proactive approaches to prevention? Does your school provide physical education programs for preschool to grade 12? Does your school have adequate school nursing and counseling services? These proactive approaches aren't cheap, but they are cost-effective and provide a tremendous benefit to our society.

What do health and wellness mean to ATOD prevention specialists or classroom teachers? Basically, when health and wellness are viewed as the integration of mind, body, and spirit into a whole self, ATOD prevention becomes a piece of a larger system. ATOD prevention does not stand alone—it is an integral part of wellness. Children and adolescents can learn to integrate the mind, body, and spirit into their whole self and remain healthy by making health-promoting decisions and avoiding or eliminating health-compromising behaviors.

Health Education

Health education is the cornerstone of health promotion efforts. Health education has been defined as a discipline, a profession, a process, and an outcome. As a discipline, health education has roots established in medicine, public health, the social and behavioral sciences, and education. As a profession, the roles and responsibilities of health educators have been defined by the Role Delineation Project. (See the FYI box.) As a process, health education encourages voluntary behavior change that can be supported and encouraged by environmental, organizational, and economic policies. As an outcome, health education results when a science-based curriculum (e.g., Teenage Health Teaching Modules) that addresses the National

Health Education Standards is implemented successfully. Health education should not claim to do more, nor be expected to do more, than support voluntary (noncoercive) change.

The Joint Committee of Health Education Terminology has defined health education as

> A continuum of learning which enables people, as individuals and as members of social structures, to voluntarily make decisions, modify behaviors, and change social conditions in ways which are health enhancing.[9]

ATOD Education

Like health education, ATOD education encourages and supports voluntary choices that are conducive to healthy living in a nonmanipulative, noncoercive way. Like health education, ATOD education is the cornerstone of ATOD prevention. Effective ATOD education (preK–12) is based on the risk factors, protective factors, and developmental assets identified as affecting individual choices and behaviors. Risk factors place individuals at greater risk for ATOD use and abuse, while protective factors buffer a child or adolescent from initiating or continuing use.

The CSAP conceptual framework classifies risk and protective factors within the social context of six life domains: individual, family, peer, school, community, and society/environmental. The relationship and interaction of these factors is explored more closely in Chapter 9 when we discuss curriculum development and school/community partnerships in the coordinated school health program. To give a brief example, the primary risk factors researchers have identified in the individual domain are lack of knowledge regarding the harms of substance use, attitudes favorable toward use, early use, biological or psychological dispositions, antisocial behavior, sensation seeking, and lack of supervision.[10] When addressing ATOD use and abuse in children and adolescents, the school focuses many efforts on the individual.

The National Institute of Drug Abuse offers fourteen principles to guide school personnel and prevention specialists in their programming efforts.[11]

1. Prevention programs should be designed to enhance protective factors and move toward reversing or reducing known risk factors.

2. Prevention programs should target all forms of drug abuse, including the use of tobacco, alcohol, marijuana, and inhalants.

3. Prevention programs should include skills to resist drugs when offered, strengthen personal commitments against drug use, and increase social competency (e.g., in communications, peer relationships, self-efficacy, and assertiveness), in conjunction with reinforcement of attitudes against drug use.

4. Prevention programs for adolescents should include interactive methods, such as peer discussion groups, rather than didactic techniques alone.

5. Prevention programs should include a parents' or caregivers' component that reinforces what the children are learning—such as facts about drugs and their harmful effects—and that opens opportunities for family discussions about use of legal and illegal substances and family policies about their use.

6. Prevention programs should be long-term, over the school career, with repeat interventions to reinforce the original prevention goals. For example, school-based efforts directed at elementary and middle school students should include booster sessions to help with critical transitions from middle to high school.

7. Family-focused prevention efforts have a greater impact than strategies that focus on parents only or children only.

8. Community programs that include media campaigns and policy changes, such as new regulations that restrict access to alcohol, tobacco, and other drugs, are more effective when they are accompanied by school and family interventions.

9. Community programs need to strengthen norms against drug use in all drug abuse prevention settings, including the family, the school, and the community.

10. Schools offer opportunities to reach all populations and also serve as important settings for specific subpopulations at risk for drug abuse, such as children with behavior problems or learning disabilities and those who are potential dropouts.

11. Prevention programming should be adapted to address the specific nature of the drug abuse problem in the local community.

12. The higher the level of risk of the target population, the more intensive the prevention effort must be and the earlier it must begin.

13. Prevention programs should be age-specific, developmentally appropriate, and culturally sensitive.

14. Effective prevention programs are cost-effective. For every dollar spent on drug use prevention, communities can save four to five dollars in costs for drug abuse treatment and counseling.

These fourteen principles provide guidance to prevention specialists in their efforts to assist community partnership development. These principles can be implemented within the context of theoretical models for effecting health behavior change, including ATOD behavior.

The next sections cover the planning models for health behavior change and ATOD prevention. As you read about these models, analyze how you would incorporate the fourteen principles of effective prevention and the characteristics of effective community partnerships into the various models. How would you apply the principles and characteristics to Lakeville's task force?

Planning Models for Health Behavior Change

A number of health behavior change planning models have been developed and evaluated for community health promotion. Readers can find more in-depth discussion of these models in health promotion textbooks.[12] The models discussed in this section are included because they have had an impact on ATOD planning and development. These models include the public health model (discussed previously), the Health Belief Model, the

PRECEDE-PROCEED model, the PATCH model, and the transtheoretical model.

Health Belief Model

The Health Belief Model (HBM) states that behaviors are chosen on the basis of (1) individual readiness to minimize health risks, (2) the environmental influences to make change possible, and (3) individual behaviors and skills to facilitate the change.[13] Readiness is based on the individual's perceived susceptibility ("It can happen to me"), perceived severity ("It has potentially serious consequences"), and the desire to change ("This behavior's benefits outweigh its costs"). Environmental factors, behaviors, and skills are assessed to determine if the planned course of action is possible. Effective health promotion programs are based on the individual's knowledge of the behavior, his or her personality, and the environmental factors that affect him or her. (See **Figure 8.9**.)

PRECEDE-PROCEED Model

The PRECEDE-PROCEED model consists of two components of health promotion planning: a diagnostic (needs assessment) component and a developmental component.[14] PRECEDE is an acronym for Predisposing, Reinforcing, and Enabling Constructs in Educational/Environmental Diagnosis and Evaluation. PROCEED is an acronym for Policy, Regulatory, and Organizational Constructs in Educational and Environmental Development. (See **Figure 8.10**.)

Social diagnosis (Phase 1) determines the factors that affect a community's quality of life. This phase requires input from all sectors of the community. People can discuss their problems, perceived needs, values, and priorities for addressing community issues.

Epidemiological diagnosis (Phase 2) provides an objective assessment of a community's health status. Risk and protective factors (social, behavioral,

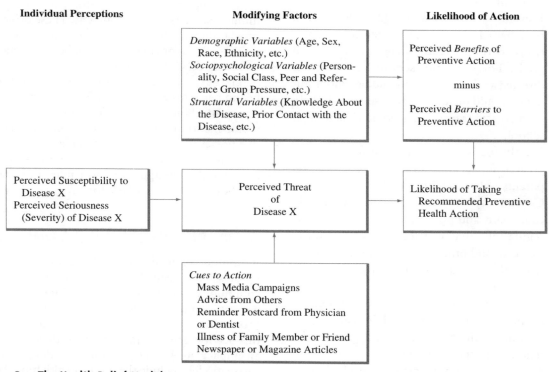

Figure 8.9 **The Health Belief Model**

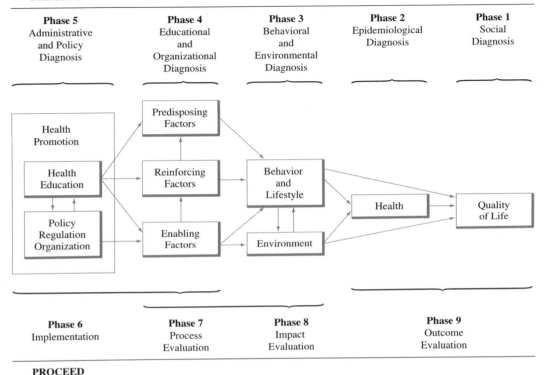

PRECEDE

Phase 5	Phase 4	Phase 3	Phase 2	Phase 1
Administrative and Policy Diagnosis	Educational and Organizational Diagnosis	Behavioral and Environmental Diagnosis	Epidemiological Diagnosis	Social Diagnosis

Phase 6	Phase 7	Phase 8	Phase 9
Implementation	Process Evaluation	Impact Evaluation	Outcome Evaluation

PROCEED

Figure 8.10 **The PRECEDE-PROCEED Model**

Source: Reprinted from *Health Promotion Planning: An Educational and Environmental Approach* by Lawrence W. Green and Marshall W. Kreuter by permission of Mayfield Publishing Company. Copyright © 1991 by Mayfield Publishing Company.

and environmental) and health status indicators (mortality, morbidity, life expectancy, etc.) are considered.

Behavioral and environmental diagnoses (Phase 3) identify the targets for intervention. Behavioral diagnosis includes four steps: determining the behaviors related to the health problem stated in the program objective, rating the relative importance and changeability of each behavior, selecting the behavioral target(s), and stating the behavioral objective(s).[15] Environmental diagnosis includes the same steps as listed for behavioral diagnosis; environmental factors are delimited as those with a strong relationship to the health problem or those having an overall impact on the community.

Educational and organizational diagnoses (Phase 4) identify the motivational, organizational, and social conditions associated with the health behavior. The predisposing, enabling, and reinforcing factors are

assessed to determine why an individual behaves in a particular way. By asking the following questions, the health promotion planning team can determine these factors: What factors predispose (motivate) an individual to behave in a particular way? What factors enable (assist) an individual to act this way? What factors reinforce (reward) the behavior?

Phase 5 is the *administrative and policy diagnosis*, whereby organizational aspects and the rules and regulations are assessed to determine how these factors facilitate or hinder the program objectives. Availability of resources to support the program are assessed.

Phase 6 initiates the *implementation component* of the model. Program implementation occurs concurrently with the diagnosis of the health problem, so drawing an arbitrary line between diagnosis and implementation is counterproductive.

Planning Models for Health Behavior Change   **151**

The direction of the health promotion effort and implementation is determined by ongoing evaluation.

Phases 7, 8, and 9 are the *evaluation components* of the model. The degree of planning done in phases 1 through 6 determines the quality of evaluation. Good planning facilitates valid and reliable evaluation. *Process evaluation* occurs during the diagnostic and implementation phases, and assesses whether the program should continue as planned or if a change is necessary. *Impact evaluation* measures the immediate effect of the health promotion program on behavioral, environmental, educational, and organizational factors. *Outcome evaluation* determines the long-term effect of the health promotion program by evaluating changes in health status or quality of life. The PRECEDE-PROCEED model for health promotion planning gives the community a well-designed process for building a strong school/community coalition.

PATCH Model

The Planned Approach to Community Health (PATCH) model was developed by the Centers for Disease Control and Prevention (CDC) and was piloted in six states and communities during the mid-1980s. Its primary focus is chronic diseases, but its approach is applicable to all health issues. PATCH uses a bottom-up rather than a top-down approach to community development, with community **empowerment** as a fundamental component. PATCH helps community groups plan, implement, and evaluate health promotion programs based on a community needs assessment. Once a community coalition is formed, professional health educators are called upon to provide technical support. However, the process is directed and guided by the coalition, usually composed of local voluntary agencies, agriculture extension programs, boards of education, and health care providers. By 1998, several hundred PATCH programs had been implemented across the United States, addressing issues such as violence and injury prevention, postneonatal mortality, improved cardiovascular health, and tobacco use reduction.

Bogan and colleagues provide several recommendations for communities thinking about implementing a community program:[16]

- Involve key local political leaders in the process.
- Assess community readiness, health indicators, and turf issues before beginning.
- Choose leadership that reflects the community's diversity.
- Use community groups to define health promotion and establish goals.
- Allow ample time for implementation (2 to 3 years).
- Prepare for the necessary time and effort commitment.
- Include funding for a full-time local coordinator.

These recommendations are appropriate in addressing a wide array of health issues, including ATOD use.

Green and Kreuter stated that PATCH inspired the expansion of PRECEDE (the first version of the model) to PRECEDE-PROCEED (the current version of the model). Their summation holds true for ATOD prevention as well as for health promotion:

> Finding the resources and political will to tackle all these fronts with comprehensive programs and communitywide interventions will remain problematic until the cost-benefit potential of community health promotion is more widely and deeply appreciated. Until local communities have resources to devote to such comprehensive health promotion, the task of state and national organizations is to find ways to supply technical assistance and other resources without usurping the initiative communities should take to control their own programs.[17]

Transtheoretical Model

The transtheoretical model, commonly referred to as the *stages of change model*, conceptualizes behavior change as a five-step process or continuum based on the individual's readiness for change. The five stages are precontemplation, contemplation, preparation, action, and maintenance.[18] *Precontemplation* is the period of time prior to an individual's thoughts or actions about changing a behavior.

This timeframe of at least six months prior to contemplation is marked by unawareness or underawareness of the need to change. The second stage is *contemplation*, the period of time during which the individual is seriously contemplating a change in behavior. This period is marked by the individual's awareness of the problem behavior, but no commitment to take action. The third stage, *preparation*, is marked by the intention to take action and an evaluation of past unsuccessful efforts. The fourth stage, *action*, is the time when an individual takes overt action to overcome an unwanted behavior. This stage is the most visible to outsiders and receives the most reinforcement. The last stage, *maintenance*, includes the steps that an individual takes to sustain the desired behavior change. The beginning of this stage is marked by at least six months of making the overt change.[19] An individual may move through the stages of change a number of times before reaching maintenance. (See Figure 8.11.)

The processes for change include consciousness raising, dramatic relief, self-reevaluation, environmental reevaluation, self-liberation, helping relationships, counterconditioning, contingency management, stimulus control, and social liberation. The decisional balance hinges on the pros and cons or gains and losses of change. *Self-efficacy* is the perceived ability to perform a task and can predict lasting change if adequate skills and incentives exist. For example, most smoking cessation programs have success rates of 20% to 50%. However, the more times an individual attempts to quit, the greater the likelihood of being successful (measured as one year of not smoking). An individual may require several attempts because success comes with learning how to do the right things at the right times. The prevention specialist should note that interventions are more likely to be successful if they are tailored to the individual's readiness or stage of change. Numerous applications of the transtheoretical model can be found on the Internet.

ATOD Prevention Models

Community-wide prevention efforts and research continue to proliferate. In addition to the community health planning models, six planning models show promising results in the ATOD prevention literature. These models, the social development model, the ecological model, the psychosocial model, the peer resource programming model, the social context model, and the developmental assets model, focus on community-wide prevention efforts and offer communities an opportunity for increased success in modifying and changing ATOD use behavior.

Social Development Model

The social development model focuses on reducing risk factors and increasing protective factors. Social learning theory, social control theory, and the subculture theory form the foundation for this model. Social learning theory suggests that behavior is molded by reward and punishment, or reinforcement.[20] Substances are used or avoided depending on the extent to which one behavior (perceived as more desirable) is differentially reinforced over another behavior (perceived as less desirable).[21] A young person, after drinking alcohol for the first time, may feel more comfortable at a party. Thus, the drinking behavior is reinforced and defined as desirable. Conversely, an adolescent who drinks too much may get physically ill or embarrassed from inappropriate behavior and thus decide to avoid

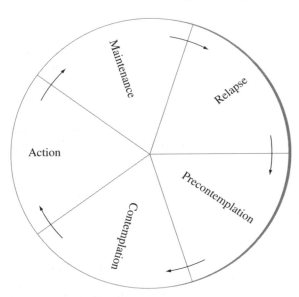

Figure 8.11 **The Transtheoretical Model**

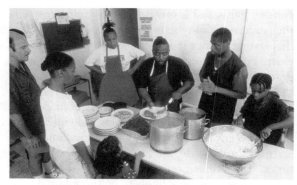

Figure 8.12 A Family Works Together to Improve Their Community   Youth who are bonded to a family and to their community are less likely to abuse drugs.

(© Michael Newman/PhotoEdit)

drinking the next time. According to social learning theory, adolescents who experience social crises (e.g., feeling uncomfortable at a party) are less able to set appropriate goals in social situations and are inept at creating options to achieve appropriate goals. Thus, social competence is a skill that can help adolescents cope more positively with social situations.

Social control theorists look at why some adolescents don't use ATOD and postulate that drug use results when the social control that causes conformity is absent.[22] Most adolescents and adults with strong bonds to conventional, mainstream social institutions do not engage in deviant or criminal acts. (See **Figure 8.12**.) Adolescents and adults who lack ties to the conforming, mainstream culture feel more free to use drugs. A young person who identifies with nondrinking parents is more likely to avoid alcohol. A young person who rebels against parental authority and school rules experiences fewer constraints and may be more likely to try ATOD.

Subculture theorists suggest that adolescents involved in social groups with attitudes favorable to drug use are more likely to use drugs.[23] The more involved these adolescents are with the drug subculture, the more they are socialized by it, influenced by its values, and engaged by its activities. According to Goode, "the most powerful factors related to drug use among adolescents are selective peer group interaction and socialization."[24]

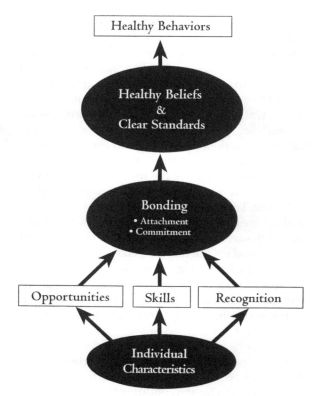

Figure 8.13 The Social Development Model

Reprinted with permission from Developmental Research and Programs, Inc. All rights reserved.

The social development model, which is widely used in prevention today, builds on these three theories. The primary tenet of the model is that increasing protective factors (e.g., prosocial bonding) increases resiliency.[25] (See **Figure 8.13**.)

The FYI box lists the risk factors that contribute to ATOD use and the protective factors that deter ATOD use, using the six life domains of CSAP as an organizing framework.

Ecological Model

The ecological model focuses on the interaction of environmental and individual factors and provides another promising prevention approach. The ecological approach recognizes that a supportive environment is equally as important as the development of social skills. The ecological

Key Risk and Protective Factors in the Six Domains

Individual Domain

Protective Factors

- Positive personal characteristics, including social skills and social responsiveness, cooperativeness, emotional stability; positive sense of self, flexibility, problem-solving skills, and low levels of defensiveness
- Bonding to societal institutions and values, including attachment to parents and extended family, commitment to school, regular involvement with religious institutions, and belief in society's values
- Social and emotional competence, including good communication skills, responsiveness, empathy, caring, sense of humor, inclination toward pro-social behavior, problem-solving skills, sense of autonomy, sense of purpose and of the future, and self-discipline

Risk Factors

- Inadequate life skills
- Lack of self-control, assertiveness, and peer-refusal skills
- Low self-esteem and self-confidence
- Emotional and psychological problems
- Favorable attitudes toward substance abuse
- Rejection of commonly held values
- School failure
- Lack of school bonding
- Early antisocial behavior, such as lying, stealing, and aggression, particularly in boys, often combined with shyness or hyperactivity

Family Domain

Protective Factors

- Positive bonding among family members
- Parenting that includes high levels of warmth and avoidance of severe criticism; sense of basic trust; high parental expectations; and clear and consistent expectations, including children's participation in family decisions and responsibilities
- An emotionally supportive parental/family milieu, including parental attention to children's interests, orderly and structured parent-child relationships, and parent involvement in homework and school-related activities

Risk Factors

- Family conflict and domestic violence
- Family disorganization
- Lack of family cohesion
- Social isolation of family
- Family attitudes favorable to drug use
- Poor child supervision and discipline
- Unrealistic expectations for development

Peer Domain

Protective Factors

- Association with peers who are involved in school, recreation, service, religion, or other organized activities
- Strong internal locus of control

Risk Factors

- Association with delinquent peers who use or value dangerous substances
- Association with peers who reject mainstream activities or pursuits
- Strong external locus of control

School Domain

Protective Factors

- Caring and support; sense of "community" in classroom and school
- High expectations from school personnel
- Clear standards and rules for appropriate behavior
- Youth participation, involvement, and responsibility in school tasks and decisions

Risk Factors

- Ambiguous or inconsistent rules and sanctions regarding drug use and student conduct
- Favorable staff and student attitudes toward substance use
- Harsh or arbitrary student management practices
- Lack of school bonding

Community Domain

Protective Factors

- Caring and support
- High expectations of youth
- Opportunities for youth participation in community activities

Risk Factors

- Lack of community bonding
- Lack of cultural pride
- Lack of competence in majority culture

- Community attitudes favorable to drug use
- Ready availability of illegal substances

Society Domain

Protective Factors

- Media literacy (resistance to pro-use messages)
- Decreased accessibility
- Increased pricing through taxation
- Raised purchasing age and enforcement

Risk Factors

- Impoverishment
- Discrimination
- Pro-drug/alcohol/tobacco messages in the media
- Unemployment and underemployment

Source: Substance Abuse and Mental Health Services Administration, *Here's Proof Prevention Works: Understanding Substance Abuse Prevention Toward the 21st Century*, DHHS Publication No. (SMA) 99-3300 (Washington, DC: DHHS, 1999).

model uses the following determinants: intrapersonal factors, interpersonal factors and primary groups, institutional factors, community factors, and public policy. Health promotion and ATOD strategies can be developed from these five domains.[26] A similar model was advanced by the Centers for Disease Control and Prevention that included three levels (individual, organizational, and governmental) in four settings (schools, worksites, health care institutions, and communities).[27] Interventions focused on multiple levels and multiple settings appear to provide greater and longer-lasting change.

Communities can affect the supply and availability of ATOD by the following actions:[28]

- Taxing
- Controlling hours for sale of alcohol
- Restricting locations for sale of drugs through zoning laws or other ordinances (e.g., prohibiting tobacco vending machines in locations frequented by young people)
- Implementing and enforcing minimum ages for tobacco and alcohol use

- Regulating pro-ATOD advertising and developing and disseminating anti-ATOD counteradvertising campaigns
- Controlling the severity of sanctions for ATOD use

Research supports the positive impact of legal interventions. Raising taxes on liquor, thus raising the price of alcohol, effectively reduced consumption[29] and alcohol-related traffic fatalities.[30] Raising the drinking age lowered the number of alcohol-related deaths;[31] conversely, lowering the drinking age increased the number of teenagers who drove while intoxicated and the number of alcohol-related deaths.[32] (See **Figure 8.14.**)

Two ecological aspects of a community, economic deprivation and violence, have received considerable attention and deserve further research. Wallace and Bachman report that higher levels of ATOD use by Native American youth may be linked to their relatively disadvantaged socioeconomic status (SES).[33] Furthermore, African American and Hispanic youths from higher SES groups demonstrate even lower levels of ATOD use than their

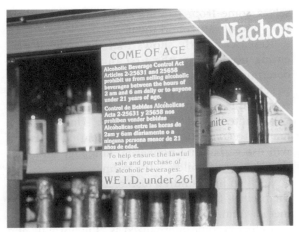

Figure 8.14 **Legal Restrictions on Alcohol to Minors**
Restricting youth's access to alcohol and tobacco is an
important prevention strategy. (© Tony Freeman/PhotoEdit)

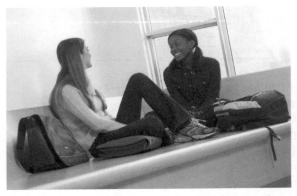

Figure 8.15 **Most Adolescents Enjoy Social Interactions
with One Another** Communication skills are encouraged in the psychosocial prevention model. (© AbleStock)

white counterparts. The relationship of economic
deprivation, including overcrowding, poverty, and
inadequate housing, to ATOD use and other health
issues must continue to be studied.

Although sociodemographic, background, and
lifestyle factors appear to have a greater influence
on ATOD use than ethnicity, the impact of ATOD
use on minority racial and ethnic groups is another
matter. Native American adolescents experience high
rates of delinquency, learning and behavior problems, and suicide. One in two Native American
youths never finishes high school. Compared with
white adults, African American adults are more
likely to be victims of alcohol-related homicide,
arrested for drunkenness, and sent to prison rather
than to treatment facilities.[34] Violence, including
child abuse, spouse abuse, suicide, and homicide,
in relationship to ATOD abuse also needs continued study.

Psychosocial Model

The psychosocial model emphasizes life skills training and peer refusal techniques. This approach
arose from the research conducted on programs
designed to reduce smoking by youth. The theory of
"psychological inoculation" suggests that tobacco
behavior spreads from one person to the next, just
as disease does. By learning resistance skills, youth

can stop the spread of "disease" (smoking). The
psychosocial approach focuses on factors that promote or deter ATOD use and the coping and lifestyle
skills necessary to avoid ATOD use.

Flay notes that these programs typically use a
combination of information and skill-building
strategies that include the following:[35]

- Developing problem-solving and decision-
  making skills
- Developing cognitive skills for resisting interpersonal and media-based pro-smoking and
  pro-drinking messages
- Increasing self-awareness and self-esteem
- Learning non-ATOD-use skills for dealing
  with anxiety and stress
- Enhancing interpersonal skills such as the ability to initiate a conversation (see **Figure 8.15**)
- Developing assertiveness skills such as the
  ability to express displeasure and anger and
  to communicate needs
- Drawing the relationships among smoking,
  ATOD use, and health concerns

Research indicates that ATOD use among all
ethnic and racial groups is related more to psychosocial factors that they share in common than
to any inherent subcultural differences. The results
of using current psychosocial approaches based on
social influence to reduce ATOD use are mixed.

ATOD Prevention Models   **157**

Sequential Steps for Building Self-Esteem

1. **Security:** Children can handle change, be spontaneous, and show self-assurance.

2. **Selfhood:** Children have an accurate and realistic description of their roles and attributes. They recognize their uniqueness and special contributions to family and community. (See Figure 8.16.)

3. **Affiliation:** Children have a sense of connection and belonging. They maintain friendships, cooperate, and show compassion.

4. **Mission:** Children know what they want and can define a process to achieve it. They set realistic and achievable goals, and follow through in meeting these goals.

5. **Competence:** Children feel capable and accept their strengths and weaknesses (areas for improvement). Mistakes are viewed as learning opportunities rather than dead ends. They feel empowered.

Source: M. Borba, *Esteem Builders: A K–8 Curriculum for Improving Student Achievement, Behavior and School Climate* (Rolling Hills Estates, CA: Jalmar Press, 1989).

Asian and African American youth appear to be at relatively low risk from peer influences. However, personal and social skills programs that are specifically modified for cultural sensitivity appear to be more successful than other approaches.[36]

Prevention programs based on the psychosocial model focus on life skills development as well as factual information. The psychosocial skills most often taught in the schools include self-esteem, decision making, refusal or assertiveness skills, communication, and coping skills. Background information regarding these life skills can be helpful to school/community teams that choose a science-based commercial curriculum (see Chapter 9).

Self-esteem

Self-esteem is the foundation of emotional well-being. Children are born with a temperament that affects their processing of information, but most of the fundamental images they receive about themselves come from parents and significant others who initially surround them.

Research clearly shows that the style of parenting used during the first three to four years determines the extent of self-esteem a child brings to school. If children are lucky, the messages they receive are internalized as "I'm okay," "I'm loved," "I'm wanted," and "I'm important." Unfortunately, many caregivers lack adequate parenting skills and will use verbal and nonverbal language and cues that damage a child's self-esteem.

Early in life, children also receive images about themselves from society, particularly from mass media. Again, if they are lucky, they receive messages that become internalized as "I'm normal" and "I have rights." Unfortunately, influenced by the media, children and adolescents often perceive these societal standards and images as unattainable, beyond their reach (just as they are for most of us).

Children and adolescents filter these images and verbal cues from parents, significant others, peers, and society through their own perceptions. This inner picture of their total attributes becomes their self-concept, their internal image of "self." One part of the self-concept is self-esteem, which is measured by the degree to which the real self (the "as is" self) and the ideal self (based on filtering the images and cues) differ. The closer together they are, the higher the level of self-esteem.[37]

How can the classroom teacher help? The first step is to establish a relationship with the child. The authors realize that this is a formidable task for teachers with a classroom of 20 to 30 students. Nevertheless, a caring, honest, supportive, and accepting relationship between the teacher and child is an essential building block in helping a child build self-esteem. The teacher serves as a mirror for the child; how the child is comforted, spoken to, loved, and accepted are lessons in self-worth. The teacher's level of self-esteem also determines her or his ability to mirror love and acceptance.

Borba states that self-esteem can be learned in a sequential order.[38] The five steps are security, selfhood, affiliation, mission, and competence (see the FYI box). Self-esteem is an important life skill for children and adolescents to learn. Self-esteem itself may not be instrumental in directly decreasing the

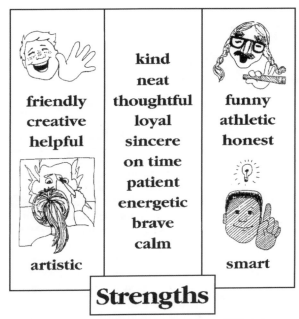

friendly
creative
helpful

artistic

kind
neat
thoughtful
loyal
sincere
on time
patient
energetic
brave
calm

Strengths

funny
athletic
honest

smart

Listed above are some qualities that most people would like to have.
Which of these do you have? Which would you like to have?

Figure 8.16 **Qualities (Strengths) That Most People Would Like to Have**

Reprinted from the *Here's Looking at You, 2000*® Teacher's Guide, © 1986 Comprehensive Health Education Foundation (C.H.E.F.®), Seattle, WA. All rights reserved.

likelihood of ATOD use, but self-efficacy (a component of self-esteem) has been found to contribute to a decrease in ATOD use.

Refusal and Assertiveness Skills

Assertiveness is the free expression of a child's desires, needs, values, and beliefs from a place of genuineness.[39] Children can learn to express their thoughts freely and retain their right to think or feel differently from another person. They also learn to accept the right of others to freely express feelings and thoughts.

Children interact with others from a very young age. When they grow up in an environment where boundaries are honored and differences in desires, needs, values, and beliefs are accepted, their interactions assume an assertive tone—they communicate in a direct, spontaneous, and honest manner. When they live in an environment where differences are not tolerated, their interactions tend to be passive or aggressive. They learn negative self-talk, self-criticism, and indirect modes of communication. (See Figure 8.17.)

Fortunately, teachers can teach children and adolescents the skills to interact assertively, regardless of their home environment. Students can learn to set boundaries. They can determine when their boundaries have been violated by asking themselves, "Do I feel beaten down, angry, depressed, used, violated?" They can learn assertive skills such as broken record, calling time out, delivering an assertive no, and delivering "if-then" messages.[40] They can learn the skills for responding to criticism and fair fighting.[41]

Butler provides a skill progression and activities for practicing assertive skills.[42] The skill progression includes (1) expressing positive feelings, (2) expressing negative feelings and protective feelings when others violate or intrude on our boundaries, (3) setting limits, and (4) practicing self-initiation (expressing what one wants).

Patterson provides another model called the Refusal Skill for Self-Control.[43] The steps for refusal are as follows: (1) Stop what you're doing, (2) name the trouble, (3) state the consequences, (4) think of something else to do and move away from the situation ("Instead, why don't I…"), and (5) give yourself credit for staying in control (e.g., "I did a good job"; "I stayed in control"; "I stayed safe").

Children and adolescents need to practice saying "no" to ATOD use. They need to learn to "stand still" for themselves when their genuine thoughts and feelings are challenged. The classroom is an ideal, safe environment for practicing the art of refusal and setting boundaries. In addition, students need opportunities outside the classroom to bridge the gap between classroom practice and real-life situations. (See Hints & Tips box.)

Decision Making and Critical Thinking

Every day children and adolescents make numerous health-related decisions that affect their wellness. Some decisions can safely be spontaneous or spur-of-the-moment (deciding to go shopping with a friend, choosing a particular food), whereas others (using birth control pills, cheating on a test) require careful consideration, additional input, and critical

Ways to Say "No"

Principle	Application	Principle	Application
Say "No, thanks"	"Would you like a drink?" "No, thanks."	Change the subject	"Let's smoke some marijuana." "I hear there's a new video game at the arcade."
Give a reason or excuse	"Would you like a beer?" "No, thanks. I don't like the taste."	Avoid the situation	If you know of places where people often use drugs, stay away from those places. If you pass those places on the way home, go another way.
Say "no" as many times as necessary (broken record)	"Would you like a hit?" "No, thanks." "Come on!" "No, thanks." "Just try it!" "No, thanks."	Give the cold shoulder	"Hey! Do you want a beer?" Just ignore the person.
Walk away	"Do you want to try some marijuana?" Say "no" and walk away while saying it.	Have strength in numbers	Hang around with nonusers, especially where drug use is expected.

Source: CASPAR.

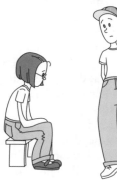

Unsure/Passive
Sound unsure
Avoid eye contact
Speak softly
Show poor posture

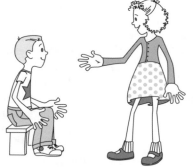

Confident/Assertive
Sound confident and calm
Make good eye contact
Speak clearly
Stand up straight

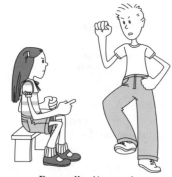

Demanding/Aggressive
Speak loudly
Stare
Sound angry or sarcastic
Stand stiffly

Figure 8.17 **Response Styles**

thinking. The basic process of critical thinking has been described as "knowledge through inquiry."[44]

With knowledge comes responsibility. Nickerson and colleagues expressed the importance of and responsibility for choices we make as follows:

Most of us who live in developed countries in the free world have a much greater range of options than did our grandparents, whether we are choosing what to have for dinner, what to do for entertainment, where to go for a vacation, or how to spend a life. It seems reasonable to expect this freedom of choice to continue to increase. But options imply the burden of making decisions and living with them; and the ability to choose wisely assumes the ability to assess the alternatives in a reasonable way.[45]

Know Your Stuff

Grade: 8, 9
Topic: Learning to make responsible decisions

Preliminary Considerations

Young people must learn to make responsible decisions about alcohol. In this lesson, we develop and practice a simple five-step model of the decision-making process called "ABCDE," which is easy for students to remember. Practicing this method of decision making has proven successful in helping adolescents approach the difficult choices they must make every day, especially those about alcohol and drugs. While abstinence from alcohol is the decision we always support with adolescents, this les-son also examines what is meant by "responsible drinking" and the factors that go into such a decision.

Description of Activity

Presenting a Model for Responsible Decision Making
The ABCDE Model

Brainstorm on the blackboard: What are the steps in making a decision?
Assess the problem.
Brainstorm alternatives.
Consider the consequences.
Decide and act.
Evaluate the consequences.

Source: CASPAR.

Critical thinking is a key component of choosing wisely. Children inevitably make decisions regarding ATOD use. These decisions are influenced by parental standards and use patterns, community standards and messages, knowledge of the health-compromising aspects of the drug, media portrayal, and peer influence. The key for teachers is to provide a safe, supportive environment in which to explore these influences. Decision making regarding ATOD use is not value-free: Choices entail consequences. Jones and Safrit suggest several activities to promote decision making: critical analysis of the source of health information, debate teams, dramatization, journal writing, creative visualization, socratic questioning, inventing, critical incidents, and using quotations or cartoons.[46] The Hints & Tips box provides an example of the decision-making process.

Elias and Kress state that the social decision-making approach can serve as a framework for integrated learning.[47] They provide a basic structure for an approach that enhances skills in self-control, social awareness and group participation, and critical think-ing. (See the FYI box.) The social decision-making model increases student involvement even for those students who often feel excluded or unengaged.

Adolescence is characterized by rapid developmental changes, and decision making is often intensified by conflicting demands of parents, peers, schools, and jobs. The complexity involved in making wise decisions has led to a recognition that the "Just Say No" philosophy is inappropriate for adolescents. "Knee jerk prescriptions such as just say no, while perhaps appropriate developmentally speaking for the 5–10-year-old, are unlikely to fortify developing early adolescents against unhealthy behavior, nor give him (her) the tools to function autonomously…the just say no approach fails to respect the child as an active processor of experience."[48] Scales states that "Just Say No" is inconsistent with critical thinking, particularly if it is viewed as an attitude as much as a skill. A neat, tight demarcation is incompatible with the premise of critical thinking, which is "to challenge, test, push, argue, doubt, and question."[49]

The Social Decision-Making Model

When children or adults use their social decision-making skills, they

1. Use self-control skills
   a. Listen carefully and accurately
   b. Follow directions
   c. Calm themselves down when upset or under stress
   d. Approach and talk to others in a socially appropriate manner

2. Use social awareness and group participation skills
   a. Recognize and elicit trust, help, and praise from others
   b. Understand others' perspectives
   c. Choose friends wisely
   d. Participate appropriately in groups
   e. Give and receive help and criticism

3. Use critical-thinking skills for decision making and problem solving
   a. Notice signs of feelings
   b. Identify issues or problems
   c. Determine and select goals
   d. Generate alternative solutions
   e. Envision possible consequences
   f. Select the best solution
   g. Plan and make a final check for obstacles
   h. Notice what happened and use the information for future decision making and problem solving

Source: *Journal of School Health*, 64, 2 (February 1994): 63.

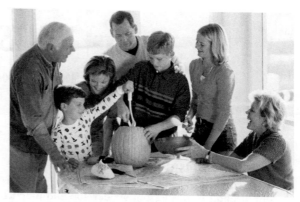

Figure 8.18 My Support System (© ThinkStock)

Coping Skills

Children learn to handle stress by emulating the adults in their lives. Many children learn that stress is natural and expected in their lives, and that talking it through, laughing with friends and family, and crying make them feel better. They watch adults confront problems and set clear boundaries to protect themselves and learn to handle stress in the same way. (See **Figure 8.18**.)

Some children watch the adults in their lives cope ineffectively with the pressures of daily living, thus succumbing to "dis-ease," rage, and distress. These adults overreact and react, rather than act. They perceive stress as a negative, rather than a positive, force to effect change. Children growing up in this environment may have a difficult time handling routine stressors.

Childhood and adolescence can be stressful times if adequate coping skills have not been learned. Teachers can help students learn to cope with expected and unexpected events in their lives. The first step in teaching effective coping is to help students recognize and identify the stressors in their lives. Then they can choose a course of action based on the three *As*— whether to alter the stressor, accept the stress, or alleviate the stressor. If alleviation is chosen, relaxation techniques such as autogenic training (relaxing with self-talk), biofeedback, and progressive muscle relaxation can be learned. In addition, natural techniques such as talking, laughing, exercising, praying, deep breathing, and other coping strategies can be used to deal with unwanted stressors.

Children can learn about the benefits of stress, and how to cope effectively. They can be taught about the consequences of excessive stress and the impact of ineffective or nonproductive coping strategies, for example, excessive alcohol consumption, smoking cigarettes, and raging. Again, the classroom is an ideal, safe environment in which to learn about coping with life's stressors.

HINTS & TIPS

Peer Resources: A Sample Activity

Objective

To develop an understanding of the importance of helping people, especially young children

Background

Children in grades 4 through 6 want to be helpful. They demonstrate this in school by responding to teachers and rules and showing interest in schoolwork, and at home by helping younger siblings. It is important for children at this age to develop a commitment to helping others. One way to instill the importance of volunteering in the community is to encourage children in grades 4 through 6 to help children in grades K through 3 adjust to school and schoolwork, learn new recreational skills, develop friendships, and experiment in art and music. At this age, children respond to praise for being helpful, and their volunteer experiences enhance their feelings of self-confidence.

Activities

In cooperation with other teachers, develop a pool of volunteers in grades 4 through 6 to help younger students. Explain to these students that they can help the younger ones with schoolwork, such as reading or math; show them how to use the library; assist in music lessons or arts and crafts; teach them a new game or sport; or be a "big brother" or "big sister."

Allow students to select the activity they would like to help with. Establish a schedule for volunteering (e.g., once a week or two afternoons a week after school).

Once the projects are under way, meet periodically with volunteers to assess what they are doing and how it affects them and the students they are helping. Ask for their suggestions on ways to improve their volunteering experience or for other project ideas.

At the end of a term (or year), give each volunteer a merit badge or certificate congratulating the volunteer on his or her service. Offer extra academic credit for volunteering or arrange a school ceremony honoring the volunteers.

Resources

A group of teachers who are willing to oversee student volunteering projects; a list of volunteering ideas

Teacher Tips

Create a list of volunteering possibilities with other teachers; encourage all students who want to participate in the volunteering project to do so; make sure teachers or other adults supervise the volunteer activity so that it proves worthwhile for both volunteers and younger students.

Source: U.S. Department of Education, *Learning to Live Drug Free: A Curriculum Model for Prevention* (Washington, DC: Government Printing Office, 1991).

Additional Life Skills

In addition to these skills, at-risk youth can benefit from training to control impulses, manage hostility and anger, structure leisure time, achieve in school, and cope with authority.

Peer Resource Programming Model

Children and adolescents can serve as positive role models by demonstrating the benefits of a healthy, drug-free lifestyle. Hill, Piper, and King found that students make better health behavior choices when they have peer leaders.[50] Effective strategies and activities "(1) actively engaged them, (2) were delivered by peers, (3) allowed them to discuss health-related

behaviors in a safe environment, and (4) involved them in planning for community wide health promotion events."

Benard advocates the adoption of a peer resource programming model of education.[51] She defines *peer resource* as "any program that uses children and youth to work with and/or help other children and youth." Peer resource programming provides children and adolescents with an opportunity to serve as caring, productive resources for each other. (See the Hints & Tips box.)

Research on this type of prevention programming is encouraging and supports the effectiveness of peer resource programs on academic and social development.[52] The peer resource programming model has been addressed within many disciplines and by many names. These programs can include youth services, cooperative learning, peer tutoring, peer helping, and dispute resolution and mediation. Youth can be trained to be peer resources by establishing a pleasant training atmosphere, by role playing and rehearsing the material and activities, and by offering public acknowledgement or monetary incentives to the participants.

Social Context Model

The social context model builds on the concept of "reciprocal determinism" that is found in social learning theory.[53] Behavior is shaped by the reciprocal interaction of cognitive, behavioral, and environmental factors. In the ATOD literature, this model has been applied primarily to teenage drinking patterns.

Social context research shows that teenage drinking behavior is influenced by specific motivational contexts and the social environment of the community. Teenagers who drink display different patterns in alcohol intake and in where, when, and why they drink. Researchers have found that adolescent drinking most often occurs away from school, on the weekends, and at unsupervised events.

> Given these conditions, it is difficult to imagine that classroom activities, student assistance programs, or other solely school-based interventions can possibly stand alone and be successful. Schools play a role in comprehensive alcohol abuse prevention programs, but coordinated community-based efforts are needed to effectively address complex problems.[54]

Developmental Assets Model

The developmental assets model has emerged as a strategy that focuses on the internal and external factors influencing students. The strategy was developed by the Search Institute, and research has shown an association between the number of developmental assets a child or adolescent perceives himself or herself to have and the health choices he or she makes.

This model focuses on building or enhancing the assets and strengths of the individual rather than eliminating the risks. This approach complements the risk and protective factors approach and can be used to help communities focus their efforts on the external factors that support youth in making positive choices. Promising findings of this approach with adolescents include better leadership skills, more respect for diversity, better health choices, and less alcohol, tobacco, and illegal drug use with increasing assets. Table 8.1 lists the 40 developmental assets used to develop school and community programs using the asset/strengths approach.

Common Elements of Successful Programs

The onus of providing successful community prevention efforts has shifted from health professionals to community members. This **paradigm shift** requires communities to become empowered, include all groups, and value diversity. With this approach, community members develop, implement, and evaluate programs, and professionals provide assistance as requested. (See **Figure 8.19**.)

The shift to include all members requires added effort to ensure all factions of the community are

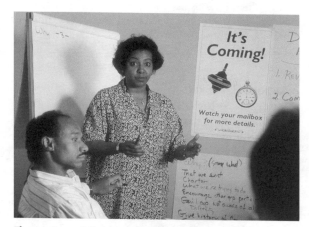

Figure 8.19 A Community Task Force Wide participation and collaboration are often more successful in community drug abuse prevention than professionally led groups. (© Mark Richards/PhotoEdit)

Table 8.1

Forty Developmental Assets

Asset Type	Asset Name	Definition
External Assets		
Support	Family support	Family life provides high levels of love and support.
	Positive family communication	Young person and her or his parent(s) communicate positively, and young person is willing to seek advice and counsel from parent(s).
	Other adult relationships	Young person receives support from three or more nonparent adults.
	Caring neighborhood	Young person experiences caring neighbors.
	Caring school climate	School provides a caring, encouraging environment.
	Parent involvement in schooling	Parent(s) are actively involved in helping young person succeed in school.
Empowerment	Community values youth	Young person perceives that adults in the community value youth.
	Youth as resources	Young people are given useful roles in the community.
	Service to others	Young person serves in the community one hour or more per week.
	Safety	Young person feels safe at home, at school, and in the neighborhood.
Boundaries and expectations	Family boundaries	Family has clear rules and consequences, and monitors the young person's whereabouts.
	School boundaries	School provides clear rules and consequences.
	Neighborhood boundaries	Neighbors take responsibility for monitoring young people's behaviors.
	Adult role models	Parent(s) and other adults model positive, responsible behavior.
	Positive peer influence	Young person's best friends model responsible behavior.
	High expectations	Both parent(s) and teachers encourage the young person to do well.
Constructive use of time	Creative activities	Young person spends three or more hours per week in lessons or practice in music, theater, or other arts.
	Youth programs	Young person spends three or more hours per week in sports, clubs, or organizations at school and/or in community organizations.
	Religious community	Young person spends one hour or more per week in activities in a religious institution.
	Time at home	Young person is out with friends "with nothing special to do" two or fewer nights per week.
Internal Assets		
Commitment to learning	Achievement motivation	Young person is motivated to do well in school.
	School engagement	Young person is actively engaged in learning.
	Homework	Young person reports doing at least one hour of homework every school day.
	Bonding to school	Young person cares about her or his school.
	Reading for pleasure	Young person reads for pleasure three or more hours per week.

(Continued)

Table 8.1

Forty Developmental Assets (*Continued*)

Asset Type	Asset Name	Definition
Positive values	Caring	Young person places high value on helping other people.
	Equality and social justice	Young person places high value on promoting equality and reducing hunger and poverty.
	Integrity	Young person acts on convictions and stands up for her or his beliefs.
	Honesty	Young person "tells the truth even when it is not easy."
	Responsibility	Young person accepts and take personal responsibility.
	Restraint	Young person believes it is important not to be sexually active or to use alcohol or other drugs.
Social competencies	Planning and decision making	Young person knows how to plan ahead and make choices.
	Interpersonal competence	Young person has empathy, sensitivity, and friendship skills.
	Cultural competence	Young person has knowledge of and comfort with people of different cultural/racial/ethnic backgrounds.
	Resistance skills	Young person can resist negative peer pressure and dangerous situations.
	Peaceful conflict resolution	Young person seeks to resolve conflict nonviolently.
Positive identity	Personal power	Young person feels he or she has control over "things that happen to me."
	Self-esteem	Young person reports having a high self-esteem.
	Sense of purpose	Young person reports that "my life has a purpose."
	Positive view of personal future	Young person is optimistic about her or his personal future.

involved, for example, businesses, parents, neighborhood leaders, religious leaders, agencies, law enforcement, schools, youth, media, and ethnic and civic groups. Involving diverse community members with service providers enhances the effectiveness of the prevention program.

Valuing diversity ensures that all cultural groups and special populations will have opportunities to provide input on the solution of ATOD use in their community. Compromise and cooperation are essential in order for all groups to have a voice to reach solutions. The FYI box contrasts the service delivery model and the community empowerment model.

Lessons from Successful Programs

Teachers and school administrators are involved in prevention in a variety of ways—as community leaders, educators, and parents. To be effective participants, they need to know the important lessons

Community Empowerment Model: A Contrast in Paradigms

Delivery of Services	Community Empowerment
Professionals are responsible (doing *for* the community).	Responsibility is shared (doing *with* the community).
Power is vested in agencies.	Power resides with community.
Professionals are seen as experts.	Community is the expert.
Planning and services are responsive to each agency's mission.	Services and activities are planned and implemented on the basis of community needs and priorities.
Planning and service delivery are fragmented.	Planning and service delivery are interdependent and integrated.
Leadership is external and based on authority, position, and title.	Leadership is from within the community, is based on ability to develop a shared vision, and maintains a broad base of support to manage community problem solving.
Ethnic and cultural differences are denied.	Ethnic diversity and special populations are valued.
External linkages are limited to networking and coordination.	Cooperation and collaboration are emphasized.
The decision-making process is closed.	Decision making is inclusive.
Accountability is to the agency.	Accountability is to the community.
The primary purpose of evaluation is to determine funding.	Evaluation is used to check program development and decision making.
Funding is categorical.	Funding is based on critical health issues.
Community participation is limited to providing input and feedback.	Community is maximally involved at all levels.

Source: U.S. Department of Health and Human Services, *The Future by Design: A Community Framework for Preventing Alcohol and Other Drug Problems Through a Systems Approach*, DHHS Publication No. (ADM) 91-1760 (Washington, DC: DHHS, 1991).

learned from successful, as well as unsuccessful, community-based prevention programs. Chapter 7 discussed the lessons from unsuccessful programs. Goplerud summarized the important lessons learned from successful community-based ATOD prevention programs.[55] The Department of Health and Human Services has provided a similar summary (see the FYI box entitled "Lessons from Successful Prevention Programs").

Summary

Community-wide prevention efforts must be inclusive, not exclusive, and community institutions and organizations must collaborate. Youth service organizations can offer jobs, job training, and recreation for young people. Schools can help create positive results by teaching academic and interpersonal skills to preschool and early childhood

1. Put first things first—prevention may not be your client's top priority.
2. High-risk, hard-to-reach people will not flock to your program just because you open your doors.
3. There must be a comprehensive array of services.
4. Access to services must be easy and direct.
5. Staff must know their clients.
6. Resources must be concentrated; a watered-down program is likely to be ineffective.
7. Only risk and resiliency factors that can be changed should be targeted.
8. Intervention must start early and be sustained.
9. The focus of programs must narrow as youth get older.
10. There must be stable, caring adult role models and surrogate parents.
11. The extent of parental involvement in child and adolescent programs deserves scrutiny.
12. Involvement of the school system is a part of almost every successful program.
13. Effective school-based prevention programs have attributes that may be generalizable to other settings.
14. Staff must be worthy of trust and respect.
15. Success depends on recruiting and training a committed staff.
16. A high level of program structure is consistently related to program effectiveness.
17. Environmental policy changes can significantly affect prevention program outcomes.

Source: U.S. Department of Health and Human Services, *The Future by Design: A Community Framework for Preventing Alcohol and Other Drug Problems Through a Systems Approach*, DHHS Publication No. (ADM) 91-1760 (Washington, DC: DHHS, 1991).

youth. Families can accept more responsibility, such as making more time for their children and providing clear guidelines for behavior. In all instances, effective prevention programs require a combined effort from the community, the schools, and families.

Scenario | Analysis and Response

As a prevention specialist, you recognize that Lakeville can benefit from a community coalition to address local ATOD problems. First, choosing a diverse task force is a key element for future success. (Review the section on successful health promotion programs and common elements of successful programs for further suggestions.) Next, the task force may choose to follow the seven steps for building a successful prevention program. (Check the following website for a suggested format: www.open.org/~westcapt/.) The concerned citizens must answer several key questions once they form an initial task force.

What will your primary role as a prevention specialist be on the task force? (Review the community empowerment model to see if you are following suggested prevention practice.)

Learning Activities

1. Locate a journal article describing a program based on a prevention model discussed in this chapter. How could this model be applied to an ATOD program in Lakeville?
2. Contact a local community health agency. Ask them about a program they provide to the community. Evaluate whether the program

is based on a traditional delivery of health services or on the community empowerment model.

3. Review the lessons from successful prevention programs found in the FYI box. In small groups, discuss additional implications each of these lessons has for your community ATOD program. What activities is your community presently doing to apply these lessons?

4. Identify several websites that provide information on successful community partnerships. Review their recommendations for success and report your findings to the class.

Notes

1. L. W. Green, *Community Health* (St. Louis: Times Mirror/Mosby College Publishing, 1990), 4.

2. G. Rose, *The Strategy of Preventive Medicine* (Oxford: Oxford University Press, 1992).

3. P. J. Brounstein, J. M. Zweig, and S. E. Gardner, "Science-Based Practices in Substance Abuse Prevention: A Guide," working draft, SAMHSA, Center for Substance Abuse Prevention, Division of Knowledge Development and Evaluation, December 1998.

4. "Prevention Works! Community Partnerships Work in Preventing Substance Abuse," *Prevention Alert*, 3, 14 (2000). Available: http://www.health.org/pubs/qdocs/prevalert/v3i14.html.

5. World Health Organization, "Constitution of the World Health Organization," *Chronicle of the World Health Organization*, 1 (1947): 29–34.

6. Halbert L. Dunn, *High Level Wellness* (Arlington, VA: R. W. Beatty, 1961).

7. W. Hettler, "Wellness Promotion on a University Campus," *Family and Community Health*, 3, 1 (May 1980).

8. D. Ardell, "The History and Future of the Wellness Movement," remarks at the First Annual Kaiser Permanente Health Promotion Strategies Conference entitled "New Roles/New Directions," Portland, Oregon, June 28, 1983.

9. 1990 Joint Committee on Health Education Terminology, "Report of the 1990 Joint Committee on Health Education Terminology," *Journal of School Health*, 61 (August 1991): 251–254.

10. Brounstein et al., "Science-Based Practices in Substance Abuse."

11. National Institute of Drug Abuse, "Prevention Principles for Children and Adolescents," in *Preventing Drug Use Among Children and Adolescents: A Research-Based Guide*. Publication PHD 734 (Washington, DC: NIDA, 1997). Available: http://www.nida.nih.gov/Prevention/ PrevPrinc.html.

12. R. W. Patton, J. M. Corry, L. R. Gettman, and J. S. Graf, *Implementing Health/Fitness Programs* (Champaign, IL: Human Kinetics, 1986); J. T. Butler, *Principles of Health Education and Health Promotion* (Englewood, CO: Morton, 1994); J. F. MacKenzie and J. L. Jurs, *Planning, Implementing, and Evaluating Health Promotion Programs* (New York: Macmillian, 1993).

13. M. H. Becker, "The Health Belief Model and Personal Health Behavior," *Health Education Monographs*, 2 (1974): 324–473.

14. L. W. Green and M. W. Kreuter, *Health Promotion Planning: An Educational and Environmental Approach* (Mountain View, CA: Mayfield, 1991).

15. Ibid.

16. G. Bogan, A. Omar, R. S. Knobloch, L. C. Liburd, and T. W. O'Rourke, "Organizing an Urban African American Community for Health Promotion: Lessons from Chicago," *Journal of Health Education*, 23 (April 1992): 157–159.

17. L. W. Green and M. W. Kreuter, "CDC's Planned Approach to Community Health as an Application of PRECEDE and an Inspiration for PROCEED," *Journal of Health Education*, 23 (April 1992): 140–144.

18. J. O. Prochaska, C. C. DiClemente, and J. C. Norcross, "In Search of How People Change: Applications to Addictive Behaviors," *American Psychologist*, 47, 9 (1992): 1102–1114.

19. Ibid.

20. A. Bandura, *Social Learning Theory* (Englewood Cliffs, NJ: Prentice Hall, 1977).

21. M. Radosevich, L. Lanza-Kaduce, R. L. Akers, and M. D. Krohn, "The Sociology of Adolescent Drug and Drinking Behavior: Part II," *Deviant Behavior*, 1 (1980): 145–169.

22. M. Argyle, *Social Interaction* (London: Methuen, 1969).

23. E. Goode, *Drugs in American Society* (New York: Alfred A. Knopf, 1989), 66–67.

24. Ibid., 74.

25. J. D. Hawkins, D. M. Lishner, R. F. Catalano, and M. O. Howard, "Childhood Predictors of Adolescent Substance

Abuse: Toward an Empirically Grounded Theory," *Journal of Children in Contemporary Society,* 18 (1985): 1–65.

26. K. R. McLeroy, D. Bibeau, A. Steckler, and K. Glanz, "An Ecological Perspective on Health Promotion Programs," *Health Education Quarterly,* 15, 4 (1988): 351–377.

27. CDC, 1988.

28. R. J. Bonnie, "Discouraging the Use of Alcohol, Tobacco, and Other Drugs: The Effects of Legal Controls and Restrictions," *Advances in Substance Abuse,* 2 (1981): 145–184.

29. D. Levy and N. Sheflin, "The Demand for Alcoholic Beverages: An Aggregate Time-Series Analysis," *Journal of Public Policy and Marketing,* 2 (1985): 47–54.

30. H. Saffer and M. Grossman, "Beer Taxes, the Legal Drinking Age, and Youth Motor Vehicle Fatalities," *Journal of Legal Studies,* 16 (1987): 351–374.

31. R. W. Hingson et al., "Impact of Legislation Raising the Legal Drinking Age in Massachusetts from Age 18 to Age 21," *American Journal of Public Health,* 73 (1983): 163–170.

32. P. J. Cook and G. Tauchen, "The Effect of Minimum Drinking Age Legislation on Youthful Auto Fatalities, 1970–1977," *Journal of Legal Studies,* 13 (1987): 169–190.

33. J. Wallace and J. G. Bachman, "Explaining Racial/Ethnic Differences in Adolescent Drug Use: The Impact of Background and Lifestyle," *Social Problems,* 38, 2 (1991): 333–354.

34. B. Benard, "Moving Toward a 'Just and Vital Culture': Multiculturalism in Our Schools," Western Regional Center for Drug-Free Schools and Communities, Far West Laboratory, April 1991.

35. B. R. Flay, "What We Know About the Social Influences to Smoking Prevention: Review and Recommendations," in *Prevention Research: Deterring Drug Abuse Among Children and Adolescents,* C. Bell and R. Battjes, eds. (Rockville, MD: National Institute on Drug Abuse, 1985), 67–112.

36. G. Austin and J. A. Pollard, "Substance Abuse and Ethnicity: Recent Research Findings," *Prevention Research Update,* 10 (Summer 1993), Western Regional Center for Drug-Free Schools and Communities, Southwest Regional Laboratory.

37. L. T. Sanford and M. E. Donovan, *Women and Self-Esteem: Understanding and Improving the Way We Think and Feel About Ourselves* (New York: Viking Penguin, 1988).

38. M. Borba, *Esteem Builders: A K–8 Curriculum for Improving Student Achievement, Behavior and School Climate* (Rolling Hills Estates, CA: Jalmar Press, 1989).

39. R. E. Alberti and M. L. Emmons, *Your Perfect Right: A Guide to Assertive Living* (San Luis Obispo, CA: Impact Publishers, 1986).

40. J. G. Woititz and A. Garner, *Life-Skills for Adult Children* (Deerfield Beach, FL: Health Communications, 1990).

41. Ibid.

42. P. E. Butler, *Self-assertion for Women* (New York: HarperCollins, 1992).

43. B. Patterson, "The 'How' of Health Education: Introducing Social Skills to Students," *Journal of Health Education* (November/December Supplement, 1993).

44. L. E. Young, "Critical Thinking Skills: Definitions, Implications for Implementation," *NASSP Bulletin,* 76 (1992): 548.

45. P. S. Nickerson, D. N. Perkins, and E. E. Smith, *The Teaching of Thinking* (Hillsdale, NJ: Lawrence Erlbaum Associates, 1985).

46. J. Jones and R. D. Safrit, "Critical Thinking: Enhancing Adolescent Decision Making," *Journal of Home Economics* (Fall 1992).

47. M. J. Elias and J. S. Kress, "Social Decision-Making and Life Skills Development: A Critical Thinking Approach to Health Promotion in the Middle School," *Journal of School Health,* 64, 2 (1994).

48. M. Zamansky-Shorin, R. L. Selman, and J. B. Richmond, *A Developmental Approach to the Investigation of Links Between Knowledge and Action in the Domain of Children's Healthful Behavior,* position paper prepared for the Carnegie Council on Adolescent Development Workshop (New York: Carnegie Corp., 1988).

49. P. C. Scales, "The Centrality of Health Education to Developing Young Adolescents' Critical Thinking," *Journal of Health Education* (November/December Supplement, 1993): 10–14.

50. H. Hill, D. Piper, and M. King, "The Nature of School-Based Prevention in Experiences for Middle School Students," *Journal of Health Education* (November/December Supplement, 1993).

51. B. Benard, "The Case for Peers," Western Center for Drug-Free Schools and Communities, Northwest Regional Laboratory, December 1990.

52. K. Klemp, A. Halper, and C. L. Perry, "The Efficacy of Peer Leaders in Drug Abuse Prevention," *Journal of School Health,* 56 (1986): 407–411; N. S. Tobler, "Meta-analysis of 143 Adolescent Drug Prevention Programs: Quantitative Outcome Results of Program Participants Compared to a Control or Comparison Group," *Journal of Drug Issues,*

16 (1986): 537–567; R. Bangert-Drowns, "The Effects of School-Based Substance Abuse Education," *Journal of Drug Education,* 18 (1988): 243–264.

53. K. H. Beck, D. L. Thombs, and T. G. Summons, "The Social Context of Drinking Scales: Construct Validation and Relationship of Indicants of Abuse in an Adolescent Population," *Addictive Behaviors,* 18 (1993): 159–169.

54. D. L. Thombs, K. H. Beck, C. A. Mahoney, M. D. Bromley, and K. M. Bezon, "Social Context, Sensation Seeking, and Teen-Age Alcohol Abuse," *Journal of School Health,* 64, 2 (1994): 73–79.

55. E. Goplerud, "Technical Assistance Guide for Prospective Demonstration Grant Applicants," unpublished manuscript, Office for Substance Abuse Prevention, March 1989.

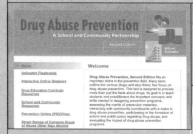

Drug Abuse Prevention
A School and Community Partnership
Second Edition

web resources

The Web site for this book offers many useful resources for educators, students, and professional counselors and is a great source for additional information. Visit the site at **http://healtheducation.jbpub.com/drugabuse/.**

Chapter Learning Objectives

Upon completion of this chapter, students will be able to:

1. Describe the components of a coordinated school health program.

2. Discuss state, district, and local school requirements for alcohol, tobacco, and other health-related issues.

3. Differentiate the levels of cognitive learning according to the cognitive educational taxonomy.

4. Differentiate the levels of affective learning according to the affective educational taxonomy.

5. Compare and contrast effective and ineffective ways to deliver grade-appropriate ATOD information.

6. Examine the components of life skills development.

7. Demonstrate the interactive methods and techniques used in ATOD education.

8. Evaluate science-based commercially prepared curricula for possible adoption.

Scenario

Rick, a former fifth-grade teacher, is currently a prevention specialist with the Family Resource Center. He has been asked to present a two-hour professional development program at Martin Luther King Elementary School. The principal wants him to address interactive teaching strategies for alcohol and drug education. What strategies should Rick present? What curricula should he use to model the various interactive strategies? How should he convince teachers that using interactive strategies is important for reducing ATOD abuse?

Chapter 9

Planning and Implementing an ATOD Curriculum

Introduction

Selecting an appropriate comprehensive ATOD curriculum is the most critical task of the school-based component of the school/community committee. The committee's first responsibility is to bridge the gap between what researchers have found to be best practices and what teachers are currently doing in the classroom. Evaluation of commercially designed ATOD curricula has proliferated during the past 10 years, making the selection of a curriculum more science based. Science-based curricula and programs are those that have been evaluated through summative research and substantiated by expert consensus. Studies have shown that most curricula demonstrate significant knowledge gains by students; however, research on the impact and outcome on changes in students' attitudes and behaviors appears to show mixed results. Some curricula show significant changes in drug use attitudes and behaviors, while others show no change or brief patterns of change. Current commercial products, particularly those that address risk and protective factors, are marked improvements over their predecessors.

Another task of the school/community committee is to decide what students need to know and be able to do. Then, the committee can select a science-based curriculum that provides the desired outcomes. The best way to bridge the gap between what researchers know based on impact and outcome evaluation (science-based information) and actual use patterns by educators is to create a better awareness of current prevention practices that work.

Most commercially prepared curricula have recognized strengths and weaknesses. The curricula have been developed, implemented, and evaluated with a tremendous output of monetary and human resources. Given the limited resources available to schools, the authors support the position that only science-based curricula should be funded at the district level. At the federal level, promising and newly developed programs should receive continued financial support for development, implementation, and evaluation. At the district level, schools can use their limited resources for training teachers and staff to implement recognized successful programs and gain experience in interactive teaching methods. We encourage school district teams to determine their unique local issues and supplement existing curricula with additional programs. Although environmental factors will vary from community to community, most successful ATOD curricula have common components, which are discussed in this chapter.

As health educators, we support the integration of the ATOD curriculum into a comprehensive health education program. The Carnegie Council on Adolescent Development stated, "Schools could do more than perhaps any other single institution in society to help young people, and the adults they will become, to live healthier, longer, more satisfying, and more productive lives." ATOD prevention education is an integral component of helping students live healthier lives, but it is only one component of a broader program. This chapter discusses coordinated school health programs (CSHPs) because ATOD curricula are taught primarily within comprehensive school health education. The chapter reviews science-based practices, particularly those related to commercially prepared curricula, and the nature of ATOD education. It continues with a discussion of the selection of a science-based curriculum to meet the local district's needs and provides a number of partial lessons from commercial products.

Coordinated School Health Program

The school environment is an essential key to ATOD prevention efforts. This setting supports teachers' efforts to educate students to be positive contributors to society, and it is the only setting where health educators have a captive audience.

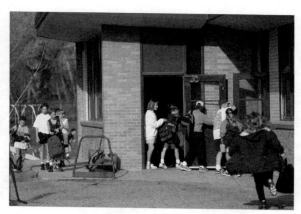

Figure 9.1 School Provides a Setting for Health Education The school should be a focal point for health promotion. (© PhotoDisc)

The school, as a social structure, provides an educational setting in which the total health of the child during the impressionable years is a priority concern. No other community setting even approximates the magnitude of the grades K–12 school education enterprise, with an enrollment of [46.9 million] in nearly [16,000] school districts comprising more than [92,000 public elementary and secondary] schools with some 2.1 million teachers.[1]

Nearly 57% of these schools are located in large or midsize cities. Thus, the school should be regarded as a social unit that provides a focal point to which health planning for all other community settings should relate. (See **Figure 9.1.**)

A coordinated school health program emphasizes the collaborative effort between schools and communities. Traditionally, health services, health instruction, and a healthful school environment composed the school health program. Kolbe proposed that the school health program be expanded to include physical education, food services, guidance and counseling services, and a faculty/staff worksite health promotion program. He called this expanded program the *comprehensive school health program*.[2] His influence was reflected in the Joint Committee on Health Education Terminology's definition:

A comprehensive school health program is an organized set of policies, procedures, and activities designed to protect and promote the health

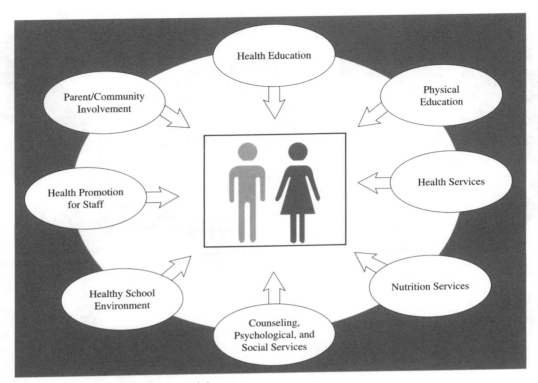

Figure 9.2 Coordinated School Health Model

Source: Centers for Disease Control and Prevention, "A Coordinated School Health Program: The CDC Eight Component Model of School Health Programs."

Available: http://www.cdc.gov/nccdphp/dash/cshpdef.htm.

and well-being of students and staff which has traditionally included health services, healthful school environment, and health education. It should also include, but not be limited to, guidance and counseling, physical education, food service, social work, psychological services, and employee health promotion.[3]

In 1992, the House Appropriations Committee commended the Centers for Disease Control and Prevention on its HIV prevention education efforts and recommended that programs be provided for encouraging schoolchildren to adopt healthy lifestyles. The CDC responded by establishing a national framework for a coordinated school health program; it currently supports 20 states' efforts to implement CSHPs. In 1998, Congress urged the CDC to expand its coordinated school health efforts. In 2002, Congress appropriated $11 million for the CDC to continue its efforts. One goal of the CDC is to extend the eight components of school

health to all American children. Figure 9.2 shows the components of an expanded CSHP, which are discussed briefly in the following sections. Figure 9.3 shows the states funded by the CDC for coordinated school health programs.

Health Services

A registered nurse, school nurse practitioner, or physician directs school health services and works to improve and monitor students' health status. School-based clinics serve the needs of students by being easily accessible. Often, community clinics are unavailable or inaccessible to high-risk students. Health educators strongly recommend the reinstatement of school nurses in the school setting.

Health concerns such as teen pregnancy, sexually transmitted diseases, and adolescents' underutilization of community health services have contributed to the increased emphasis on school-based clinics.

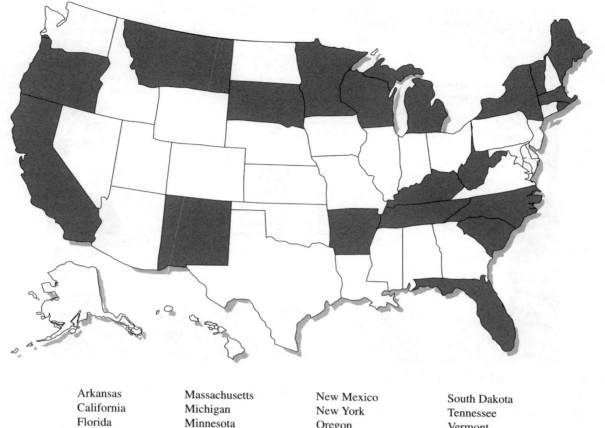

Arkansas	Massachusetts	New Mexico	South Dakota
California	Michigan	New York	Tennessee
Florida	Minnesota	Oregon	Vermont
Kentucky	Montana	Rhode Island	Wisconsin
Maine	North Carolina	South Carolina	West Virginia

Figure 9.3 States Funded by CDC for Coordinated School Health Programs

Source: Centers for Disease Control and Prevention, "Health Youth: An Investment in Our Nation's Future." Available:

http//www.cdc.gov/nccdphp/dash/about/healthyyouth.htm.

Healthy School Environment

Administrative policy sets the tone for a healthful school environment. The school environment includes personal safety (physical, emotional, and social) and structural conditions (lighting, ventilation, sanitation). A school environment must be a place that is conducive to learning and where students are free from fear of violence, physical and emotional abuse, and environmental hazards. Safe schools continue to be a primary concern of all school personnel.

Physical Education

The physical fitness of children and adolescents is enhanced by a comprehensive P–12 physical education program. Research shows that students benefit from daily vigorous activity. Unfortunately, many schools have eliminated elementary physical education because of budgetary constraints. Without daily planned physical activity in the curriculum, many schools have attempted to include physical activity in their before- and after-school programs to engage students in positive lifestyle behaviors. (See **Figure 9.4.**)

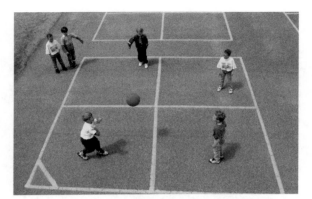

Figure 9.4 PE Programs Provided Before or After School Physical activity is an important part of the school health program. (© PhotoDisc)

The School Health Policies and Programs Study found that a mere 8.0% of elementary schools, 6.4% of middle/junior high schools, and 5.8% of senior high schools provide daily physical education or its equivalent (150 minutes per week for elementary schools; 255 minutes per week for middle/junior high and senior high schools) for the entire school year for students in all grades in the school. Only 71.4% of elementary schools provide regular recess for K–5 students, while 99.2% of co-ed middle/junior and senior high schools offer interscholastic sports. Unfortunately, interscholastic sports involve a limited number of students and leave behind many students who really need physical activity. The best way to ensure all students receive adequate physical activity is through physical education. Health educators strongly support a P–12 comprehensive physical activity program and recognize that schools have a long way to go to meet this recommendation.

Nutrition Services

Schools should adhere to the USDA/DHHS dietary guidelines when planning and serving school lunches. Often, the decisions on food selection and preparation are left to minimally qualified individuals. The School Health Policies and Programs Study found that only 15.7% of states offered

—— [**Table 9.1**] ——

Dietary Guidelines for Americans: ABCs for Good Health

A. Aim for Fitness
  • Aim for a healthy weight.
  • Be physically active each day.

B. Build a Healthy Base
  • Let the Pyramid guide your food choices.
  • Eat a variety of grains daily, especially whole grains.
  • Eat a variety of fruits and vegetables daily.
  • Keep food safe to eat.

C. Choose Sensibly
  • Choose a diet that is low in saturated fat and cholesterol and moderate in total fat.
  • Choose beverages and foods that limit your intake of sugars.
  • Choose and prepare foods with less salt.
  • If you drink alcoholic beverages, do so in moderation.

Source: U.S. Department of Agriculture, Agricultural Research Service, *Report of the Dietary Guidelines Advisory Committee on Dietary Guidelines for Americans, 2000.* Available: http://www.ars.usda.gov/dgac.

and 9.8% required certification for school-level food service managers. Students should be encouraged to select foods that meet the dietary guidelines established by the USDA, thus promoting healthy, nutritional choices. In reality, many school lunch programs provide students with fast-food choices that often are high in saturated fat, sodium, and added sugars. They offer selections to compete with off-campus sites or to encourage students to eat on-campus. Students who receive free meals through governmental subsidies should be encouraged to make healthy, rather than convenient, food choices. Lunch programs can help students select healthy foods by providing a nutritional breakdown of the various foods and offering a variety of healthy choices. A rising prevalence of obesity and a continuing emphasis on body image are two nutrition health issues that school personnel should be addressing. Table 9.1 lists some of the 2000 USDA/DHHS guidelines for Americans.

Counseling, Psychological, and Social Services

Traditionally, counselors found themselves serving as administrative assistants—checking attendance records, dealing with truancy, and serving as school "nurses"—and seldom had time to practice the skills for which they were trained. Today the primary role of school counselors has shifted from that of administrative assistant and career counselor to that of intervention and prevention specialist. Progressive schools establish student assistance programs, train peer educators, initiate primary prevention programs, and deliver individual and group counseling services for students. The School Health Policies and Programs Study found that 34.0% of states and 51.2% of districts required schools to offer student assistance programs to all students, and 62.8% of schools offered such programs. Health educators support the vital role of school counselors in establishing a comprehensive intervention and treatment plan for students.

Health Promotion for Faculty and Staff

Worksite health promotion programs give teachers and staff opportunities to practice health-promoting behaviors in an easily accessible and affordable environment. Teachers and staff members serve as role models for children and adolescents, who observe the health behaviors of school personnel. Participation in healthy lifestyle choices by administration, teachers, and staff contributes greatly to the success of a comprehensive health promotion program. (See **Figure 9.5**.) During the 12 months preceding the School Health Policies and Programs Study, 24.4% of districts provided funding for or sponsored employee assistance programs, and 37.1% of schools offered such programs.

Parent/Community Involvement

Chapter 8 discussed the movement from a service delivery model to a community empowerment model. This paradigm shift can apply to schools. Successful school health programs will incorporate the current design of community development programs, in which all members of the school

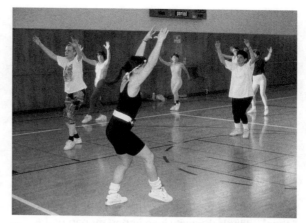

Figure 9.5 A Fitness Class for the Staff School-based worksite wellness programs can complement health promotion efforts for students.

(© David Young-Wolff/PhotoEdit)

and community accept responsibility and feel empowered to implement a coordinated school health program.

The key to a successful CSHP is the integration of community and school services and health instruction to meet the multiple needs of the faculty, staff, and students. This integration can only occur with support from central administration. Teachers and staff can conduct a self-study of existing school health components and offer suggestions for addressing missing components. Schools have many services available but seldom integrate them into a coordinated program. Allensworth and Wolford have provided a more thorough discussion of comprehensive school health and suggested methods for integrating instruction.[4]

Throughout this discussion of curricular issues, remember that sensitivity to factors such as race, SES, ethnicity, sexual orientation, and gender are important. Prevention efforts must (1) actively include youth in community development, (2) enhance cultural consciousness and pride, (3) include public awareness campaigns that counter the alcohol and tobacco industries' advertising, (4) encourage the restructuring of schools to provide opportunities for academic success, and (5) incorporate educational interventions that allow youth to develop bicultural and bilingual competence.[5]

Health Education

The purpose of health instruction is to encourage all students to attain a certain level of health knowledge (including ATOD information), develop attitudes conducive to healthy lifestyle choices, and practice healthy lifestyle behaviors. Currently students' average exposure to health education is approximately 2.5 weeks total from kindergarten through 12th grade. Today, teachers seldom have the credentials to teach health education, particularly at the elementary school level, where attitudes and behaviors are being formed.[6] (See **Figure 9.6.**) Health instruction is the foundation of the CSHP and an area in which teachers can have a profound impact. Studies show that students who receive health instruction report more knowledge and better health behaviors than those who receive no health instruction.[7] Research studies of planned, sequential health education have found a 37% reduction in the onset of smoking in seventh-grade students, a decrease in the prevalence of obesity among girls in grades 6 to 8, and less likelihood of using tobacco, alcohol, or marijuana.

In 1990, the Joint Committee on Health Education Terminology defined health instruction as follows:

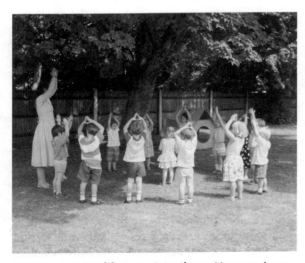

Figure 9.6 A Health Demonstration   Many students receive only limited exposure to health instruction, including drug education. (© PhotoDisc)

Comprehensive school health instruction refers to the development, delivery, and evaluation of a planned curriculum, preschool through 12, with goals, objectives, content sequence, and specific classroom lessons which include, but are not limited to, the following major content areas: community health; consumer health; environmental health; family life; mental and emotional health; injury prevention and safety; nutrition; personal health; prevention and control of disease; and substance use and abuse.[8]

Today, the CDC defines the key elements of comprehensive health education as follows:[9]

1. A documented, planned, and sequential program of health instruction for students in grades kindergarten through twelve.
2. A curriculum that addresses and integrates education about a range of categorical health problems and issues at developmentally appropriate ages.
3. Activities that help young people develop the skills they need to avoid: tobacco use; dietary patterns that contribute to disease; sedentary lifestyle; sexual behaviors that result in HIV infection, other STDs, and unintended pregnancy; alcohol and other drug use; and behaviors that result in unintentional and intentional injuries.
4. Instruction provided for a prescribed amount of time at each grade level.
5. Management and coordination by an education professional trained to implement the program.
6. Instruction from teachers who are trained to teach the subject.
7. Involvement of parents, health professionals, and other concerned community members.
8. Periodic evaluation, updating, and improvement.

Ideally, health instruction should be comprehensive and sequential for grades P–12 and be provided by qualified teachers. In addition to the traditional content areas, a health education curriculum should focus on the National Health Education Standards and the risk behaviors identified by the Centers for Disease Control and Prevention. The School Health Policies and Programs Study demonstrates that many states and districts fall short in providing comprehensive school health education. A summary of 22 topical areas required at the elementary school level by state can be found at the CDC website.[10]

ATOD Classroom Instruction

Classroom instruction is the foundation of the educational component of an ATOD prevention program. ATOD education usually is taught by the health educator, whether as a self-contained unit within the planned instruction, correlated with other subjects, integrated across the curriculum, or as incidental learning. Students typically receive ATOD instruction to increase their knowledge, develop and assess attitudes and beliefs, and build skills to voluntarily make health-promoting choices. ATOD education, like health education, encourages voluntary behavior change. Its aim is to promote, without manipulation or coercion, choices that are conducive to healthy living. ATOD abuse is only one of many health-compromising behaviors to which adolescents are exposed. Therefore, ATOD instruction should be integrated into the coordinated health education program at all grade levels.

As teachers, we use noncoercive strategies to encourage positive behavior choices. We also recognize the necessity of environmental, organizational, and economic support in encouraging ATOD nonuse and health-promoting behavior. These factors do not necessarily fall within the domain of schools, yet they are essential to the success of the school health program. Cooperation among school personnel, community agencies, media, law enforcement, and parents is imperative for successful health behavior change. In addition to voluntary changes, ATOD use and abuse prevention can occur through coercive strategies, a topic that is discussed in the next chapter.

When members of a school district select a science-based curriculum, they should consult a number of health education textbooks to review detailed descriptions of the curriculum design process. The next section provides an abbreviated discussion of the key steps in ATOD curriculum design and can be used to review existing science-based curricula.

Selecting an ATOD Curriculum

The first task in selecting an ATOD curriculum is to form a school/community curriculum committee. Suggested members include an ATOD prevention specialist, a curriculum specialist, teachers, a parent, students, a principal, and key community members who represent the community's diverse population. The initial task of the school/community committee is to become familiar with the ATOD literature on science-based curricula. Once committee members are familiar with the literature, they can begin to evaluate the curricula (universal, selective, indicated) appropriate for their needs. Committee members often assume differing roles and tasks as the curriculum selection process unfolds.

Step 1: Select a Prevention Model

The curriculum committee's first step is to choose a prevention model that fits most closely with its goals, objectives, and expected outcomes. The prevention model chosen determines the philosophy and direction of the entire ATOD educational component. A key question from an educational perspective is, "Does the current literature support this approach, and will it work?" A key question from a community perspective is, "Will the community support this approach?"

Committees often select curricula based on the activities or strategies that teachers are interested in delivering, rather than the philosophy of the program. The prevention model determines the direction of the entire program, whether the approach is based on risk reduction, social development, persuasion, decision making, life skills development, or some combination of these approaches. (See Table 9.2 for a review of prevention models.)

Step 2: Set Goals and Objectives

What does the committee hope the curriculum will achieve? Are the goals and objectives based on outcome, performance, or competency? Do the goals and objectives align with state expectations and the National Health Education Standards? **Goals** are the long-range, hoped-for results, whereas **objectives** are the steps to achieve the goals. How will the committee measure the curriculum's impact and outcomes? The **impact** is the immediate result of the specific curriculum. The **outcome** is the actual action or behavior that results from the program and is usually measured longitudinally. What types of assessment will be used to determine changes in

Educational Taxonomy of the Cognitive Domain

1. **Knowledge:** Recall of specific factual information
   state, copy, locate, choose, select, name, identify, list, recall

   Given a scenario for decision making, students write down the steps in making a wise decision.

2. **Comprehension:** Know what is being communicated
   order, rename, collect, calculate, convert, match, measure, compute, explain

   After viewing the video, students verbally explain the difference between short-term and long-term consequences of tobacco use.

3. **Application:** Recall of data and use of the data in a particular situation
   solve, construct, draw, illustrate, reproduce, extract, infer, annotate, verify

   Given a role-play of an opportunity to use ATODs, students demonstrate the five-step refusal process.

4. **Analysis:** Breakdown of material into its constituent parts
   deduce, differentiate, investigate, analyze, diagram, subdivide, separate, illustrate, distinguish

After class discussion, students diagram on graph paper four aspects of the cost of drug use to society.

5. **Synthesis:** Combine component parts into a pattern or structure
   connect, build, predict, synthesize, invent, relate, create, assemble, design

   After viewing the video on pregnancy and ATOD abuse, students summarize on a worksheet the key concepts of fetal development and maternal ATOD use.

6. **Evaluation:** Make qualitative and quantitative judgments
   criticize, evaluate, decide, prove, compare, hypothesize, judge, contrast, delineate

   After conducting informal interviews, students compare the ATOD use patterns of students in fifth and eighth grades.

Source: B.S. Bloom et al., *Cognitive Domain*, bk. 1 of *Taxonomy of Educational Objectives* (New York: David McKay Company, 1956).

[**Table 9.2**]

Prevention Models and Theories

Health belief model	Social development model
PRECEDE-PROCEED model	Ecological model
Psychosocial model	Social decision-making model
Risk reduction model	Social context model
PATCH model	Peer resource programming model

student's knowledge, attitudes, and behaviors? Is this assessment or evaluation reliable and valid?

Reviewing the Curricular Goals and Objectives

Two educational taxonomies that address the cognitive and affective domains can be beneficial when the committee begins to review the curricular goals and objectives of commercially prepared curricula.[11] (See the accompanying Hints & Tips boxes.) These taxonomies are hierarchically ordered and designed to elicit developmentally appropriate responses to learning. As committee members review the curricula, they should pay particular attention to the level of learning being addressed by the providers.

Selecting Appropriate Themes

The U.S. Department of Education suggests that certain themes be present at all levels of instruction, K through 12. These themes are listed in the Hints & Tips box on page 183. The curriculum selection committee can use these themes as guidelines in reviewing the curricular goals and objectives. (How might these themes be addressed by Rick when he provides the professional development inservice on interactive strategies?)

Step 3: Assess the Content

Classroom instruction is the foundation of a school's prevention effort. The content selected by curriculum developers should provide clear and consistent support for healthy choices. The information should be factual, up-to-date, and sensitive to the differences and needs of diverse groups (e.g., culture, gender, and families with chemical dependency). Table 9.3 provides suggestions for delivering ATOD information.

If misconceptions about peer norms exist, as they often do, they need to be corrected. Consistent messages of ATOD nonuse by children and adolescents and a clear sense of right and wrong should be conveyed through direct instruction. Content should be developmentally appropriate and presented with student involvement, using interactive teaching methods and techniques whenever possible.

Delivering ATOD Education to Special-Needs Students

Does the curriculum provide suggestions for special-needs students? In most school districts, special education students, except for the most severely mentally handicapped, are mainstreamed for health, the class in which ATOD education is usually presented. (See **Figure 9.7.**) Most teachers are not adequately trained to effectively serve students with learning disabilities (who constitute approximately 12% of a typical school's enrollment), so some schools provide an opportunity for collaboration with special education teachers.

The key to adapting material to special-needs students is familiarity with the program or text format. Students are most comfortable when adaptations are not readily noticed by the rest of the class. Unobservable adaptation can be accomplished

Themes for ATOD Instruction, Grades K–12

- A clear and consistent message that the use of alcohol, tobacco, and other illicit drugs is unhealthy and harmful
- Knowledge of all types of drugs, including what medicines are, why they are used, and who should (or should not) administer them
- The social consequences of substance abuse
- Respect for the laws and values of society
- Promotion of healthy, safe, and responsible attitudes and behavior by correcting mistaken beliefs and assumptions, disarming the sense of personal invulnerability, and building resistance to influences which encourage substance abuse

- Strategies to involve parents, family members, and the community in the effort to prevent use of illicit substances
- Appropriate information on intervention and referral services, plus information on contacting responsible adults when help is needed in emergencies
- Sensitivity to the specific needs of the local school and community in terms of cultural appropriateness and local substance abuse problems

Source: U.S. Department of Education, *Drug Prevention Curricula: A Guide to Selection and Implementation* (Washington, DC: Office of Educational Research and Improvement, 1988).

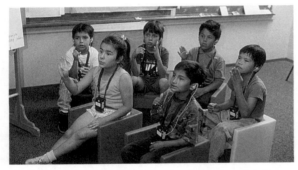

Figure 9.7 **Special Education Students Receive Drug Education**   The needs of all students should be considered in planning a drug education curriculum.

(© David Young-Wolff/PhotoEdit)

by a joint effort between the special education teacher and the regular teacher who is teaching the ATOD unit. With careful planning, special education students may be able to complete a portion of the assignments in the resource room. Two special issues of concern are readability and teaching methods.

Readability

Is the reading level of the material suitable for children with reading disabilities? Many health text-books and ATOD curricula are written at levels too advanced for the intended audience. This barrier is serious for students who can't read even at their current grade level. If the curriculum frustrates the student, learning will be minimal. If the reading level is too advanced, adaptations should be made. The teacher should determine the readability of materials by using a variety of available readability measures. One example is the Fry Readability Scale, which can be found in Edward B. Fry's *Reading Diagnosis: Informal Reading Inventories* (Jamestown Publishers, 1981). (See Figure 9.8.) This readability graph is an effective, quick way to assess reading levels.

Teaching Methods

Does the curriculum incorporate cooperative learning? Curriculum activities should be designed to give special students a better chance to learn, to experience success, and to be integrated in a desirable way with higher-functioning students. Cooperative learning tends to bond special students more effectively to school and mainstream values and establishes ties between special education students and regular students (as role models). A curriculum that is very heavily oriented to basic skills (e.g., reading and writing) may present a

Table 9.3

Effective and Ineffective Ways to Deliver Information

Age and Grade	Don't	Do
Preschool–3rd grade	Expect these children to understand cause-and-effect relationships	Focus on health promotion information that develops and helps internalize the desire to be healthy
4th–5th grade	Expect abstract reasoning, experimentation with self-image, or primary orientation to peer group	Give information that is very concrete and amenable to classifying, ordering, and reversing
		Regulate information to rules, standards, stereotypes, and exploration
		Focus on information that enhances skill mastery
6th–10th grade	Demand strict conformity	Focus information on risk-taking behaviors and range of influences on behavior
	Expect orientation to adult world authority	
		Focus on short-term efforts
	Lecture or threaten	
		Expect resistance to and questioning of information
		Use peers to help deliver information
		Give information that empowers youth, such as the names of community treatment resources
4th grade–adulthood	Expect people to depend on experts for information	Present self as a resource, encourage everyone to assume leadership and empowerment
	Focus solely on information at the expense of skill development	Use power of information as basis for discussion, interaction, and skill practice

Source: Office for Substance Abuse Prevention, *Getting It Together: Promoting Drug-Free Communities* (Rockville, MD: OSAP, 1991).

greater challenge to special education students. It is preferable to use a wider variety of learning activities that enable special education students to use their other skills (which may be normal or even superior). Suggested methods for adapting existing curricula and using cooperative learning are provided later in this chapter.

Step 4: Choose Methods and Techniques

The committee should give attention to the interactive teaching methods and techniques used in the curriculum. (See Figure 9.9.) By reviewing the following methods and techniques, the committee can determine if the methods and techniques are appropriate at each grade level.

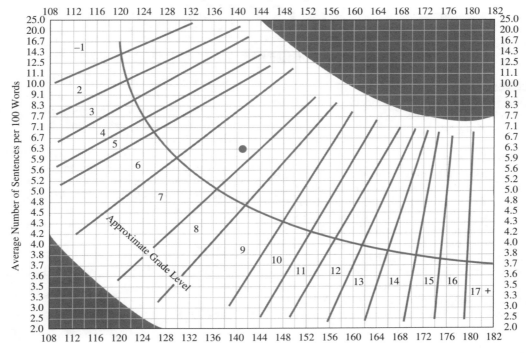

Average Number of Syllables per 100 Words

Directions:
1. Randomly select three 100-word passages from the book.
   (Count all words, numbers, and abbreviations.)
2. Count the number of sentences to the nearest one-tenth.
3. Count the total number of syllables in the 100-word passage. For example:

	Syllables	Sentences
First Hundred Words	124	6.6
Second Hundred Words	141	5.5
Third Hundred Words	158	6.8
Average	141	6.3

4. Plot averages to see grade level (see dot).

Figure 9.8 Fry's Readability Scale

Source: Edward B. Fry, *Reading Diagnosis: Informal Reading Inventories* (Providence, RI: Jamestown Publishers, 1981).

Traditional Methods and Techniques

Traditional teaching methods and techniques are found in all ATOD curricula. Suggested traditional teaching methods and techniques are found in Table 9.4. The Hints & Tips box depicts a sample lesson plan using traditional teaching methods.

Interactive Methods and Techniques

The majority of classroom time in an ATOD curriculum should be spent on interactive teaching methods, where students play a large role. Teachers who are uncomfortable with these teaching methods may need additional training. Does the commercial curriculum being considered train teachers to use interactive methods? A brief summary of interactive teaching methods (role playing, modeling, and cooperative learning) and related teaching strategies (media analysis, brainstorming, and trigger films) follows. (How might Rick incorporate the following material into his professional development in-service for teachers?)

Traditional Teaching Sample Lesson Plan: Labeling Drugs—A Lesson for K-3

Objectives

To identify and label medicines and illegal drugs. To distinguish between substances that may be helpful and those that are harmful.

Background

Young children should be made aware that there are medicines that are good for us when we are sick and illegal drugs that harm us. Children should know that medicines can be essential to our general health and well-being when they are used as directed by the person for whom they were prescribed. They should also know that medicines are given to them by a credible person, such as a parent or the school nurse, who wants them to feel better and be healthier. It's important for children to be able to distinguish between medicines and illegal drugs so that they won't resist taking medicines but will resist accepting harmful drugs.

Activities

Ask the students to help you create a list of drugs, and write the list on the chalkboard (examples: aspirin, cough syrup, tobacco). Have cut-out copies of large plus and minus signs available for the discussion.

Discuss each drug and explain whether it is a medicine (helpful) or a drug they should not take (harmful or illegal). With students' help, tape a plus sign on the chalkboard next to each medicine and a minus sign next to each illegal or harmful drug.

Discuss how each medicine on the list can help make people well and healthy (example: aspirin reduces swelling and pain; cough syrup calms a cough). Explain that medicines are accompanied by directions on how much to take and when to use them (too much medicine or the wrong medicine can make people sick).

Resources

Large paper plus and minus signs (copied and cut out), scissors, tape, chalkboard.

Teacher Tips

- For illegal drugs, provide some examples of common or street names.
- Prepare your own list of medicines and illegal drugs in case students have trouble coming up with suggestions.

Source: U.S. Department of Education, *Learning to Live Drug Free* (Washington, DC: Government Printing Office, 1992).

Table 9.4

Traditional Teaching Methods and Techniques

Bulletin boards	Case studies
Class discussion	Creative writing
Current events	Debates
Demonstrations	Direct instruction
Field trips	Games and puzzles
Group presentations	Guest speakers
Health fairs	Overhead transparencies
Slides	Valuing
Visual displays	Written reports (technical writing)

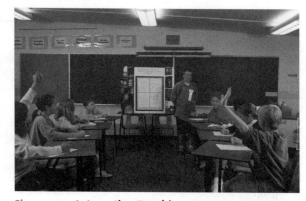

Figure 9.9 Interactive Teaching Instructors should strive to incorporate a variety of teaching methods, such as direct instruction, debate, games and puzzles, journal writing, and bulletin boards. (© PhotoDisc)

Role Playing

Role playing gives students the opportunity to take a role not normally their own or, if it is their own, in a place where the event does not normally occur.[12] Four components increase the effectiveness of role playing. First, students should have the opportunity to volunteer to participate. Second, all students should be encouraged to participate because the ability to change attitudes often relies on moving from private views to public statements. Third, situations should be believable and improvised, not canned. Finally, reward and reinforcement ensure that the benefits gained from role playing continue.[13]

Students should have the choice of participating in a role play. There are many reasons why students refrain from participation. They may be shy, they may be too emotionally involved in the scenario despite the change of location, they may prefer to see how others might handle a situation, or they may feel they are too "cool" to participate. When the teacher creates a nonthreatening environment, students are more likely to participate in role plays.

The situations selected for the role play should be realistic and easy to understand. Improvising their roles, rather than reading from a canned program, enhances students' learning. However, when students have limited exposure to role playing, canned programs can ensure that the appropriate values or concepts are learned. When students first learn a new skill, such as refusal, **assertiveness,** or conflict resolution, teachers and peers can provide assistance to the role players as the scenario is enacted. Each student should have the opportunity to enact the new skill. Remember: Students who practice the role play are more likely to be affected by the event.[14] Through role play, they have the opportunity to move from a private view to a public statement. Role playing empowers them and increases the likelihood that the lessons will affect their attitudes and make learning more effective. Students who have difficulty verbalizing their views may prefer other techniques, such as writing the script, directing the role play, or acting in front of a video camera.

Rewarding positive experiences, reinforcing learned behaviors with praise, approving and encouraging, and critiquing and retraining are all important components of the role play.[15] Role players need feedback from the teacher and their peers regarding how well they have done because attitude changes and skill mastery are more likely to last with reinforcement. The Hints & Tips box describes a role-play exercise.

Modeling

Modeling is learning through imitation. While modeling occurs from a very early age (children learn behaviors and skills from their parents and siblings), teachers are concerned with modeling that occurs among peers. (See the Hints & Tips box "A Classroom Modeling Activity.") Peers can be trained to model appropriate behaviors or skills and demonstrate these skills to others. Modeling is enhanced when peers are the same sex, age, and social status, and when the model is viewed as an expert or held in high regard.[16]

Modeling is most effective "when the modeling display shows the behaviors to be imitated (1) in a clear and detailed manner; (2) in the order from least to most difficult behavior; (3) with enough repetition to make overlearning likely; (4) with as little irrelevant (not to be learned) detail as possible; and (5) when several different models, rather than a single model, are used."[17] Peers who model appropriate behaviors and skills, as well as those who rehearse them, need rewards when they successfully demonstrate their learning. Reinforcement motivates them to continue the modeled and rehearsed behaviors and skills. Some curricula refer to modeling as *rehearsal*, while others refer to demonstrating the skill as *modeling* and practicing the skill as *rehearsal*. Both aspects of skill learning are important so that training can transfer from one situation or environment to another.

Students must be taught that using new skills is easy in some situations and environments and difficult in others. Practicing skills in a nonthreatening environment increases the likelihood of success in other, more difficult situations, but transfer of training does not always occur. Therefore, evaluating how a situation was handled and how the student might handle it differently the next time is an important aspect of mastering a new skill.

Example of a Role-Play Exercise: Member of the Family

Level: Grade 8
Topic: Attitudes Toward Family Alcoholism
Objective: To differentiate between constructive and destructive responses to family alcoholism.

Preliminary Considerations

The teacher should be familiar with role-play directions. Except for dramatizing the futility of talking to someone who is drunk, students should be discouraged from developing scenarios in which one character is drunk. One teacher comments, "As expected, volunteers were reluctant at first. However, students did enjoy the role play and I even got boy volunteers to do a father-son scene."

Materials Needed

A role-play scenario.

Description of Activity

1. Students develop and role-play scenarios in which a member of their family has a drinking problem, and students must decide how to cope with him or her in specific situations. A sample scenario is given below. Students should be encouraged to create their own scenarios and role profiles. Participants discuss the feelings they had while role playing.

2. After the role plays, the teacher lists on the board ways in which students responded to each problem drinker. Class discussion is then held on which responses students and teacher feel were most constructive and why.

Sample Role-Play Scenario

One morning before school, a student and her mother are discussing the issue of the mother meeting with her daughter's teacher.

Student

Your mother has been asked to meet with your teacher and guidance counselor, but now she tells you she's not going because she was drinking yesterday and doesn't feel well today. She tells you to go to school and tell the teacher that she has visitors and won't be able to make the meeting. This is the third time she has canceled her appointment. You really want her to talk to your teacher because you feel she has been unfair in giving you poor grades. You may have to stay back a year if your grades aren't changed. What do you do?

Mother

You have been drinking heavily for several months now, but you feel this is none of your daughter's business. You know what you're doing and you're going to quit drinking any day now. You are supposed to meet with your daughter's teacher and guidance counselor about her poor grades but you just don't feel up to it today. You're angry at your daughter because she gets bad marks—she doesn't seem to try at all. You are also annoyed with the school for not forcing your daughter to do her work, so you tell your daughter to tell them you have visitors and can't make the meeting. This is the third time you have canceled.

Source: CASPAR.

Cooperative Learning

Cooperative learning is presented in different forms depending on whether the teacher's focus is on achievement, process skills, or both.[18] Successful cooperative learning experiences have four basic components: (1) student-student interaction; (2) working with each other in small groups while performing a task (thus, group process skills are understood and practiced); (3) positive interdependence, in which group responsibility outweighs self-interests; and (4) accountability, so that each student is evaluated individually to determine his or her level of mastery. (See Figure 9.10.)

Cooperative learning groups consist of three to five students and remain intact to accomplish a particular task. Each student in the group has a different task, such as recorder, reader, summarizer, materials gatherer. Facilitators usually are not assigned by the teacher (but all students should have opportunities to practice leadership skills). Cooperative learning offers students increased involvement in a cooperative, rather than competitive, environment. As students interact and learn more about each other, they build leadership skills in cooperation, enhance their self-esteem, and increase their respect for others. Cooperative

HINTS & TIPS

A Classroom Modeling Activity

Suggest an alternative to drug use or another risky behavior. (A key phrase to use in this exercise is "Instead, why don't we . . . .") Point out that suggesting an alternative lets the troublemaker know that students are rejecting the activity, not the person. Have the group brainstorm a list of healthy, fun alternatives. Put the ideas on butcher paper and title the list "Alternatives." Make the alternatives specific to the situation, and point out that they can be simple, like "going for a walk in the mall" or "sitting and talking."

Use the risky behaviors and alternatives from the butcher paper to model with students how to ask questions, name the trouble, identify the consequences, and suggest an alternative. Don't pressure the students during the lesson; let them get used to the idea that their responses work. Here is an example of how you might model the first four steps of the skill:

Student: "Hey, [teacher's name], do you want to go down to the store?"

Teacher: "What for?"

Student: "I want to get some tapes."

Teacher: "I thought you were broke; isn't that what you told me?"

Student: "I *am* broke, but it's easy to sneak out some tapes."

Teacher: "[Student's name], that's theft. If I do that, I can end up arrested. At the very least, my folks would ground me for the rest of the year, and I know I'd never be able to see you again. Listen, instead why don't we ask Joshua to loan us some of his tapes?"

Student: "Hey, that's not a bad idea; Joshua has great tapes!"

Model the step again, this time "thinking out loud." For example, set up a situation in which you and a student are in a mall one evening:

Student: "I just tried this stuff; you should, too."

Teacher: "Oh, yeah, what is it?"

Student: "Everyone's using it, and it's totally harmless."

Teacher: (Looking at class while student "freezes") "When [student's name] says 'totally harmless,' it usually means that there's some risk involved. I better ask what exactly is 'totally harmless.' (To student) What is this great stuff?"

Student: "Chewing tobacco. Chew. It's smooth and it's cool, and it just relaxes you."

Teacher: (Looking at class while student "freezes") "Well, I don't have to ask any more questions. Chewing tobacco is trouble for me. I want to tell [student's name] that chewing tobacco would make me feel both stupid and sick, and that in any case I told my folks I'd stay away from nicotine. (To student) [Student's name], that doesn't appeal to me at all. If I chew that, it'll make me sick, plus it looks disgusting. That stuff can give you cancer of the mouth."

Source: Here's Looking At You, 2000.

---

learning activities also can help special education students integrate more easily into the health classroom. Teachers can establish the groundwork for cooperative learning by following these guidelines:

1. *Decide when to use cooperative learning.* Any activity that requires brainstorming, problem solving, discussion, or peer editing provides an excellent opportunity for cooperative groups. (See the Hints & Tips box "Some Quick Cooperative Learning Starters.")

2. *Set rules.* Teachers and students should develop their own rules based on the classroom atmosphere and the teacher's style of presenting material. Post the rules and remind

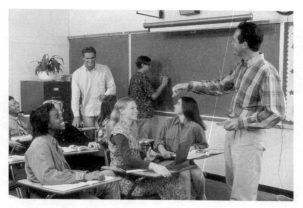

Figure 9.10 A Cooperative Learning Group
Cooperative learning reinforces self-esteem, teamwork, and a spirit of mutual helpfulness. (© Tom McCarthy/PhotoEdit)

students about them before each session. Some suggested rules are the following:

- Contribute to the team.
- Follow directions.
- Disagree politely; state why.
- Don't be bossy.
- Be positive; encourage all team members.
- No put-downs.

3. *Make group decisions.* Teachers must decide on the format and arrangement of the groups for activities. The following criteria may be applied:

- Arrange groups effectively (physical arrangement).
- Decide on group size and blend (different abilities within a group work best).
- Decide how long (minutes, days) the group will stay together.
- Form new groups. Allow time for students to get to know each other. Change group memberships from time to time to allow all students to get to know each other.
- Assign group responsibilities. Reader—may use more than one; recorder—takes notes for the group; questioner—gains the teacher's attention and asks questions; materials organizer—obtains books, equipment, and so forth; leader—facilitates the group activity.

- Determine responsibilities according to group size and activity.

4. *Encourage responsibility.* The teacher can select a number of ways to ensure the group is on task and completing the assignment. They include the following:

- Peer influence works quite well to maintain discipline in the group.
- Give group rewards for completing each criterion (point system).
- Consider giving the group an identity beyond the specific learning activity, such as an additional classroom responsibility; for example, straightening shelves and desks, watering plants, running errands, cleaning boards.
- Choose a new team leader each week. The team leader sees that all team members complete their assignments, puts their names on the work, and turns in the group's work to the teacher.

5. *Encourage effective social skills.* Use prompts and cues (e.g., thumbs down) to point out when a group is distracting other teams. Also, point out things you like about what the group is doing. Discuss the importance of social skills. Ask the students to create a class list of social skills that are necessary for successful groups. Post the list of social skills in your room, next to the rules.

6. *Actively participate.* The teacher should be an active figure in monitoring and encouraging groups. This time is not an opportunity to catch up on other work. Children need guidance in effective team learning, particularly in the initial stages.

Brainstorming
Unlike the teaching methods described previously, brainstorming is a technique students can use to generate a list of ideas during class discussion or in a small group. The teacher or an assigned recorder writes down all ideas and statements given as answers to a particular question. For example, students are asked to list responses to questions such

HINTS & TIPS

Some Quick Cooperative Learning Starters

1. *Turn to Your Neighbor:* Ask students to turn to a neighbor and ask him or her something about the lesson, for example, to explain a concept you have just taught, to explain the assignment, to explain how to do what you have just taught, to summarize the three most important points of the discussion, or whatever fits the lesson. (Three to five minutes.)

2. *Reading Groups:* Students read material together and answer the questions provided by the teacher. One person is the reader, another the recorder, and the third the checker (who checks to make certain everyone understands and agrees with the answers). They must come up with three possible answers to each question and circle their favorite one. When they are finished, they sign the paper to certify that they all understand and agree on the answers.

3. *Jigsaw:* Each person reads and studies part of an assigned reading material and then teaches what he or she has learned to the other group members. Each student then quizzes the group members until satisfied that everyone knows his or her part thoroughly.

4. *Focus Trios:* Before a film, lecture, or reading, have students form groups of three, summarize together what they already know about the subject, and come up with questions they have about it. Afterward, the trios answer questions, discuss new information, and formulate new questions.

5. *Drill Partners:* Have students drill each other on the facts they need to know until they are certain both partners know and can remember them all. This drill works for spelling, vocabulary, math, grammar, test review, and so forth. Give bonus points on the test if all group members score above a certain percentage.

6. *Reading Buddies:* In lower grades, have students read their stories to each other, getting help with words and discussing content with their partners. In upper grades, have students discuss their books and read their favorite parts to each other.

7. *Worksheet Checkmates:* Have two students, each with a different job, complete one worksheet. The reader reads, then suggests an answer; the writer can write it.

8. *Homework Checkers:* Have students compare homework answers, discuss any they have not answered similarly, then correct their papers and add the reason they changed an answer. They make certain everyone's answers agree, then staple the papers together. The teacher grades one paper from each group and gives group members that grade.

9. *Test Reviewers:* Have students prepare each other for a test. They get bonus points if every group member scores above a preset level.

Source: Material adapted from D. W. Johnson, R. T. Johnson, and E. J. Holubec, *Cooperation in the Classroom* (Edina, MN: Interaction Book Co., 1991), 1:19, 20.

---

as "Why do people use drugs?" or "What are some ways to get high without using drugs?" (See the Hints & Tips box.) No value judgments or discussion occurs during the brainstorming session. Brainstorming with a large group continues until all possible responses have been elicited. With small groups, the teacher may want to set a time limit and then collate all responses.

Media Analysis

Advertising of tobacco, alcohol, and other drugs is a multibillion dollar business paid for by consumers via the increased costs of products. Legislation enhances this process by making adver-

tising a tax-exempt business.[19] Despite the ban on television advertising of tobacco products, the tobacco industry has maintained a presence by promoting tobacco products with actors and sponsoring sporting entities (e.g., Marlboro race cars).

Tobacco is the most heavily promoted commercial product in America despite restrictions placed on the industry as a result of the Master Settlement Agreement with the state attorneys general. The agreement required tobacco companies to phase in restrictions on use of outdoor and transit advertising and brand-name sponsorships, distribution of free samples, and distribution and sale of products with brand-name logos. These restrictions had a measurable impact on the tobacco industry. The Federal Trade Commission found that cigarette sales fell by 10.3% from 1998 to 1999, but total advertising and promotional expenditures rose 22.3% to $8.24 billion, the most ever reported to the Commission. The tobacco industry increased expenditures for advertising via newspapers (up 73.0%), magazines (up 34.2%), sampling (up 133.5%) and direct mail (up 63.8%). However, these increases (only 10% of all advertising and promotional costs) were miniscule compared with the $3.54 billion spent in promotional allowances (i.e., payments made to retailers to facilitate sales).[20]

Although less money is spent on advertising alcohol than tobacco products, alcohol advertisers enjoy the luxury of getting their message to consumers through television. Again, sporting events are a popular forum for alcohol advertisements.

The alcoholic beverage industry spent nearly $1.2 billion on advertising in 1998. Nearly 75% of major concerts have beer company sponsors, despite the majority of the audience being under the age of 21. The industry's advertising and promotional campaigns parallel the tobacco industry in disproportionately targeting young people and ethnic minorities.[21]

The pharmaceutical industry is currently under attack for the high price of prescription drugs, yet it remains a key player in the advertising of drugs. Prescription and ethical drug advertising, a $25 billion business, supports highly profitable medical and pharmaceutical journals and other forms of promotion to health professionals. Ten of the biggest drug companies control the $7 billion-plus nonprescription proprietary, or OTC, drug market. More than $1.5 billion in this market is spent on advertising.[22] Check the following website for the top 200 prescriptions for 2001: www.rxlist.com/top200.htm.

Persuasion Techniques in Advertising

How do advertisers persuade people to buy something? Here are a few ways:

1. *Testimonial:* The ad uses important or famous people to testify about the product. These people say that the product is good, even though they actually know nothing about the product. Example: A former star baseball player testifies about an electric coffee maker.

2. *Transfer:* A good-looking or successful person sells the product. You don't know this person, but the ad tries to get you to think that if you buy the product, you will be good-looking or successful, too. The advertiser hopes that you will transfer the person's good qualities to the product, and then to yourself. Example: A pretty woman in a beautiful dress sells cars.

3. *Bandwagon:* The ad pretends that everyone is using the product. It tries to get you to jump on the bandwagon with everyone else and buy the product. Example: An ad shows people in different parts of the country all drinking a type of cola.

4. *Humor:* The ad is funny, and the advertiser hopes that you remember feeling good when you see the product again. Example: An airline company exaggerates how uncomfortable it is to fly with other airlines.

5. *Statistics:* The ad uses numbers and figures to impress you, even though it may leave important information. Example: Eight of ten doctors recommend using a certain painkiller, but you never know who the doctors are or what choices they were given when they recommended it.

6. *Card Stacking:* The ad "stacks the cards" in favor of its product. It tells you only the good things about the product, not the bad. Example: An ad shows people enjoying chewing tobacco, but neglects to mention that chewing tobacco can cause cancer.

7. *Public Good:* The ad shows you all the good things its product does for the public but neglects to mention any harm it does to the public. Example: An oil company shows you that it uses a new way to detect oil without drilling, but it doesn't mention oil spills that have polluted beaches and killed birds.

8. *Appeal to the Senses:* The advertiser presents high-tech images and sounds, hoping that they make you feel good and think well of the product, even though you may know nothing about the product. Example: An advertisement for a stereo system shows fantastic scenes while someone listens to the system.

9. *Plain Folks:* The ad shows an interview of someone "off the street" who says he uses the product all the time. The ad wants you to think that the person represents everybody else, even though the person is a paid actor. Example: Someone with an Italian accent claims that the product—a tomato sauce—is better than homemade sauce.

10. *Catch Phrases:* The ad repeats a certain phrase, hoping that you will remember it when you are shopping and buy the product. The phrase may give you no information about the product, but you remember it because you have heard it so many times. Example: A bartender reminds people always to ask for the beer by name, and not just "any light beer."

Source: Here's Looking At You, 2000.

Focus groups conducted by the Comprehensive Health Education Foundation show that teens are greatly influenced by media and current news stories.[23] Children and adolescents are bombarded with ads for tobacco, alcohol, and OTC drugs. A key component of an ATOD curriculum must be the inclusion of lessons that address media literacy. Students must understand the persuasion techniques used by advertisers to sell their products. (See the FYI box.) Marketers, despite their denial of such tactics, often appeal to students' fear of not belonging or aspirations for sophistication.

They perpetuate the myth that only those who use their products will be accepted. The Amercian Academy of Pediatrics believes parents must help children distinguish between fact and fiction. For example, the fictions include the following: Alcohol use is a right of passage. Drinking alcohol is normal. Everybody's doing it. Alcohol is relaxing in social settings. The facts include the following: Someone dies in an alcohol-related car crash every 31 minutes. More than 43% of teenagers who began drinking before the age of 14 became alcoholics. Alcohol abuse by adults contributes to as many as 70% of child abuse cases.[24]

Trigger Films

Trigger films are short clips, lasting anywhere from 2 to 15 minutes, that incite discussion or reinforce skill building. They can be clips from television or movies that illustrate a key component of adolescent development. Trigger films may conclude with a question for the students to discuss, such as "What would you do if you were Mike's friend?" or participants may be asked to role play an ending to the problem presented in the video. Trigger films can be used to introduce a topic, reinforce a key concept, or evaluate the level of learning.

Step 5: Use Existing Resources

The curriculum committee should compile a list of existing resources in the school and community. Teachers often feel overwhelmed by time constraints for planning and teaching a variety of essential subjects. It is beneficial for students to have adequately trained facilitators. Curricula that provide in-service training (or professional development) for teachers will be taught more uniformly throughout the district. The selection committee can alleviate teachers' stress by providing ancillary resources. Teachers seldom feel they have the time to locate recommended external resources. If the selection committee believes a resource is important, it should provide the materials for classroom use.

Step 6: Evaluate and Compare Existing Curricula

The most important components of any curriculum are the philosophy, prevention model, content, mode of delivery, and assessment protocol. The U.S. Department of Education has suggested a number

[**Table 9.5**]

Factors to Be Considered When Selecting a Commercial Curriculum

Ease of use
Appropriate and clearly defined goals and objectives
Longevity and regular updating
Flexibility and adaptability to different teaching styles and needs
Completeness, timeliness, and accuracy of materials
Ability to be integrated with other subjects
Proven track record of success (if purchased from a publisher)
Readily available customer service (if purchased)
Cost-effectiveness (considering published materials plus training and other prevention program components)

Source: U.S. Department of Education, *Drug Prevention Curricula: A Guide to Selection and Implementation* (Washington, DC: Office of Educational Research and Improvement, 1988).

of other factors to be considered by the selection committee, which are listed in Table 9.5. In addition, Appendix A provides an evaluation process for curriculum selection. You may want to practice using this form with several different commercial curricula. If you are serving on a curriculum selection team, this evaluation tool or a similar format is beneficial as a starting point for discussion of the various curricula being considered for adoption.

Funds and existing resources are usually limited, so schools must make hard decisions about how best to use them. Decisions about whether to use a prepared curriculum or create a local curriculum are also influenced by a district's available money and time. Once a selection committee has chosen a curriculum, budgetary constraints should be considered, but a sound educational rationale rather than the budget should direct the selection process.

Science-Based Practices and Curricula

Science-based **best practices** are strategies, activities, or approaches that effectively delay or prevent ATOD use. These practices serve as the foundation for achieving success and accountability in prevention programs. A number of federal agencies publish their lists of best practices (e.g., the Office of Juvenile Justice and Delinquency Prevention's *Blueprints*). According to the National Clearinghouse for Alcohol and Drug Information, two questions are the starting point for selecting appropriate programs:

1. What sources and resources for science-based and best-practice programs are available in your content area?
2. How do the results of these programs and practices fit with your program's goals and objectives?

This section briefly reviews some nationally recognized commercially prepared school-based curricula. We start with two comprehensive health education curricula. These curricula differ from specific ATOD programs in that their focus is broader, in line with the coordinated school health effort. We include a variety of ATOD-specific curricula, with a primary focus on social skills development, resistance skills development, risk reduction, and protective enhancement. We include the DARE program because of its continued use in school settings and the developers' commitment to expanding its focus. In addition, the authors recognize that school climate approaches, community partnership approaches, and parent involvement approaches are equally as important.

Growing Healthy

Growing Healthy, also known as the School Health Curriculum Project or the Berkeley Project, began partly as an effort to address ATOD use by youth. This comprehensive health curriculum addresses health issues from a body systems approach. All health topics are integrated across the curriculum, and the multimedia resources facilitate an experiential approach to learning. The teaching materials include audiovisuals, models, workshop materials, and strategies to involve parents. Schools send a team of two classroom teachers per grade level, one principal, and one staff member for approximately 30 hours of intensive training. Ten major content areas are addressed at every grade level: growth and development; mental and emotional health; personal health; consumer health; personal safety and first aid; disease prevention and control; family life and health; nutrition; alcohol, tobacco, drugs, and other hazardous substances; and community and environmental health management. Research shows reduced ATOD use by ninth graders who received all or part of the curriculum.[25]

Teenage Health Teaching Modules

Teenage Health Teaching Modules (THTM) is a comprehensive health education curriculum for middle and high school students. THTM was developed by Education Development Center, Inc., to provide an organizing framework for adolescent health education. THTM originally consisted of 16 developmentally appropriate instructional modules and was founded on the concept of health tasks (physical, emotional, and social) that adolescents must perform to develop their full health potential. All modules are designed to develop skills in five areas: self-assessment, communication, decision making, health advocacy, and healthy self-management. Each "framing" module addresses a critical adolescent health issue and provides from 4 to 15 hours of instruction. Some modules are suitable for any grade between 6 and 12; others are recommended for either middle or high school. Sample module titles include "Health Is Basic," "Understanding Growth and Development," "Planning a Healthy Future," "Locating Health Resources," "Protecting Oneself and Others," and "Communication in Families."

A large-scale controlled study involving approximately 5,000 secondary students and 150 teachers, conducted by Macro Systems between 1986 and 1989, found that THTM contributed to self-reported reductions in drug use, alcohol consumption, and cigarette smoking among middle and secondary students. Also, teachers who were trained before using THTM felt more prepared and implemented the curriculum with greater fidelity than those who were not trained.[26]

Life Skills Training

Life Skills Training (LST) is a universal program designed to address a variety of risk and protective factors. It focuses on reducing pressure to smoke cigarettes, drink, or use drugs; developing personal competence to meet the challenges of adolescence; and practicing specific skills for resisting peer pressure.[27] The curriculum has three major components: drug resistance skills and information, self-management skills, and general social skills. LST consists of a 15-session Level 1 curriculum, a 10-session Level 2 curriculum, and a 5-session Level 3 curriculum. A one-day training session, although not mandatory, is available for classroom teachers. The teacher's manual is user friendly and easy to implement. Older peers (11th and 12th graders) receive intensive training to assist as instructors. Results of research studies found significantly lower smoking, alcohol, and marijuana use six years after the initial baseline assessment.

Project Alert

Project Alert is a prevention program for seventh and eighth graders that is designed to reach them before they start experimenting with alcohol, tobacco, and marijuana. The program, largely video based, places heavy emphasis on resistance skills. The videos portray real-life situations to which students respond in discussion and role play. There are 10 weekly lesson plans for seventh graders, and 3 additional booster sessions for eighth graders. A two-day teacher training session is required before a school can implement the program. Project Alert has been developed and tested over a 10-year period by the Rand Corporation and has demonstrated positive results in preventing cigarette and marijuana use in many school systems with both high- and low-risk students.

Quest

Skills for Adolescence is a curriculum for students in grades 6 through 8. Skills for Living was developed for students in grades 9 through 12. A youth development model, called Skills for Growing, was developed later for use in grades K through 5. These curricula are all included under the umbrella name

Quest. Quest is endorsed by Lions International, the American Association of School Administrators, and the National PTA. The curriculum consists of 80 lesson plans for a semester course. Materials include a student workbook, teacher training manual, and a notebook for student reflection. The lessons are designed to help students acquire competence in self-discipline, responsibility, good judgment, and the ability to get along with others. In addition, students perform community service as part of the curriculum. The parent component includes a book about adolescent development, *The Surprising Years*. A school/community team of four to eight members receives a three-day training program.

Adolescent Alcohol Prevention Trial

Adolescent Alcohol Prevention Trial (AAPT) is a universal classroom program designed for fifth-grade students, with booster sessions in seventh grade. The program uses a combination of resistance skills training and normative education. The program focuses on social and behavioral skills, correcting erroneous perceptions about peer use, and bonding to prosocial norms.

Seattle Social Development Project

The Seattle Project is a universal program for grades 1 through 6 that focuses on reducing risk factors and enhancing protective factors. The training program for teachers focuses on active classroom management, interactive teaching strategies, and cooperative learning. Long-term results indicate reductions in antisocial behavior, improved academic skills, greater commitment to school, reduced levels of alienation, better bonding to prosocial others, less misbehavior in school, and fewer incidents of drug use.

Project STAR

Project STAR (Support and Training for Assessing Results) is a universal program that encompasess the entire community population. The middle school–based component is a social influence curriculum designed for a two-year implementation cycle. Teachers are trained to implement the program. Students showed significantly less use of marijuana, alcohol, and cigarettes than adolescents who did not participate in the program.

Drug Abuse Resistance Education

The DARE curriculum is used extensively throughout the United States. On April 11, 2002, President George W. Bush proclaimed National D.A.R.E. Day and stated: "The Drug Abuse Resistance Education (D.A.R.E.) curriculum plays an important role in helping our young people understand the many reasons to avoid drugs."[28] The National School Board Association (a nationwide federation of school boards) has joined with DARE to reinforce the junior high and middle school curricula.

The DARE curriculum originated in 1983 as a collaborative effort between the Los Angeles Police Department and the Los Angeles Unified School District. This curriculum is taught by uniformed law enforcement officers who have had two weeks of training. The officers teach students resistance to peer pressure, self-management skills, and alternatives to drug use. The curriculum was initially taught to fifth- or sixth-grade students, depending on the exit year from elementary school. These sessions consisted of 15 weekly one-hour lessons. Research showed delayed onset of tobacco use in students trained with this DARE curriculum; however, long-term behavior change has been minimal.[29]

Recognizing a need for follow-up and a more comprehensive approach, developers expanded the program to serve students who are exiting from middle school (junior high school), using nine weekly one-hour lessons. Parental involvement is encouraged, particularly at the graduation session for fifth- and sixth-grade students. (See **Figure 9.11**.) The curriculum continues to be modified based on current research findings.

Summary

Health instruction is the foundation of the CSHP. The goals of instruction are to increase students' knowledge of health, develop appropriate attitudes toward healthy living, and practice healthy lifestyle choices. This instruction occurs by implementing a planned, sequential P–12 curriculum. A school and community curriculum team should evaluate

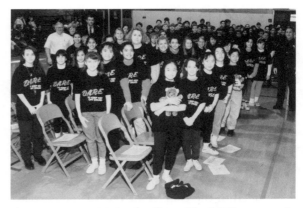

Figure 9.11 A DARE Graduation   The DARE program is one of the most widely used drug education curricula. (Photograph courtesy of Park View School District 70 sixth-grade class, Morton Grove, IL.)

curricula by science-based practices. Evaluation at the local level is an essential component of the instruction regardless of whether the curriculum showed promising results at the national level.

Scenario | Analysis and Response

Rick may want to begin the professional development presentation by reminding teachers of the heavy toll ATOD abuse has on children and adolescents. Next, he may want to review the reasons for using a science-based curriculum (bridge the gap between research and practice). Elementary teachers are the first line of the school's efforts to reduce ATOD use. They need to feel comfortable using interactive teaching methods in the classroom. Rick will want to involve them in a number of opportunities to practice using interactive methods. He can use science-based curricula lessons for the demonstrations. Can you prepare the presentation for Rick?

Learning Activities

1. Divide the class into groups of three to five students. Each group should receive two to three curriculum guides that cover a particular age group (early childhood, and elementary, middle, and high school). For example, Group 1 could receive copies of materials from Project Alert and THTM (middle school).

Group 2 could receive copies of materials from DARE and the Seattle Project (elementary students). Each group should use the evaluation form in Appendix A to compare and contrast the different curricula.

2. Using the guidelines provided in *Learning to Live Drug Free: A Curriculum Model for Prevention* or those at www.healthteacher. com, write several goals, objectives, and performance outcomes for a specific grade level.

3. Select one of the life-skills lesson plans provided in the chapter or one of the curriculum guides. With a group of three to five students, practice delivering the lesson. (Videotape your presentation, if possible.) Critique (reflect on) your own performance.

4. Review the curricula described as "best practices" at the following CSAP website: www.samhsa.gov/centers/csap/modelprograms/matrix.cfm?compare=yes. Compare model programs on the basis of a variety of factors such as cost, target setting, and key outcomes. What criteria are most important to you? What criteria would you use in the selection of a program?

Notes

1. American Public Health Association, "Education for Health in the Community Setting," *American Journal of Public Health*, (1975): 65. Statistics updated with data from the National Center for Education Statistics, http://www.ed. gov/ccd.

2. L. J. Kolbe, "Indicators for Planning and Monitoring School Health Programs," in *Health Promotion Indicators and Actions*, S. B. Kar, ed. (New York: Springer, 1989).

3. 1990 Joint Committee on Health Education Terminology, "Report of the 1990 Joint Committee on Health Education," *Journal of School Health*, 61 (August 1991): 251–254.

4. D. D. Allensworth and C. A. Wolford, *Achieving the 1990 Health Objectives for the Nation: Agenda for the Nation's Schools* (Bloomington, IN: Tichenor Publishing, 1988).

5. B. Benard, "Moving Toward a 'Just and Vital Culture': Multiculturalism in Our Schools," Western Center for Drug-Free Schools and Communities, Portland, Oregon, April 1991.

6. P. C. Scales, "The Centrality of Health Education to Developing Young Adolescents' Critical Thinking," *Journal of Health Education* (November/December Supplement, 1993).

7. P. M. Kingery, B. E. Pruitt, and R. S. Hurley, "Adolescent Exposure to School Health Education: Factors and Consequences," *Journal of Health Education* (November/ December Supplement, 1993).

8. 1990 Joint Committee on Health Education Terminology, "Report."

9. Centers for Disease Control and Prevention, "School Health Defined: Comprehensive Health Education Curriculum." Available: http://www.cdc.gov/nccdphp/dash/about/comprehensive_ed.htm. Accessed 17 March 2002.

10. Centers for Disease Control and Prevention, "School Health Policies and Programs Study: State-Level Summaries, School Health Policies and Practices." Available: http://www.cdc.gov/nccdphp/dash/shpps/summaries/index.htm. Accessed 17 March 2002.

11. B. S. Bloom et al., *Cognitive Domain*, bk. 1 of *Taxonomy of Educational Objectives: The Classification of Education Goals* (New York: David McKay Company, 1956); D. R. Krathwohl et al., *Affective Domain*, bk. 2 of *Taxonomy of Educational Objectives: The Classification of Education Goals* (New York: David McKay Company, 1964).

12. J. H. Mann, "Experimental Evaluations of Role Playing," *Psychological Bulletin*, 53 (1956): 227–234.

13. A. P. Goldstein et al., *Skill Streaming the Adolescent: A Structured Learning Approach to Teaching Prosocial Skills* (Champaign, IL: Research Press Company, 1980).

14. Ibid.

15. Ibid.

16. Ibid.

17. Ibid., 17.

18. W. Egginton, "Approaches to Cooperative Learning: Everyone Has a Part to Play," University of Louisville, *Cardinal Principles*, 4, 2 (Fall 1989).

19. G. Gerbner, "Stories That Hurt: Tobacco, Alcohol, and Other Drugs in the Mass Media," in *Youth and Drugs: Society's Mixed Messages*, H. Resnick, ed. OSAP Monograph 6, DHHS Publication No. (ADM) 90-1689 (Rockville, MD: DHHS, 1990).

20. Federal Trade Commission, "Cigarette Report for 1999 [issued 2001]." Available: http://www.ftc.gov/reports/cigarettes/1999cigarettereport.pdf. Accessed June 10, 2002.

21. Center for Science in the Public Interest, "Alcohol Advertising: Its Impact on Communities, and What Coalitions Can Do to Lessen That Impact," *Strategizer* 32. Available: http://www.cspinet.org/booze/Alcohol_Advertising.pdf. Accessed June 10, 2002.

22. G. Gerbner, "Stories That Hurt."

23. G. Tanaka, J. Warren, and L. Tritsch, "What's Real in Health Education?" *Journal of Health Education* (November/December Supplement, 1993).

24. American Academy of Pediatrics, "Alcohol Advertising: Fiction vs. Fact." Available: http://www.aap.org/advocacy/chm98fac.htm. Accessed June 10, 2002.

25. D. B. Connell, R. R. Turner, and E. F. Mason, "Summary of Findings of the School Health Education Evaluation: Health Promotion Effectiveness, Implementation, and Costs," *Journal of School Health*, 55, 8 (1985): 316–321.

26. M. T. Errecart et al., "Effectiveness of Teenage Health Teaching Modules," *Journal of School Health*, 61, 1 (1991): 26–30; R. S. Gold et al., "Summary and Conclusions of the THTM Evaluation: The Expert Work Group Perspective," *Journal of School Health*, 61, 1 (1991): 39–42.

27. G. Botvin, "Substance Abuse Prevention Efforts: Recent Developments and Future Directions," *Journal of School Health,* 56 (1986): 369–374.

28. George W. Bush, "National D.A.R.E. Day, 2002: A Proclamation." Available: http://www.dare.com/ NewsRoom/StoryPage.asp?N=NewsRoom&M=14&S=34&RecordID=15. Accessed June 20, 2002.

29. W. DeLong, "A Short-Term Evaluation of Project DARE: Preliminary Indicators of Effectiveness," *Journal of Drug Education,* 17 (1987): 279–294.

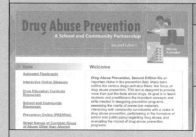

web resources

The Web site for this book offers many useful resources for educators, students, and professional counselors and is a great source for additional information. Visit the site at **http://healtheducation.jbpub.com/drugabuse/.**

Chapter Learning Objectives

Upon completion of this chapter, students will be able to:

1. Describe the process by which statutes are made.

2. Differentiate between regulatory and nonregulatory agencies.

3. Recognize the primary government agencies involved in demand-reduction programs.

4. Discuss aspects of the intent of law.

5. Compare the Drug-Free Schools and Community Act of 1986, the Safe and Drug-Free Schools and Community Act of 1994, and the Elementary and Secondary Education Act (the No Child Left Behind Act) of 2001.

6. Analyze the components of a local school ATOD policy.

7. Discuss students' legal protection against search and seizure.

8. Describe students' legal protection regarding suspension.

Scenario

Rashid, a middle school health teacher, has been nominated by the teachers of Western Middle School to serve on the school policy panel for Safe and Drug-Free Schools. The current administration wants to implement a drug-testing protocol for middle and high school student-athletes. Parents of the student-athletes are upset because their children are being targeted for participating in athletics. They believe all students should be randomly selected. Some parents and teachers are concerned that the cost of testing will take away valuable resources from other areas. What recommendations would you make if you were Rashid? What resources are available to Rashid?

Policy Issues in ATOD Education

Introduction

Schools actively and comfortably conduct **noncoercive** strategies such as direct instruction, and have begun to implement rigorous **coercive** strategies such as zero tolerance and drug testing. (See **Figure 10.1.**) Zero tolerance, a drug-free policy implemented in some schools, prohibits the use of tobacco and other drugs by students, faculty, and staff on school property. Drug testing of students, while proving to be controversial, has received approval from the Supreme Court. Previous chapters explored how a multiple-strategy approach is more effective than a single-focus approach in reducing ATOD use; similarly, a combination of noncoercive and coercive strategies is more effective than either used alone. Although classroom teachers traditionally provide limited input into school **policy**, they realize that policy can be a powerful deterrent to alcohol, tobacco, and other drug use. Teachers can play a major role in helping their school and community reduce ATOD use by taking an active role in policymaking.

Classroom teachers, school administrators, and other school personnel must understand the role coercive strategies play in ATOD prevention. When evaluating the effectiveness and breadth of their policy and its effect on the school environment, school personnel need to ask the following questions: Is the school a safe environment that is free from violence, harassment, and other destructive behaviors? Are students encouraged to achieve to their highest level? Do students have dreams and aspirations for continuing their learning, for choosing a career, and for attaining a comfortable lifestyle? Policy is a key component for ensuring that students reach their goals within the school, community, state, and nation.

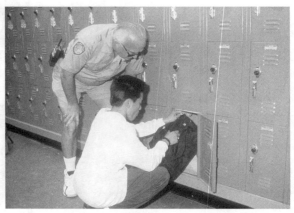

Figure 10.1 **A Police Officer Searches a School for Drugs** Coercive policies can aid drug abuse prevention and the overall educational mission of schools.

(© David Young-Wolff/PhotoEdit)

The impact of policy should not be underestimated. For classroom teachers, policy enforcement keeps the classroom safe and consistent. For example, children and adolescents constantly test the limits of classroom rules, which is one way they learn about consequences for their actions. Crossing boundaries or breaking rules means accepting the consequences that follow. Effective discipline requires clear rules and administrative and parental support for enforcement of those rules. If contradictory messages are given by any of the providers, students may try to test the limits even more. Clearly defined and consistent enforcement of policies and **regulations** ensures the maintenance of a stable, safe classroom environment. The final report by the National Commission on Drug-Free Schools states:

> Policies form the foundation for a disciplined, safe school environment. Policies send an explicit message about the rules of the school and an implicit message about the rules of society. The best school policies are clear, direct, firmly and consistently applied, and perceived as fair and appropriate by students and staff. The most promising drug prevention program is undermined if school policies are not consistent with the program.[1]

This chapter discusses some important current laws, regulations, and policies that affect ATOD prevention in schools and communities. School personnel do not need a complete understanding of federal, state, and local statutes, regulations, and other procedural policy. However, some knowledge of policy issues will help them understand how to effect change and evaluate the current school policy and understand how they are affected directly and indirectly by school laws, regulations, and policy. This chapter provides a brief overview of national, state, and local school and community laws, regulations, and policies.

A Review of U.S. Governmental Structure

Living in a democracy, U.S. citizens view individual freedom as one of the cornerstones of their heritage, yet the laws we abide by to maintain a civil society are numerous, complex, and often seem unfair. As pointed out in the introduction to this chapter, laws are coercive strategies designed to punish and protect as well as to set up codes of desirable behaviors.

We have all been taught the basic structure of the U.S. government's branches, but many of us have not been taught how laws are made, particularly as they apply to schools. This section reviews the role of governmental branches regarding the law and discusses some of the ATOD laws of importance to teachers and school administrators.

The Branches of Government

The legislative, executive, and judicial branches of federal government were created in the U.S. Constitution in Articles I, II, and III. Article I states: "All legislative Powers herein granted shall be vested in a congress of the United States, which shall consist of a Senate and House of Representatives."[2]

From this starting point, Article I determines how a bill becomes law and enumerates the specific powers of Congress.[3] In other words, Congress can make and repeal laws that are binding on all citizens. The laws of Congress are compiled in the U.S. Code, and a particular law is referred to as a **statute**.

Article II establishes the executive branch and states in part: "The executive Power shall be vested in a President of the United States of America."[4]

Undoubtedly, the president has a great deal of power and authority, yet a close reading of Article II reveals that the president's ability to *create* law is very limited. The president's role in the area of law and policy is nevertheless important. The president's personal views shape the mood of the citizenry and affect the election of members of Congress (who make laws). The president is also responsible for appointing many people to positions of power.

The executive branch controls the federal agencies, such as the Department of Education and the Department of Health and Human Services. Federal agencies have become increasingly powerful over the past several decades, with the power to create rules and regulations that have the force and effect of any other law.

Article III addresses the judicial branch. The U.S. Supreme Court is the only court created in the Constitution. Congress is given power to establish other inferior courts as necessary, which it has done to create our current federal court system.

Early in the history of the United States, the Supreme Court delineated its role in deciding the rights of individuals, with the Constitution as the paramount law. Thus, by interpreting the Constitution and other laws, the courts create, in effect, "judge-made" law. A good example of a judge-made law is that which resulted from *Brown v. Board of Education of Topeka*, 347 U.S. 483 (1954), wherein the Supreme Court found segregated education to be unconstitutional. There was no written law governing segregated education at the time of the Brown decision, but the Court's decision essentially outlawed segregated schools.

An example of how courts can affect drug use can be found in *United States v. Oakland Cannabis Buyers' Cooperative*, 532 U.S. 483 (2001). This case held that because marijuana is a schedule I controlled substance under the Controlled Substances Act, there was no "medical necessity" exception to the act available to the cooperative. The cooperative distributed marijuana to qualified patients for medical purposes. The Supreme Court stated that in the Controlled Substances Act, Congress had determined that marijuana had no medical benefits and no currently accepted medical use. Therefore, the courts could not broaden the clear language of the legislation. The *Oakland* case will most likely affect the laws of some states that allow the use of marijuana for medicinal purposes, since state laws cannot override federal laws. In some instances, Congress responds to Supreme Court decisions concerning particular laws by amending, repealing, or passing legislation to change the impact of the law in question.

As shown by these cases, courts have a significant role in shaping the rules of society and, consequently, our schools. What recent decision by the Supreme Court might affect Western Middle School's decision regarding drug testing of students?

State Governments

Powers not delegated to the federal government by the Constitution are given to the states expressly by the 10th Amendment to the Constitution. The role of individual states in making and implementing law and policy concerning schools, drug use, and other issues is extremely broad and very important. Teachers need to know that state governments generally mirror the federal government in structure: a state constitution and three branches of government, plus agencies for the implementation of laws. Each state has different laws and procedures, so teachers should familiarize themselves with the laws of their particular state.

Although the federal government is responsible for funding and developing many programs that affect schools, implementation of such programs is often accomplished by state agencies or at the local level.

The Important Role of Agencies

Administrative agencies exist at both the state and federal levels. Although it is not necessarily important for educators to know how agencies are created or how they operate, it is important to understand the broad-based powers vested in them. In American government, agencies have executive, legislative, and judicial powers, and their actions affect our lives in ways most people would never suspect.

Two Types of Agencies

Agencies can be regulatory or nonregulatory. **Regulatory agencies** have authority to regulate the economic activities of individuals and businesses; these agencies can restrict the actions of persons and mandate actions in certain situations. As such, these agencies shape behavior and therefore affect policy, but their actions tend to be coercive in nature. Examples of federal regulatory agencies include the Interstate Commerce Commission, the National Labor Relations Board, and the Securities and Exchange Commission.

Educators are generally more interested in the activities of **nonregulatory agencies**, particularly those that promote social and economic welfare. On the national level, agencies increasingly are used to further social and ethical policies and goals. While these agencies also have the power to make rules and regulations that have an impact on behavior (e.g., the Equal Employment Opportunity Commission [EEOC]), they are also responsible for dispersing substantial sums of money for programs that promote particular goals, such as the prevention of drug abuse among school children.

Public policy is widely shaped by the actions of federal agencies such as the Department of Education, the Department of Health and Human Services, the Department of Justice, and others. The next subsection presents some federal agencies and discusses what contribution they make to ATOD abuse prevention.

Federal Agencies Involved in ATOD Prevention

Nearly 50 federal agencies are involved in the drug control effort, and most are engaged in demand-reduction programs. These agencies include the following:

- Department of Health and Human Services
- Department of Transportation
- Department of Justice
- Department of the Treasury
- Department of Education
- Department of Labor
- Department of Housing and Urban Development
- Department of Veteran Affairs
- Department of the Interior
- Department of Defense

Administration for Children and Families

The Administration for Children and Families (ACF) promotes services and programs to support the economic and social well-being of children, families, individuals, and communities. The ACF provides direct services and assistance; it also conducts research, collects and analyzes data, publishes various reports, and develops the Annual Government Performance and Results Act (GPRA) Plan. The ACF provides grants to community-based public and private agencies for services to runaway and homeless youth and their families. The National Runaway Switchboard has a toll-free number: 1-800-621-4000.

Administration for Native Americans

The Administration for Native Americans (ANA) promotes the economic and social self-sufficiency of American Indians, native Alaskans, and native Hawaiians through the provision of grants, training, and technical assistance. Its efforts include prevention efforts targeting this population. ANA is the only federal agency serving all Native Americans.

Centers for Disease Control and Prevention

The Centers for Disease Control and Prevention (CDC) is the federal agency charged with protecting the nation's health. Through its Planned Approach to Community Health (PATCH) program, the CDC works with state and local health departments and community members to organize local intervention programs. The CDC provides materials and technical assistance, and communities invest time and resources to make the programs work. PATCH programs have focused on such areas as smoking cessation and alcohol problems.

Center for Substance Abuse Prevention

The mission of the Center for Substance Abuse Prevention (CSAP) is to decrease substance use and

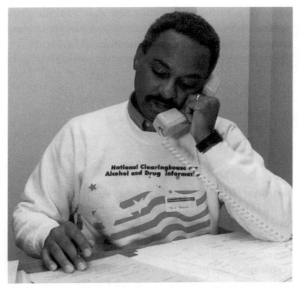

Figure 10.2 The National Clearinghouse for Alcohol and Drug Information Is Sponsored by the Center for Substance Abuse Prevention

(Photograph courtesy of National Clearinghouse for Alcohol and Drug Information. For information contact 1-800-729-6686.)

abuse by bringing effective prevention to every community. It is the sole federal organization with responsibility for improving the accessibility and quality of substance abuse prevention services. CSAP provides leadership in developing policies, programs, and services to prevent the onset of illegal drug use and underage alcohol and tobacco use, and to reduce the negative outcomes of using ATOD. (See **Figure 10.2.**)

Department of Defense

The Department of Defense (DOD) implements prevention and education efforts worldwide through education, training, and public service announcements on Armed Forces radio and television, posters, and pamphlets.

Department of Education

The Department of Education (DOE) provides the largest block of federal funds devoted to the prevention of alcohol and other drug problems. Title IV of the Elementary and Secondary Education

Act as reauthorized by the No Child Left Behind Act of 2001 authorizes the Safe and Drug-Free Schools and Communities program.

The Safe and Drug-Free Schools program consists of two major components: state grants for drug and violence prevention programs, and national programs. Among the initiatives are direct grants to school districts and communities with severe drug and violence problems, evaluation of programs, and dissemination of information.

Department of Housing and Urban Development

The Department of Housing and Urban Development (HUD) operates the HUD Drug Information and Strategy Clearinghouse, which deals specifically with alcohol and other drug problems in public housing projects. HUD established the Office of HIV/AIDS to manage the Housing Opportunities for Persons with AIDS (HOPWA) program. Other programs include homeless assistance programs, programs for persons with disabilities, and the HOME Initiative. Youthbuild provides grants to assist high-risk youth between the ages of 16 and 24 to learn housing construction skills and complete high school.

Department of Justice

The Department of Justice forms partnerships with state and local governments to help policymakers, practitioners, and citizens understand what crime costs in terms of public safety and the social and economic health of communities. It awards formula grants to states and to specific crime prevention programs.

The Office of Juvenile Justice and Delinquency Prevention (OJJDP) within the Department of Justice provides national leadership, coordination, and resources to prevent and respond to juvenile delinquency and victimization. The OJJDP supports states and local communities in their efforts to develop and implement effective and coordinated prevention and intervention programs.

Department of Labor

Through the Substance Abuse Information Database (SAID), the U.S. Department of Labor provides employers, and those organizations that work with employers, with information that assists them in developing workplace substance abuse programs. The Department of Labor provides information related to federal and state legislation, as well as information on studies and surveys on how drugs and alcohol affect the workplace.

Department of Veterans Affairs

Formerly the Veterans Administration, the Department of Veterans Affairs (VA) became a cabinet-level department in March 1984. The primary mission of the VA with regard to alcohol and other drug problems is to provide treatment services to eligible veterans with dependence disorders. Because of the VA's treatment focus, prevention activities are mainly secondary and tertiary. Most treatment programs, offered through academic affiliates and community outreach activities, also involve primary prevention.

Drug Enforcement Administration

The Drug Enforcement Administration (DEA) is responsible for enforcing federal drug laws and regulations. It conducts prevention programs in conjunction with numerous national organizations, including the National High School Athletic Coaches Association, the Ladies Professional Golf Association, the National Youth Sports Coaches Association, and the Boy Scouts of America. The DEA also develops and distributes a variety of publications and videos on prevention.

Federal Bureau of Investigation

The Federal Bureau of Investigation (FBI) is the lead federal investigative agency within the Department of Justice. In addition to other prevention activities, the FBI disseminates drug demand-reduction materials to appropriate organizations, makes public presentations on drug awareness, and works closely with demand-reduction specialists of other organizations. The FBI headquarters and field offices work with citizens across the country who are actively involved in drug prevention and education efforts.

Indian Health Service

The Alcoholism and Substance Abuse Program Branch of the Indian Health Service (IHS) has initiated a number of programs that provide prevention services to members of American Indian and native Alaskan communities. IHS funds 34 Indian health organizations that provide outreach and referral services, including alcohol and drug abuse prevention, education, and treatment; AIDS and sexually transmitted disease education and prevention services; mental health services; nutrition education and counseling services; and health education.

National Highway Traffic Safety Administration

A major focus of the National Highway Traffic Safety Administration (NHTSA) is the prevention of impaired driving. NHTSA is responsible for reducing deaths, injuries, and economic losses resulting from motor vehicle crashes. The NHTSA provides resources to state and community law enforcement agencies, as well as impaired driving programs, and has developed a range of prevention publications.

National Institute on Drug Abuse

The National Institute on Drug Abuse (NIDA) is the lead federal agency for drug abuse research. NIDA's mission is to bring the power of science to bear on drug abuse and addiction. Its charge has two critical components: to provide strategic support and conduct of research, and to ensure rapid and effective dissemination of research results to improve prevention, treatment, and policy.

Office of Personnel Management

The Office of Personnel Management (OPM) is an independent agency in the executive branch that oversees and regulates matters pertaining to the management of civil service personnel. OPM's primary function related to alcohol and other drug prevention focuses on workplace employee assistance programs. OPM provides regulatory and policy guidance in the *Code of Federal Regulations*; the *Federal Personnel Manual*; and through publications, conferences, and seminars regarding employee assistance programs (EAPs) for federal civilian employees. Additionally, OPM is required to report annually to Congress on programs to prevent problems for federal civilian employees.

Substance Abuse and Mental Health Services Administration

The Substance Abuse and Mental Health Services Administration (SAMHSA) administers service-related programs for alcohol, other drug, and mental health problems. SAMHSA's focus is on prevention, intervention, and treatment services, and its primary role is to coordinate the delivery of these services to health professionals and the general public.

U.S. Coast Guard

The U.S. Coast Guard (USCG) is a branch of the Armed Forces and an agency of the Department of Transportation. (See **Figure 10.3**.) Preventing drug smuggling into the United States is one of the Coast Guard's highest priorities, and it is expanding its educational programs in this area. The USCG also develops and directs a national boating safety program that encourages recreational boaters to avoid alcohol and other drugs. The five strategic goals of the USCG are maritime safety, maritime mobility, maritime security, national defense, and protection of natural resources.

White House Office of National Drug Control Policy

The Office of National Drug Control Policy (ONDCP) is a component of the executive office of the president. It was established by the Anti-Drug Abuse Act of 1988. The ONDCP establishes policies, priorities, and objectives for the nation's drug control program. The director of the ONDCP (the drug czar) is charged with producing the National Drug Control Strategy, which establishes a program, a budget, and guidelines for cooperation among federal, state, and local entities.

State and Local Agencies

Just as states mirror the federal government with three branches of government, so state agencies have responsibilities much like federal agencies. State agencies may regulate everything from highways to school curricula, and though they must operate within the constitutional framework (not unlike federal agencies), their power is still very broad.

The most significant local agency for education is probably the board of education or a similar body. A board of education is often responsible for making policy that directly affects the conduct of students, teachers, and administrators. Local boards also can direct policy by emphasizing particular programs over others. For example, if a local board is concerned about ATOD abuse among students, it may give incentives for teachers to develop programs to combat abuse or encourage administrators to try to secure state or federal funding. The local board's role and its impact on policy should not be underestimated. Without local support, it is futile to seek help from state or federal agencies to effect change.

Some Important Laws

This section gives some examples of how the federal government attempts to affect ATOD use and abuse in schools and local communities. This overview does not detail the entire scope of ATOD law and policy, but instead is included to give educators an idea of (1) the process of law making and implementation and (2) the issues identified by the government as important in the fight against ATOD abuse.

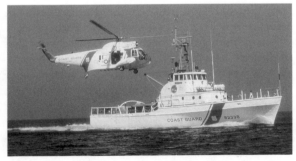

Figure 10.3 A Coast Guard Boat Patrols for Illegal Drug Smuggling The U.S. Coast Guard has the responsibility of restricting the flow of drugs by boat into the country. (© Michael Newman/PhotoEdit)

Additionally, a review of these laws and regulations provides a good basis for discussion about whether the government's actions are indeed affecting ATOD abuse. Many people take the position that these laws do little to solve the ATOD dilemma and are merely political "fluff." Others believe that the government is doing all it can because ATOD issues must be addressed at the local level or within the family structure. Whatever your position, it is important to look behind the mere words of a law and try to discover its intent. Laws generally arise out of society's demand for change or control.

It is also important to remember that law is not static; the statutes and regulations identified here may change. It is extremely important to seek out resources that include the most current laws. While it is not necessary to know how to perform legal research, it is important to identify sources of help and expertise in your area to keep abreast of changes in the law.

The relatively straightforward federal statute found in the FYI box provides a good example of Congress's methods for ensuring compliance with ATOD prevention laws. Subpart (a) of this legislation threatens to withhold all federal monies if an institution is in noncompliance; this threat is probably the most coercive action imaginable for state-supported colleges and universities. Therefore, the "enforcement" of this law lies primarily in its threat of lost federal funds.

This statute also demonstrates the broad roles of federal agencies. Note that all subsections make reference to the "Secretary," which refers to the Secretary of Education, head of the federal Department of Education. In its broadest sense, the DOE acts as the police (compliance), judge (interpretation by the publication of regulations), and jury (determination of compliance or noncompliance). Giving such broad power to an agency is common in our current governmental structure. A familiarity with the workings of federal, state, and local agencies is imperative to understanding the scope of the rules that affect education.

Now we turn to how the legislation is actually implemented. Do you see this law at work at your college or university? Some universities comply with this law by distributing assorted printed materials during class registration; these materials are most likely discarded immediately. For these institutions, compliance with the law does little to affect drug and alcohol abuse on college campuses. Other universities use this law as an opportunity to have an impact on ATOD abuse on their campus. They take a comprehensive approach to implementation that includes peer-led programs; stringent policies regarding ATOD use on campus; enforcement of the existing policies; support groups for students, faculty, and staff who are addicted; support groups for those living with someone who is addicted; support groups for those who grew up with someone who is addicted; and screening of promotional materials prepared by advertisers and sponsors of student events. Again, what is the intent of this legislation? What goals did Congress have in mind? Does this law accomplish those goals at your institution?

Those who are skeptical of the impact of such laws as the Federal Guidelines on Drug and Alcohol Abuse Prevention in Higher Education should remember that the laws set *minimum* standards for action or behavior. Thus, the problem may not be with the actual legislation but rather with the institutions that are content with minimal compliance and, in fact, seek to circumvent the intent of the law. In general, policy sets limits of acceptable and unacceptable behavior, dictates how individuals are held accountable, and guides how rules and regulations are communicated. If drug and alcohol abuse is a problem on our campuses, who should be most responsible for addressing the problem? Should Congress or the Department of Education bear such responsibility? Perhaps university administrators need to reevaluate what can be done at the local level, not simply to comply with the law but to go beyond and create programs and methods that seriously address such problems.

Drug-Free Schools and Communities Acts

The Drug-Free Schools and Communities Act of 1986 was part of comprehensive federal legislation known as the Anti-Drug Abuse Act. Many provisions of this act did not actually become effective until 1988. Unlike some other laws, Congress

Federal Guidelines on Drug and Alcohol Abuse Prevention in Higher Education

a. Notwithstanding any other provision of law, no institution of higher education shall be eligible to receive funds or any other form of financial assistance under any Federal program, including participation in any federally funded or guaranteed student loan program, unless it certifies to the Secretary that it has adopted and has implemented a program to prevent the use of illicit drugs and the abuse of alcohol by students and employees that, at a minimum, includes—

1. The annual distribution to each student and employee of—
   A. standards of conduct that clearly prohibit, at a minimum, the unlawful possession, use, or distribution of illicit drugs and alcohol by students and employees on its property or as part of any of its activities;
   B. a description of the applicable legal sanctions under local, State, or Federal law for the unlawful possession or distribution of illicit drugs and alcohol;
   C. a description of the health risks associated with the use of illicit drugs and the abuse of alcohol;
   D. a description of any drug or alcohol counseling, treatment, or rehabilitation or reentry programs that are available to employees or students; and
   E. a clear statement that the institution will impose sanctions on students and employees (consistent with local, State, and Federal law), and a description of those sanctions, up to and including expulsion or termination of employment and referral for prosecution, for violations of the standards of conduct required by paragraph (1) (A); and
2. A biennial review by the institution of its program to
   A. determine its effectiveness and implement changes to the program if they are needed; and
   B. ensure that the sanctions required by paragraph (1) (E) are consistently enforced.

b. Each institution of higher education that provides the certification required by subsection (a) shall, upon request, make available to the Secretary and to the public a copy of each item required by subsection (a) (1) as well as the results of the biennial review required by subsection (a) (2).

c.
1. The Secretary shall publish regulations to implement and enforce the provisions of this section, including regulations that provide for—
   A. the periodic review of a representative sample of programs required by subsection (a); and
   B. a range of responses and sanctions for institutions of higher education that fail to implement their programs or to consistently enforce their sanctions, including information and technical assistance, the development of a compliance agreement, and the termination of any form of Federal financial assistance.
2. The sanctions required by subsection (a) (1) (E) may include the completion of an appropriate rehabilitation program.

d. Upon determination by the Secretary to terminate financial assistance to any institution of higher education under this section, the institution may file an appeal with an administrative law judge before the expiration of the 30-day period beginning on the date such institution is notified of the decision to terminate financial assistance under this section. Such judge shall hold a hearing with respect to such termination of assistance before the expiration of the 45-day period beginning on the date that such appeal is filed. Such judge may extend such 45-day period upon a motion by the institution concerned. The decision of the judge with respect to such termination shall be considered to be a final agency action.

Source: *U.S. Code*, vol. 20, sec. 1445g (1986).

The Drug-Free Schools and Communities Act of 1986

Findings

The Congress finds that:

1. Drug abuse education and prevention programs are essential components of a comprehensive strategy to reduce the demands for and use of drugs throughout the Nation.

2. Drug use and alcohol abuse are widespread among the Nation's students, not only in secondary schools, but increasingly in elementary schools as well.

3. The use of drugs and the abuse of alcohol by students constitute a grave threat to their physical and mental well-being and significantly impede the learning process.

4. The tragic consequences of drug use and alcohol abuse by students are felt not only by students and their families, but also by their communities and the Nation, which can ill afford to lose their skills, talents, and vitality.

5. Schools and local organizations in communities throughout the Nation have special responsibilities to work together to combat the scourge of drug use and alcohol abuse.

6. Prompt action by our Nation's schools, families, and communities can bring significantly closer the goal of a drug-free generation and a drug-free society.

Purpose

It is the purpose of this title [20 USCS §§3171 et seq.] to establish programs of drug abuse education and prevention (coordinated with related community efforts and resources) through the provision of Federal financial assistance—

1. to States for grants to local and intermediate educational agencies and consortia to establish, operate, and improve local programs of drug abuse prevention, early intervention, rehabilitation referral, and education in elementary and secondary schools (including intermediate and junior high schools);

2. to States for grants to and contracts with community-based organizations for programs of drug abuse prevention, early intervention, rehabilitation referral, and education for school dropouts and other high-risk youth;

3. to States for development, training, technical assistance, and coordination activities;

4. to institutions of higher education to establish, implement, and expand programs of drug abuse education and prevention (including rehabilitation referral) for students enrolled in colleges and universities; and

5. to institutions of higher education in cooperation with State and local educational agencies for teacher training programs in drug abuse education and prevention.

Source: *U.S. Code*, vol. 20, Secs. 3172–3173 (1986).

clearly identified the findings and purposes of this act, as shown in the FYI box.

Note that Congress identified drug abuse education and prevention programs as "essential components" of a "comprehensive strategy" to decrease ATOD abuse. Further, Congress identified schools as having "special responsibilities" to "combat the scourge of drug use and alcohol abuse." Such language showed that Congress indeed viewed the

issue of preventing ATOD abuse as the proverbial "war on drugs." However, strong language alone is not necessarily indicative of the law's effectiveness.

The purpose of the act, "to establish programs of drug abuse education and prevention through the provision of Federal financial assistance," tells how Congress intended to fight ATOD abuse—by providing money to states, colleges, and universities. Congress appropriated $350 million in 1989 to carry out the program portion of the act, and stipulated further provision for increased funding in subsequent years. Another $16 million was appropriated to train elementary and secondary teachers in ATOD abuse education and prevention.

Nearly eight years later, Congress enacted the Safe and Drug-Free Schools and Communities Act of 1994. The FYI box identifies the findings and purpose of the 1994 act. Funding appropriations for fiscal year 1995 were $630,000,000.

In 2001, Congress amended Title IV of the Elementary and Secondary Education Act to read as follows: 21st Century Schools—Part A, Safe and Drug-Free Schools and Communities; Part B, 21st Century Community Learning Centers; and Part C, Environmental Tobacco Smoke. The entire No Child Left Behind Act can be viewed at www.ed.gov/offices/OESE/asst.html. The FYI box entitled "21st Century Schools" identifies the purpose of the Safe and Drug-Free Schools and Communities section of this act. Authorization for appropriations for fiscal year 2002 was $650,000,000 for both state grants under subpart 1 and national programs under subpart 2.

The Role of the Department of Education

How are appropriated funds for ATOD education stipulated in an act distributed? The Department of Education is given this responsibility. Awards are given as grants, with the criteria established by the Secretary of the Department of Education. The Secretary's rules for grant applications are spelled out in the *Code of Federal Regulations* (CFR), which is a compilation of the rules and regulations of all federal agencies. Whereas Congress enacts legislation such as the No Child Left Behind Act, the Department of Education implements the law. Viewed from another perspective, Congress generally drafts broad statements and then allows the implementing agency to write specific rules and regulations. Therefore, educators should realize that knowing the particulars of actual legislation is usually not as important as gaining knowledge and a working understanding of the specific rules and regulations promulgated by the agency. It may not even be necessary for educators to know specific rules and regulations if resource personnel are available in the school or community to keep educators updated on changes in the law and opportunities for funding.

Further Policy Considerations

As just discussed, the government attempts to affect ATOD abuse through coercive means, such as withholding funding. Another coercive action is to enact state and federal criminal laws that penalize ATOD abuse. Imposing stricter penalties for possessing or selling drugs close to or on school grounds is another way legislators send the message that ATOD abuse and use in and around schools is a special concern. The government also attempts to affect the ATOD problem by allocating massive funds for state and local prevention programs.

Although it seems apparent that the government is concerned about ATOD abuse, problems continue to plague our schools. Are coercive deterrents such as criminal penalties effective? Has the coercive threat of discontinued funding made colleges and universities develop more effective ATOD prevention programs? Does a large monetary grant directly affect ATOD issues in our schools? These questions can be accurately answered "yes," "no," and "maybe," respectively. In some regions, these deterrents, coupled with funded prevention programs, work very well; other areas do not have such positive results. How, then, should ATOD policy be developed to achieve the most effective results, and who should develop it? Views are widely divergent on these issues.

School Boards and Administrators

One area that cannot be overlooked is the effort expended at the local level, because actions at this level affect the larger environment. For example, state and national organizations often are made up of local chapters, county governments are linked to state and national governments, individual churches are linked to national and sometimes international bodies, and many local television stations are affiliates of networks. In fact, it is almost impossible to be active and influential at the local level without affecting the broader environment. Prevention workers must remind the community

The Safe and Drug-Free Schools and Communities Act of 1994
Findings

The Congress finds as follows:

1. The seventh National Education Goal provides that by the year 2000, all schools in America will be free of drugs and violence and the unauthorized presence of firearms and alcohol, and offer a disciplined environment that is conducive to learning.

2. The widespread illegal use of alcohol and other drugs among the Nation's secondary school students, and increasingly by students in elementary schools as well, constitutes a grave threat to such students' physical and mental well-being, and significantly impedes the learning process. For example, data show that students who drink tend to receive lower grades and are more likely to miss school because of illness than students who do not drink.

3. Our Nation's schools and communities are increasingly plagued by violence and crime. Approximately 3,000,000 thefts and violent crimes occur in or near our Nation's schools every year, the equivalent of more than 16,000 incidents per school day.

4. Violence that is linked to prejudice and intolerance victimizes entire communities leading to more violence and discrimination.

5. The tragic consequences of violence and the illegal use of alcohol and drugs by students are felt not only by students and such students' families, but by such students' communities and the Nation, which can ill afford to lose such students' skills, talents, and vitality.

6. While use of illegal drugs is a serious problem among a minority of teenagers, alcohol use is far more widespread. The proportion of high school students using alcohol, though lower than a decade ago, remains unacceptably high. By the 8th grade, 70 percent of youth report having tried alcohol and by the 12th grade, about 88 percent have used alcohol. Alcohol use by young people can and does have adverse consequences for users, their families, communities, schools, and colleges.

7. Alcohol and tobacco are widely used by young people. Such use can, and does, have adverse consequences for young people, their families, communities, schools, and colleges. Drug prevention programs for youth that address only controlled drugs send an erroneous message that alcohol and tobacco do not present significant problems, or that society is willing to overlook their use. To be credible, messages opposing illegal drug use by youth should address alcohol and tobacco as well.

8. Every day approximately 3,000 students start smoking. Thirty percent of all secondary school seniors are smokers. Half of all new smokers begin smoking before the age of 14, 90 percent of such smokers begin before the age of 21, and the average age of the first use of smokeless tobacco is under the age of 10. Use of tobacco products has been linked to serious health problems. Drug education and prevention programs that include tobacco have been effective in reducing teenage use of tobacco.

9. Drug and violence prevention programs are essential components of a comprehensive strategy to promote school safety and to reduce the demand for and use of drugs throughout the Nation. Schools and local organizations in communities throughout the Nation have a special responsibility to work together to combat the growing epidemic of violence and illegal drug use and should measure the success of their programs against clearly defined goals and objectives.

10. Students must take greater responsibility for their own well-being, health, and safety if schools and communities are to achieve the goals of providing a safe, disciplined, and drug-free learning environment.

of the axiom "The individual makes a difference," particularly when the individual is a member of an interest group. School boards and administrators set the tone for the ATOD policy adopted at their school. Local policy issues and some sample school policies are discussed in the next section.

Components of a Local Policy

The local school board is responsibile for developing and implementing local school policies and enforcing the intent of national, state, and local regulations and guidelines. The effectiveness of a local ATOD policy depends on its comprehensiveness and administrative support.

The final report by the National Commission on Drug-Free Schools found the following.

Although most schools have policies on the use, possession, and distribution of drugs at school, these policies are not always effective because they:

- Are not enforced consistently [see Figure 10.4];
- Do not apply beyond the school day or building;
- Ignore the possession or use of tobacco; and
- Are not reinforced by parents and the community.

Many schools and colleges treat violations of law merely as violations of school policy and do not refer them to local police.

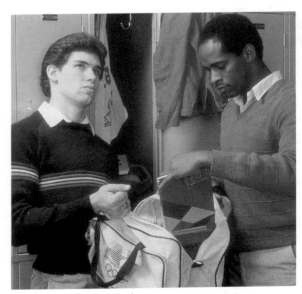

Figure 10.4 **A Teacher Searches a Student's Backpack** Many teachers do not enjoy enforcing school drug policies. (© Richard Hutchings/PhotoEdit)

21st Century Schools: Safe and Drug-Free Schools and Communities

The purpose of this part is to support programs that prevent violence in and around schools; that prevent the illegal use of alcohol, tobacco, and drugs; that involve parents and communities; and that are coordinated with related Federal, State, school, and community efforts and resources to foster a safe and drug-free learning environment that supports student academic achievement, through the provision of Federal assistance to—

1. States for grants to local educational agencies and consortia of such agencies to establish, operate, and improve local programs of school drug and violence prevention and early intervention;

2. States for grants to, and contracts with, community-based organizations and public and private entities for programs of drug and violence prevention and early intervention, including community-wide drug and violence prevention planning and organizing activities;

3. States for development, training, technical assistance, and coordination activities; and

4. public and private entities to provide technical assistance; conduct training, demonstrations, and evaluation; and to provide supplementary services and community-wide drug and violence prevention planning and organizing activities for the prevention of drug use and violence among students and youth.

The National Commission on Drug-Free Schools made six recommendations to local communities regarding ATOD policies. These recommendations are as follows:

All schools should build upon existing law and develop comprehensive policies on the possession, use, distribution, promotion, and sale of drugs, including alcohol and tobacco; specify sanctions for policy violations; and provide all students and parents copies of policies.

Colleges should develop and enforce policies that prohibit the use of all illegal drugs.

Local police departments should work with schools and colleges to develop and enforce school and college policies on drugs, including alcohol and tobacco.

Parents should work with schools and colleges to develop and enforce drug policies.

The Department of Education should monitor closely the development and enforcement of school and college antidrug policies.

All private-sector employers should enforce legal alcohol and tobacco policies on the job for employees under age 21.[6]

A local policy may include procedures and recommendations for classroom instruction, teacher training, parent training, a student assistance program, peer educators, school environment (including search and seizure and student expulsion), and an employee assistance program.

School Environment

A school policy should carry a clear message that ATOD use, possession, or distribution will not be tolerated. Provisions for search and seizure (discussed in a later section) should be stated clearly. A very important component of any policy is the procedure for informing students, staff, and teachers of existing policy and policy changes. Parents, students, and school personnel should be aware of the procedures and protocol for addressing ATOD issues. In many schools comprehensive policies have been established, but only administrators and school board members are aware of them. A policy should spell out the process for notifying all parties who may be affected by its contents.

The Hints & Tips boxes that appear on the following pages provide criteria for evaluating the

Many schools and colleges create policies in a vacuum without the involvement of students, parents, or local police, and they do not seek support for policies or inform the community about policy changes.

College drug policies often urge "responsible use" rather than "no use" of alcohol for underage students.

Some short-sighted school policies increase problems for the community by calling for suspension or expulsion of students who violate drug policies without providing reasonable alternatives.[5]

HINTS & TIPS

Evaluating School Environment in a Local School ATOD Policy

1. Includes a clear message of nonuse
2. Provides for use of law enforcement on school property
3. Delineates protocol for search and seizure
4. Delineates protocol for student expulsion
5. Gives clear statement of consequences for noncompliance
6. Describes procedures for notification of existing policy and any changes
7. Describes procedure for collaboration with community agencies
8. Describes procedure for emergency situations involving drug overdosing

Evaluating Classroom Instruction in a Local School ATOD Policy

1. Gives procedure for curriculum approval and adoption
2. Complies with minimum standards of state regulations
3. Complies with the intent of state regulations
4. Establishes curriculum from preschool through 12th grade
5. Establishes time requirements for classroom instruction

Evaluating Teacher Training in a Local School ATOD Policy

1. Provides for release time for teacher training
2. Provides for staff development/in-service
3. Provides for facilities and equipment provided by school
4. Specifies the content and/or categories of training
5. Gives protocol for intervention and referral process

Evaluating Parent Training in a Local School ATOD Policy

1. Includes a parent training component
2. Delineates responsibilities of parents
3. Provides structure for working with parents
4. Includes notification procedures if child is caught
5. Delineates parental role in the intervention and referral process

Evaluating Student Assistance in a Local School ATOD Policy

1. Includes a referral procedure for students
2. Addresses confidentiality
3. Describes types of services provided by school personnel
4. Describes types of services provided by community agencies
5. Delineates role of parents in this process
6. Delineates notification procedures if child is caught using or possessing ATOD
7. Delineates notification procedures if child is caught selling ATOD
8. Addresses choices available to the student
9. Delineates assessment process

Evaluating Peer Educators in a Local School ATOD Policy

1. Provides for peer leaders
2. Provides selection process for peer leaders
3. Describes compensation and/or release time to participate in training
4. Describes compensation and/or release time to deliver services
5. Includes responsibilities of peer leaders

Evaluating Employee Assistance in a Local School ATOD Policy

1. Delineates referral procedures for administrators, teachers, and staff
2. Delineates protocol for confidentiality
3. Describes services to be provided by school
4. Provides release time for inpatient and/or outpatient treatment
5. Provides substitutes for classroom and/or office responsibilities

components of a local school drug policy. This material is adopted from the following sources: J. V. Fetro, *Step by Step to Substance Use Prevention: The Planning Guide for School-Based Programs* (Santa Cruz, CA: Network Publications, ETR Associates, 1991); and L. J. Colker and C. H. Flatter, *Drug-Free Schools and Children: A Primer for School Policy Makers* (Rockville, MD: American Council for Drug Education).

Classroom Instruction

Many states are currently undertaking educational reform, including performance-based assessments. This process (determined by policy) affects ATOD classroom instruction. Guidelines for curriculum adoption often are determined at the state level and implemented at the local level. Local policy should adhere to state guidelines and establish criteria for classroom instruction.

Teacher Training

Teachers need up-to-date information on current ATOD trends and how to recognize ATOD use. They should be informed about what to do when ATOD use is suspected and should have an established protocol for their role in intervention and referral. The policy should establish how this training will be conducted and should specify the protocol for granting release time to attend the training. In addition, when new curriculum materials are adopted, teacher training can be beneficial in ensuring uniformity of curriculum delivery among classrooms. (Could the teachers provide a written statement for Rashid to take to the committee? What would the statement say?)

Parent Training

Parents also need up-to-date information regarding ATOD trends and information on how to recognize ATOD use. They need guidance regarding what to do when ATOD use is suspected and how to intervene. Although schools do not assume primary responsibility for parent training, they may play an active role in ensuring that parents are aware of the current school policy and their role if their child is caught using, possessing, or distributing alcohol, tobacco, or other drugs. (Would the drug-testing procedure at Western Middle School include parent training?)

Student Assistance Program

The policy should delineate a referral procedure for students who are caught using, possessing, or distributing alcohol, tobacco, or other drugs. If the school decides to play a role in the referral and intervention process, this role should be clearly defined in the policy. The assessment process should be carefully delineated.

Peer Educators

The effectiveness of peer leaders was discussed in Chapter 8. If a school decides to add this component to its comprehensive ATOD program, the policy should clearly define the role of these students and the training protocol to be followed. (See Figure 10.5.)

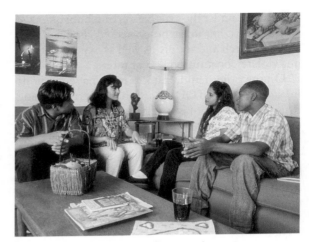

Figure 10.5 **A Peer Counseling Session** Peers can have an influential role in a school drug education program and in conflict mediation. (© Michael Newman/PhotoEdit)

Employee Assistance Program

Schools may have an elaborate system in place for addressing ATOD issues for students but no protocol for addressing ATOD issues for teachers, administrators, and staff. Schools must be sensitive to the pervasiveness of ATOD abuse and recognize the need for an established protocol to address the needs of school personnel.

Search and Seizure and Student Expulsion

Despite strong national, state, and local prevention efforts, some students will possess, use, distribute, and sell ATOD. As discussed earlier, schools must address and set policies for handling situations once alcohol, tobacco, and other drugs are found or suspected. There are legal considerations whenever students or their property are searched, or when students are expelled from school. A famous sentence from a U.S. Supreme Court decision sums up this issue: "It can hardly be argued that either students or teachers shed their constitutional rights to freedom of speech or expression at the schoolhouse gate."[7] Although the Court was deciding a case involving free expression, the reasoning is applicable to all school-related issues: Students have constitutional rights while under the supervision of school officials, and those rights must be protected. Policies that address **search** and **seizure** as well as expulsion must not violate constitutional guarantees.

On the other hand, schools must have methods in place to keep ATOD off school property. Keeping drugs out of school is an important public policy, evidenced by the law that says selling drugs within 1,000 feet of school property is a federal crime with enhanced penalties.[8] Similar state and local laws exist in most, if not all, jurisdictions. Therefore, a dilemma arises: Does the school policy go far enough to keep the school free of drugs while at the same time protecting students' constitutional rights?

Area Searches

Search of a private place is subject to constitutional scrutiny. Student lockers are areas within the school that may, in a sense, be considered private. However, courts generally uphold locker searches if a school's established written policy states that the school retains joint control of lockers and if a school advises students that it reserves the right to inspect lockers at any time.[9]

Student Searches

In support of a strong public policy to keep schools drug-free, schools may need to search a student if it is believed the student has drugs on his or her person. The U.S. Supreme Court has established a standard for such searches in light of the public policy favoring drug-free schools. In the case of *New Jersey v. TLO*, 469 U.S. 325 (1985), the Supreme Court stated that the standard for student searches is "reasonable grounds" to believe the student is violating or has violated the law or school rules. This standard is less stringent than the "probable cause" standard applicable to police searches of private citizens.

The "reasonable grounds" standard is open to interpretation. Given some reliable information, including tips from anonymous sources, courts have upheld searches of persons and pockets as reasonable.[10]

Student Suspension and Expulsion

If a student violates the law or school rules applicable to ATOD use, the school policy should provide for penalties that are suitable to the severity of the violation.

Procedurally, schools must recognize constitutional due process protections afforded to students who are faced with suspension or expulsion. Such protections include those of "notice" and "an opportunity to be heard." In other words, at a bare minimum, a student must be advised of the charges against him or her and given a chance to tell his or her side of the story.

Whether more formal proceedings are necessary depends on the severity of the possible sanction or penalty. The U.S. Supreme Court, in *Goss v. Lopez,* 419 U.S. 565 (1975), held that formal hearings are not required if a student is suspended for 10 days or less. To satisfy constitutional due process scrutiny, schools need only do the following when suspending a student for 10 days or less:

- Inform the student of the charges (either orally or in writing) against him or her and the evidence supporting the charges
- Give the student an opportunity to deny the charges and tell his or her version of the facts

However, notice and informal hearing requirements may be postponed if a student poses an ongoing threat or danger and the school wishes to remove the student immediately. The notice and hearing requirements may be satisfied soon thereafter.

Students who are suspended for more than 10 days (as well as students expelled from school) are afforded more formal proceedings. Necessary procedures include the following:

- Notifying the student in writing of the specific charges against him or her
- Informing the student of the names of all witnesses who would testify against him or her, with a report on all facts to which each witness could testify
- Providing the student an opportunity to defend against the charges and to present witnesses or testimony on his or her behalf

It should be noted that these guidelines are minimum federal constitutional rights. States may have other laws concerning student suspension and expulsion.

It is obvious that schools must provide a clear, written ATOD policy that contains an explanation of what types of violations will result in extended suspension or expulsion. Schools then must be certain to follow procedural protocol when violations occur.

Summary

Regulations and policies directly and indirectly affect the drug user, people who are within the user's environment, and society as a whole.[11] In discussing an ecological perspective on health promotion, McLeroy and colleagues said, "One of the defining characteristics of public health—apart from its emphasis on the health of populations rather than the health of individuals—is the use of regulatory policies, procedures and laws to protect the health of the community."[12] The school's role in creating, implementing, and carrying out ATOD regulatory policies and procedures designed to protect the health of the school community is significant. The teacher's role is to know and strive to uniformly enact and implement the existing school policies. In addition, evaluation of the individual and collective impact of such policies and regulations, while difficult to assess, should be carefully undertaken.

Scenario | Analysis and Response

Rashid should meet with fellow teachers and write a position statement regarding drug testing of student-athletes. He is representing the entire group and should have input from as many teachers as possible. The teachers should be aware of the need for a comprehensive drug and alcohol policy, including referrals for treatment. In addition, they need to review discrimination policy issues. Can only selected students be drug tested? A 2002 Supreme Court decision regarding drug testing upheld the right of the school district to randomly drug test all students involved in extracurricular school activities. Another issue for discussion is the use of coercive strategies by the school district. How coercive do teachers want the policy to be? How can they be sensitive to parental concerns? In writing the position statement, teachers need to be careful about the language they use to describe what they want. They should include statistical data to support their position, and they should know the interests of other community members.

Learning Activities

1. Write to your local school district and request a copy of its Safe Schools and Drug-Free policy. Evaluate the policy according to the criteria provided in the chapter.

2. Select a regulatory or nonregulatory agency in your state government. Discuss the role and responsibilities of this agency.

3. Write to another state's department of education and request a copy of its current laws regarding ATOD education. How do those laws compare with your state's laws? Compare your information with information obtained by your classmates.

Notes

1. National Commission on Drug-Free Schools, *Toward a Drug-Free Generation: A Nation's Responsibility*. (Washington, DC: U.S. Department of Education, 1990), 25.

2. U.S. Constitution, Article I, Section 1.

3. U.S. Constitution, Article I, Sections 7 and 8.

4. U.S. Constitution, Article II, Section 1.

5. National Commission on Drug-Free Schools, *Toward a Drug-Free Generation*.

6. Ibid.

7. *Tinker v. Des Moines Independent Community School District*, 393 U.S. 503 (1969).

8. See 21 U.S.C. § 845.

9. *Zamora v. Pomeroy*, 639 F. 2d 662 (10th Cir. 1981).

10. *Martens v. District No. 220*, 620 F. Supp. 29 (N.D. Ill. 1985).

11. M. S. Goodstadt and E. Mitchell, "Prevention Theory and Research Related to High-Risk Youth" in *Breaking New Ground for Youth at Risk: Program Summaries*, DHHS Publication No. (ADM) 89-1658 (Rockville, MD: DHHS, 1990).

12. K. R. McLeroy et al., "An Ecological Perspective on Health Promotion Programs," *Health Education Quarterly*, 15, 4 (1988): 351–377.

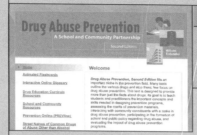

web resources

The Web site for this book offers many useful resources for educators, students, and professional counselors and is a great source for additional information. Visit the site at **http://healtheducation.jbpub.com/drugabuse/.**

Chapter Learning Objectives

Upon completion of this chapter, students will be able to:

1. Describe and characterize types of young people that are more likely to have impairment problems.

2. Describe a typical school intervention procedure.

3. Summarize the roles of school personnel in intervention.

4. Compare the purpose and services of a student assistance program with those of a family resource and youth service center.

5. Explain why school intervention isn't always effective.

Scenario

During the first week of school at Boone County East Middle School, Sasha Farouk notices that James Anders is late every day to her morning home room. She further notices that James is not well dressed, has poor hygiene, and does not seem to interact with the other students. It is now the end of the week, and she is wondering if she should take some action with respect to this student who seems to have problems. In addition to homeroom duties, Sasha has over 100 other students to whom she must attend every day. She wonders, "Can I take the time to focus on the individual needs of this student, or do I need to do my best with the routine needs of most of the students I serve as an instructor?"

Chapter 11

Early Intervention with Drug Abuse and Related Problems

Introduction

Many board games are microcosms of real life, or at least mimic limited aspects of it; for example, Monopoly represents a capitalist marketplace. Such games may be called simulations, but the game manufacturers don't usually use that word because it sounds boring. In any case, if these games have anything in common, it is that all the players start at the beginning, at the same point and time. (See **Figure 11.1.**)

If we were to design a simulation that portrayed a comprehensive program to eliminate the abuse of alcohol, tobacco, and other drugs, all the players would not start at the same place and time. Some of the players would address the causes of drug use, while others would respond to the causes of abuse. Still others would try to reduce the magnitude of drug abuse consequences. In other words, the players would have the same goal, but they would have different game rules.

The lesson of this analogy is that not all children and youth are effectively served by the same prevention activities. Some children are beyond the point of first-use prevention and need help to keep a small problem from becoming a big one. Some children have big problems that require rehabilitation, and some children have an array of interacting personal and social problems. This chapter discusses **intervention**— identifying problems in their early stages of development and resolving them while the consequences are still relatively minor.

People need intervention for several reasons. In some cases, prevention programs were not provided to them, and the ecological supports (e.g., a nurturing family) that reinforce a drug-free lifestyle were absent. In other cases, prevention programs

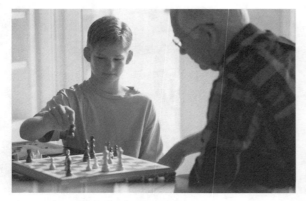

Figure 11.1 **Child Playing a Board Game** With most board games, every player starts at the same place. In contrast, drug educators must recognize that children come to school with different problems and needs; that is, they start at different places. (© ThinkStock)

were provided, but individuals failed to participate fully, for example, students who don't participate in drug-free clubs or school lock-in parties at prom time. Another common circumstance is that an individual's life is so dysfunctional or devoid of wholesome developmental supports that prevention is ineffective. Prevention programming as it is currently practiced makes only a small contribution to the wellness and development of those people most likely to develop problems. The more precursors to drug abuse an individual experiences, the less likely it is that prevention will succeed. These precursors, which are depressingly common, bring us to the concept of risk.

Teachers know intuitively that some children have a difficult time with school and adjusting to life, some children have more behavior problems than others (see **Figure 11.2**), some children are more likely to drop out, and some children are more likely to use drugs. Such problems are not randomly and equally distributed among all children, but are concentrated in a certain group of children and adolescents. These intuitions have been substantiated by many researchers, most notably Hawkins and colleagues.[1] (See the Viewpoints box.) Characteristics of risk were discussed in Chapters 1 and 8, so our focus here will be on outward manifestations of increased risk and the early development of problems.

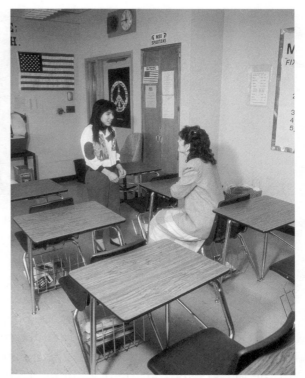

Figure 11.2 **Staying After School** Some students have more trouble than others in school, often from the very beginning. (© Dennis MacDonald/Unicorn Stock Photos)

Observing and Recognizing Impairment Problems

Before intervention is possible, signs of a problem must be recognized. Before those signs can be recognized, they must be observed. Before signs can be observed, someone must have an interest in observing them. Often teachers and other personnel are not interested. Classroom duties and class sizes may be so daunting that teachers feel they are doing well to plan and conduct lessons, much less worry about students with special problems. When a child's special problems manifest themselves in disruptive or antisocial behavior, a teacher may feel the only feasible recourse is to send the child to the principal or an alternative classroom, where the solution may be more disciplinary than rehabilitative.

I Taught Them All

I have taught in high school ten years. During that time, I have given assignments, among others, to a murderer, an evangelist, a pugilist, a thief, and an imbecile.

The murderer was a quiet little boy who sat on the front seat and regarded me with pale blue eyes; the evangelist, easily the most popular boy in the school, had the lead in the junior play; the pugilist lounged by the window and let loose at intervals a raucous laugh that startled even the geraniums; the thief was a gay-hearted Lothario with a song upon his lips; and the imbecile, a soft-eyed little animal seeking the shadow.

The murderer awaits death in the state penitentiary; the evangelist has lain a year now in the village church-yard; the pugilist lost an eye in a brawl in Hong Kong; the thief, by standing on tiptoe, can see the windows of my room from the county jail; and the once gentle-eyed moron beats his head against the padded wall in the state asylum.

All of these pupils once sat in my room, sat and looked at me gravely across worn brown desks. I must have been a great help to those pupils—I taught them the rhyming scheme of the Elizabethan sonnet and how to diagram a complex sentence.

Source: Naomi J. White, "I Taught Them All," *The Clearing House,* November 1937, 151.

Failure to observe occurs in other settings as well. A child may not receive the supervision he needs at home because he is a latchkey child, the child of a single parent, a child with many siblings, or perhaps a stepchild. Some parents are simply too preoccupied to pay attention when a child begins to experience problems.

These statements sound like they should lead up to a longing for life as it was lived in Lake Wobegon, where "all the women are strong, all the men are good-looking, and all the children are above average," or for the "good old days," when people looked out for each other, when every child had two parents and divorce was rare, when every child had a mother who stayed home, and when children were nurtured in small classes in school. However, this nostalgic view is not documented in fact; besides, the past is gone. We must deal with the here and now. There are ways that today's schools and home environments can be structured to recognize and react better to early signs of trouble with alcohol and other drugs.

One way is for teachers to respond to students' personal problems. Being responsive means (1) recognizing behavioral signs, (2) being available to listen, (3) discussing at a later time expressions of personal problems or other disclosures made in the classroom or in other settings, (4) being sensitive to confidentiality issues with children and their parents, and (5) helping students get help for problems that are beyond the teacher's role.

In reality, this list is rather heroic. If teachers are to go beyond their role as instructors, they need administrative support. Support can take the form of manageable class sizes, an expectation that teachers address needs beyond learning, intervention training, a policy that guides teachers in their relationships with troubled students and their parents and that outlines the procedures for seeking help and making referrals, and the provision of other resources within the school, such as a student assistance program.

Parents also can learn to be more responsive to children's needs, even when their families struggle with disadvantages. One way parents can learn responsiveness is from parent education courses that teach the early signs of drug abuse and related problems, and how to intervene effectively. Every community needs to redouble its efforts in providing parent training programs.

Experience has taught that increased parent training is easier said than done. Many parents are busy, won't schedule time for a parent education course, or have the misconception that attending a parenting course implies that their kids are in trouble or that they are bad parents. The parents who most need training are often those who are most difficult to reach. In spite of all these challenges,

Table 11.1
Barriers to Parent Education
Can You Give Specific Examples of These Barriers?
Stigmas about parenting skills and family needs
Schedule conflicts
Lack of childcare
Lack of cultural sensitivity in the program
Objectionable or inaccessible location
Promotion activities not well channeled to target audience
Gaps in literacy and learning skills

Table 11.2
Signs of Drug Abuse and Related Problems
Poor or declining academic performance (for children) or poor employment performance (for adults)
Withdrawal or social isolation
Disruptive, rebellious, defiant behavior
Excessive tardiness or truancy
Unusual nervousness and emotional volatility
Fatigue, sleepiness, lethargy
Neglected appearance, poor hygiene
Intoxicated demeanor (speech, ambulation, posture, emotional state, reactions)
Sudden change in friends, pastimes
Drug-related clothing and jewelry
Possession of alcohol or other drugs
Trouble with the police
Running away

schools and other community agencies (e.g., churches) should provide greater access to parent education. Barriers to participation should be removed in every way possible. (See Table 11.1.)

It is true that many attitudes and forces in Western society are antithetical to good parenting. Vigorous political debate is ongoing in America on this topic, and it is not going to end anytime soon. What has caused the deterioration of the family? What should be done about it? What is the role of government? Both Republicans and Democrats have platforms and proposals on family values. What do you think is most likely to strengthen families, the sine qua non of a healthy society and successful schools?

Guilt about troubled children and adolescents is sometimes placed on parents, sometimes appropriately so. However, it is not appropriate when environmental supports for good parenting are not present. In these cases, community services can really make a difference. Examples include "Parent's Day Out," inexpensive day care programs, parent support groups, more vigorous enforcement of child support laws, and foster grandparent programs.

Signs of Impairment

Impairment is a broad term that refers to any problem that interferes with a person's ability to carry out the responsibilities and expectations placed on her and to live in the way she would normally choose. Although impairment can refer to a physical handicap, in this context it refers to alcohol and other drug use that causes living problems. It should be mentioned that tobacco rarely, if ever, causes impairment in this sense. If smokers or chewers are impaired, it is because of problems other than tobacco use.

Although the focus of this chapter is drug impairment, it should be understood that many things can cause psychosocial impairment. In fact, the signs of impairment usually observed in school are not very specific; they can signal alcohol or other drug abuse, physical abuse, mental illness, or other individual or family problems. When **behavioral signs** are observed that deviate from the norm, a process of elimination is required to discover the real problem. However, problems often appear in clusters, for example, drug abuse with child abuse and with other family dysfunction. Table 11.2 shows behavioral signs of alcohol and drug abuse or other related problems. (See Figure 11.3.)

Human beings are not clones, and normality is a bell-shaped curve. While most people fall within two standard deviations of the median, the line between normal and abnormal is not precisely marked.

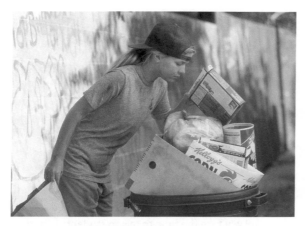

Figure 11.3 **Child with Neglected Appearance**
Does this child's appearance indicate a problem?

(© David Young-Wolff/PhotoEdit)

Judging a child, adolescent, or adult by the criteria listed in Table 11.2 is not always easy. For example, appearance and hygiene habits certainly vary greatly; poor hygiene may present problems in interpersonal relationships, but it doesn't always indicate emotional pathology. For another example, while some individuals are pliant and seek to please, others are naturally independent and unruly; rebelliousness is subjective, relative, and not always diagnostic. An important criterion not listed in the table is change. A change for the worse in any of the other criteria may be the most important indicator of a problem.

Some Barriers to Intervention

It is important to remember that intervention is not treatment; it is not even diagnosis. The first step in intervention is simply to observe, and sometimes to document in writing, specific instances of the criteria in Table 11.2 or any other changes of an undesirable nature. Often a reality check is reassuring; without violating confidentiality, observations may be shared with a neutral third party to seek corroboration of concerns.

Confidentiality also may present a barrier to intervention. Although some students jump at the chance to unload their emotional burdens, they may not want others—teachers, peers, or even parents—to know. All people concerned must make a commitment to maintain confidentiality. Teachers who make referrals should not chat casually about individual cases with other teachers or students. Student assistance program staff members should work to provide services in such a way that anonymity is assured.

Confidentiality presents a dilemma in some cases. Most of the time, parental notification is in the best interests of the child, even when the child opposes it. There may be times when law enforcement agencies must be notified, to ensure the child's welfare, even if the child and his or her parents object. Such actions should not be left to an individual staff member's discretion, but should be outlined clearly in school policy (see Chapter 10). Staff should be trained in these issues.

Intervention is often difficult. Sometimes people's intentions are misconstrued, or they are accused of nosiness or meddling. Sometimes they make exceptions, allowances, or excuses for a person's behavior out of misplaced kindness. Sometimes they doubt and blame themselves for a person's problems.

Often an individual who is targeted for intervention accuses others of meddling, exploits others' patience, and casts blame. This behavior is part of the **denial** phenomenon. Not everyone who denies he or she has an alcohol or drug problem is "in denial." Nevertheless, denial is real and significantly affects the intervention process.

Those people who take the first step in intervention should also be cautious about the "addiction industry." Agencies that provide treatment services for alcohol and drug problems or other dependency behavior have a vested interest in determining who needs treatment and who doesn't. Assessments done by these agencies may not always be unbiased, with the potential client's interest as the only consideration.

Many drug addiction treatment agencies have recruiters who network with schools, social welfare agencies, juvenile courts, and employee assistance programs. Their role is to provide **assessments** and recommend treatment as appropriate, which can be a helpful service. However, some recruiters are assigned quotas; that is, they are expected to secure a minimum number of new treatment clients per month. Although not bad in itself, this quota arrangement guarantees that some unnecessary treatment will be provided.

The U.S. General Accounting Office has estimated that 10% of the cost of illness in the United States is due to fraud, which includes rendering inappropriate or unnecessary services.[2] Although medical care in general is different from mental health services in many ways, it shouldn't surprise anyone that a measure of fraud is found in the delivery of chemical dependency services. If a treatment agency decides that someone needs treatment, a careful scrutiny of the basis for that decision should be conducted. Schools should expect a standardized assessment procedure, including a form that documents the nature of the problems and provides an objective basis for diagnosis. It may be wise to get a second opinion. Aside from the fact that chemical dependency treatment is very expensive, there is concern that adolescents unnecessarily exposed to treatment may suffer psychosocial harm.[3]

Intervention in the School

Impairment problems come to the attention of society primarily at school and at work because normative standards of behavior—one's actions and demeanor as compared with peers'—are most noticeable in these settings. Also, people are judged on their performance at work and at school, and alcohol and drug abuse interferes with their work.

In schools, teachers usually are first to notice a child's troubled behavior, but sometimes guidance counselors, coaches, other personnel, or peers notice it first. Parents may also observe problem behavior. Schools should provide training for personnel to help them recognize students with drug abuse and related problems and to know how to respond. In brief, the steps usually are as follows:

1. Observe a pattern and document it in personal notes.
2. Talk to the child about the observations.
3. Talk to the parents about the concerns.

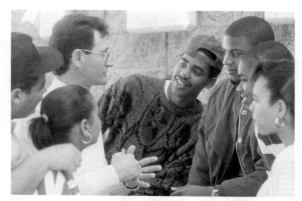

Figure 11.4 **Talking with Students** Dedicated school personnel will take the time to talk to students, including those who seem to have personal problems.
(© Mary Kate Denny/PhotoEdit)

4. Seek counsel from other personnel with expertise and responsibility for resolving such problems (e.g., a student assistance program staff).
5. Work with administrators in involving community agencies.
6. Follow up with the child to determine what is being done and if he or she feels hopeful about progress. (See **Figure 11.4**.)

Intervention may have both good and bad consequences. Sometimes drug abuse problems lead to violations of school drug policies or even criminal statutes. There may be a conflict between the need for punishment for breaking school rules and the need to nurture a troubled child. The positive side of discipline is that it may deter a child, or others who witness the punishment, from repeating the proscribed behavior in the future.[4] Furthermore, disciplinary consequences may be effective in persuading a student to accept help. The downside of discipline is that it may exacerbate the problem, particularly in the case of suspension or expulsion.

For many youth, school is the most, and perhaps only, wholesome and beneficial environment to which they are exposed. If discipline involves excluding them from the school, an action that is sometimes necessary and appropriate, they lose the one thing that is good in their life. The flip side is that if they are excluded, they are less able to adversely influence other students. It seems clear, therefore, that if discipline is part of the response to alcohol and drug problems, it should not be administered impulsively; those who are responsible for the decision should carefully consider what is best for all involved.

Teachers and coaches are typically most involved in the initial step of intervention because they have the most contact with students. Guidance counselors in many districts are fully occupied with scheduling and academic affairs and may have little time for student problems. However, many guidance counselors conduct **group guidance**, in which they teach classes on social relationships, mental health, sexuality, **conflict resolution** and violence prevention, and alcohol and drug issues. This forum may allow students to bring personal problems to the attention of guidance counselors.

Guidance counselors may become involved later, if not at the first step. Often they take the lead role in establishing a school drug policy and provide support to ensure that the policy is carried out. In addition, they may be the liaison between teachers and needed community resources.

Administrators also play a role in intervention. It is their responsibility to provide appropriate training for school personnel and to direct the development, implementation, and communication of the school drug policy. It is also their responsibility to ensure that adequate support is available in the form of budget resources, legal counsel for policy formation, intervention time in schedules, and in-service intervention training.

In some school districts, students are enlisted to play a role in intervention. The rationale is that students have the most uninhibited contact with other students; they may know what peers are doing before it is observed by adults. Also, students often speak to a peer before they reach out to an adult. There should be some apprehension about using peer helpers because they may not have the wisdom and judgment to do the right thing when a problem is presented to them. Another concern is that if a crisis results in serious consequences, such as a suicide, the peer helpers may not be able

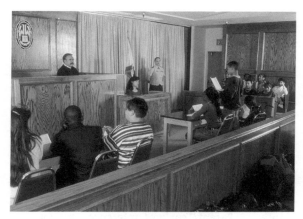

Figure 11.5 Mock Court Session Many schools have mock courts that give students an opportunity to participate in meting out discipline for violations of school policy. (© Michael Newman/PhotoEdit)

to dispel guilt feelings. Peer helpers need careful training, well-defined guidelines, close supervision, and debriefing after intervention incidents occur to appraise and refocus attitudes and feelings of guilt, remorse, fear, or depression. (See **Figure 11.5**.)

Family Relations

Another important aspect of intervention is developing a constructive relationship with the child's family. This can be accomplished in part by providing training for parents to help them become more skilled and effective. Training should be an ongoing effort, divorced from any particular incident or student problem. However, when a specific intervention begins, the family must be included from the outset.

Parents' responses to a call from a teacher or staff member vary. Some parents are concerned, glad for the call, and want to work closely with the school to help the student. Other parents are ambivalent or hostile. Unwilling to cooperate, they deny that there is a problem. In some cases, family members are part of the problem (e.g., they are abusive or have their own drug problems), and their defensiveness is an effort to conceal. For other parents, school recalls unhappy memories, or they are intimidated by teachers and other school personnel.

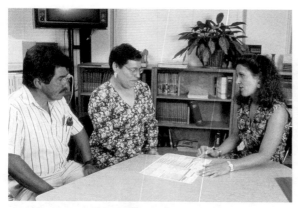

Figure 11.6 Parent/Teacher Conference School personnel must be sensitive to differences that exist between themselves and parents.

(© Michael Newman/ PhotoEdit)

It is important to be sensitive to parents' educational and cultural differences that may make them avoid the school. If a meeting is in order, a home visit or some neutral location (e.g., a church or community center) may be a better choice than the principal's office. (See **Figure 11.6**.)

Codependency

It is appropriate to present the concept of **codependency** in the context of family relations. Although the codependency behavior pattern is not new, it has been articulated as a distinct diagnosis or integrated syndrome only since the 1980s. Previously, codependency was called *maladjustment* or *neurosis*. In the mid-1980s, several influential writers began using the word *codependency* to describe a set of attitudes, response patterns, and behaviors that seemed to occur frequently in families with alcohol or drug abuse or other dependency problems. Codependency typically is seen in family members of alcoholics, but it also may be found in families with excessive behavior of any sort, including eating, gambling, anger and rage, sexual promiscuity, and shopping.

Furthermore, codependency may affect family dynamics so much that it can outlive the primary addiction, often extending into future generations. Children of alcoholics bring the codependency that developed in their childhoods into their marriages and parenting.

Some addiction treatment providers believe that everyone is codependent to some extent, that all of us have dysfunctional tendencies, and that we would benefit from at least a support group or perhaps more intensive services from mental health professionals. These claims are invalid and unnecessarily label all human problems and deficiencies as clinical pathology. The truth is that most people have remarkable resiliency and, with resource supports, have ample capacity to manage their lives in spite of their imperfections. There are many proponents of the codependency concept, particularly among therapists and clinical mental health workers. However, it is not a diagnostic label that is rigorously documented and described in the conventional ways of medical science, or even psychological science. Instead, it is founded on anecdotes and clinical perceptions. Consequently, codependency is vague, nonspecific, and ambiguous; it is a phenomenon that falls on a continuum with no clear line dividing functional pathology from normal variations of personality and social attitudes. While this can be said about much in the field of mental health, healthy skepticism is in order. The label *codependency* is riding on a bandwagon right now; the future will tell whether it will pass the test of time.

Labels aside, the behavior called codependency does occur and can be very disabling, so it is helpful for those who play a role in intervention to recognize its basic characteristics. The FYI box notes characteristics of codependency. Readers should recognize that the items included are difficult to assess and quantify. Most of the characteristics are found in every individual to some degree, and some of them are even desirable under certain circumstances. Although it may be subjective to apply these criteria to an individual when attempting to diagnose codependency, intervention professionals should recognize that the more an individual is characterized by these traits, and the more pronounced they are, the more accurate it is to consider that individual as being codependent.

The codependency literature identifies some common ways that family members, including youth, respond to an addicted person in the household. These roles are discussed in the accompanying FYI box.

Characteristics of Codependency

- We assume responsibility for others' feelings and/or behaviors.
- We feel overly responsible for others' feelings and/or behaviors.
- We have difficulty identifying our feelings.
- We have difficulty expressing our feelings.
- We tend to fear and/or worry how others may respond to our feelings.
- We have difficulty in forming and/or maintaining close relationships.
- We are afraid of being hurt and/or rejected by others.
- We are perfectionists and place too many expectations on ourselves and others.
- We have difficulty making decisions.
- We tend to minimize, alter, or even deny the truth about how we feel.
- Other people's actions and attitudes tend to determine how we respond/react.
- We tend to put other people's wants and needs first.
- Our fear of others' feelings (anger) determines what we say and do.
- We question or ignore our own values to connect with significant others. We value others' opinions more than our own.
- Our self-esteem is bolstered by outer, other influences. We cannot acknowledge good things about ourselves.
- Our serenity and mental attention are determined by how others are feeling and/or behaving.
- We tend to judge everything we do, think, or say harshly, by someone else's standards; nothing is done, said, or thought well enough.
- We do not know or believe that being vulnerable and asking for help is both okay and normal.
- We do not know that it is okay to talk about problems outside the family, or that feelings just are, and it is better to share them than to deny, minimize, or justify them.
- We tend to put other people's wants and needs before our own.
- We are steadfastly loyal—even when the loyalty is unjustified and often even personally harmful.
- We have to be needed in order to have a relationship with others.

Source: Co-dependents Anonymous, Glendale, Arizona.

It is important to recognize that the responses and personalities represented in the FYI boxes often do not indicate problems, nor are they always manifestations of codependency. Furthermore, some of the responses are harmful, destructive, or dysfunctional only when they are excessive. Still, it is helpful to understand the different ways in which youth and others may adapt to serious family problems.

The issue of codependency is important to school personnel and other prevention professionals who play a role in intervention. First, references to codependency are ubiquitous in the intervention and treatment literature. Limitations of the concept aside, those people involved in intervention need to have a working knowledge of what it is, just to be conversant.

Next, some young people exhibit dysfunctional behavior as a result of a family member's alcohol or other drug addiction. Sometimes parents are unresponsive to requests or suggestions from school staff or behave in ways that are counterproductive to a child's welfare. In such cases, understanding codependency may improve relationships with these students and parents and help one realize that they may need resources beyond those that the school can provide.

An awareness of codependency also provides a safeguard for school personnel. As they reach out to troubled youth, there is some danger that they will become emotionally entangled to such a degree that their mental health and social adjustment are adversely affected. School personnel have a role to

fyi

Dysfunctional Family Roles

Chief Enabler: Assumes responsibility for both the cause of the addict's behavior and for protecting him or her from the consequences.

Hero: Tries to compensate for the failures of the addict by becoming an overachiever, a workaholic, and a perfectionist.

Scapegoat: Responds by acting out with self-destructive behavior, including ATOD abuse, suicide, and troublemaking in school and with the police.

Lost Child: Responds by withdrawing into himself or herself in shyness and a lot of solitary activity.

Mascot: Responds by providing humor and fun, becoming the class clown.

---

play in helping young people with ATOD abuse and related problems, but they must be careful to establish boundaries to avoid overly identifying with or assuming responsibility for those problems. They must walk a fine line between heartlessly disregarding students' problems and pain and being consumed by students' needs to the neglect of the other professional and private roles they play.

Student Assistance Programs

So far we have described the most basic intervention steps: (1) school personnel are trained to observe troubled behavior, (2) they respond in some systematic way as dictated by school policy, and (3) they continue to follow the child to facilitate healing and rehabilitation. However, many schools have found that the nature and extent of problems are so staggering, and the solutions so perplexing and troublesome, that a more formal program response is necessary. In this case, a student assistance program is the most common form. (See **Figure 11.7.**)

Implementation of a student assistance program (SAP) is a recognition that many students have serious problems, that these problems have a significant deleterious impact on learning and social development, and that the community, as manifested by the school, intends to allocate resources to salvage as many troubled young people as possible.

Many of the functions carried out by SAPs can be done by informal programs, but they usually are

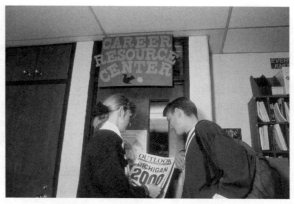

Figure 11.7 Student Assistance Program
Establishing student assistance programs is a way that schools can respond to students' drug abuse and other personal problems. (© Dennis MacDonald/Unicorn Stock Photos)

done less satisfactorily, and these informal programs usually do not have the stockpile of resources and expertise that can be gathered by a SAP.

SAPs usually target drug and alcohol abuse. However, because drug problems, teen pregnancy, child abuse, delinquency, school failure, suicide, and violence are interrelated, and because intervention procedures for all of these problems overlap, SAPs usually are concerned with the whole range of youth problems.

The structure and function of SAPs vary from school to school, but there are two primary models for their organization: the counselor model and the core team model. In the counselor model, a SAP director is the primary provider of services, establishing referral mechanisms and policies for students, parents, and school personnel; providing teacher orientation; completing crisis counseling and referral for students; and conducting student support groups and other follow-up activities. This model is most effective when it is confined to a single school or a small school system. Staffing consists of one or more full-time employees who coordinate the schoolwide program and provide direct services. Another alternative in a more limited counselor-centered program is for a coordinator to perform SAP duties only part of the time. This pattern is effective if the time allocated for SAP responsibilities in the coordinator's work load is realistic.

Table 11.3	
Components of a Core Team Student Assistance Program	
Staff	Core team
Referral procedure	Administrative support
Student participation	School drug policy

Source: B.S. Newsam, *Complete Student Assistance Program Handbook: Techniques and Materials for Alcohol/Drug Prevention and Intervention in Grades 7–12* (West Nyack, NY: Center for Applied Research in Education, 1992).

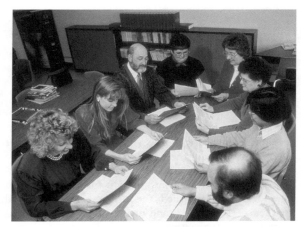

Figure 11.8 **Student Assistance Core Team** Core team SAPs usually include teachers, guidance counselors, administrators, students, and parents.

(© Dennis MacDonald/Unicorn Stock Photos)

The second way to organize SAP services is with the core team model. This model usually has the same generic components (see Table 11.3) as the counselor model, except that it has a core team of several volunteer members. Core team SAPs usually serve a group of schools in a school district. The core team model is based on the idea of assembling a number of school personnel to provide SAP services, rather than just one counselor. This approach not only generates greater schoolwide understanding and appreciation of the SAP, but also enables the SAP to serve more students at a lower unit cost because the people who serve as core team members are volunteers. That is, the work they do on the core team is considered service as part of their primary job in the school system. While a number of people may give their time to a SAP, the school system's only additional salary expense is that for the SAP coordinator. (See **Figure 11.8**.)

The central element of this type of SAP is the core team, which consists of SAP staff and other professional school personnel who have a commitment to the program. In a multischool SAP, there may be only one core team, a core team for each level (e.g., middle school, high school), or one for each school. Core teams promote awareness of SAP services and how to access them among personnel, students, and parents. When an intervention situation arises, the core team talks with students and parents and serves as a bridge to community resources. (See the Viewpoints boxes.)

SAPs are designed to identify students' personal problems and bring appropriate resources to bear. They generally do not provide treatment, but may organize support groups (called *aftercare*) for students who have completed treatment, or they may sponsor support groups for students with other problems, such as child abuse, drug-dependent parents, grief, and making adjustments as a transfer student.

SAPs work within the guidelines of a referral procedure, which is organized as a flow chart, giving direction based on the unique pattern of contingencies. A referral procedure is illustrated in **Figure 11.9**. Included with the referral procedure is an information form, illustrated in the Hints + Tips box, which documents the child's level of functioning at school, family relationships and problems, self-assessment of adjustment and happiness, drug use history, relevant physical habits, such as eating and sleeping, and the exact nature of the immediate problems that led to the referral. The completed form is then discussed with the child, parents, and, as appropriate, school officials.

Earlier in the chapter we discussed how critical administrative support is for effective intervention. This is true for SAPs as well. It may be desirable to include an administrator on the core team because, even if the administrator's contribution is more limited than other members', his or her inclusion will promote better schoolwide success. When administrators are fully informed and have

A Student Assistance Program Success Story

Danny was a high school junior when one of his teachers noticed he was withdrawn and unhappy. The teacher decided to contact the SAP in the school system. The SAP staff received feedback from all of Danny's teachers from standardized information forms. After all of the forms were returned, the SAP core team reviewed the teachers' feedback and made a decision that intervention was appropriate.

The coordinator of the core team met with Danny to discuss his problems, at which time Danny disclosed that he smoked marijuana each day, sometimes used LSD, and had been drinking alcohol since the sixth grade. In addition, he had an alcoholic stepfather who abused Danny's mother, and there had been violence between him and his stepfather. Danny agreed to join a support group conducted by the SAP. The SAP's intention was that the support group would help Danny understand the magnitude of his problems and agree to a formal chemical dependency assessment.

Danny began attending the support group. He felt inferior to other students in the group because he was from a low-SES family, was not popular at school, and had below-average grades. However, after about three sessions, he began to discuss his problems honestly, receive support, and gain insights. He also began to develop a positive relationship with the teacher who facilitated the group; in fact, she became an informal mentor for him. By session seven, Danny agreed to have a chemical dependency assessment done by a local mental health agency.

The agency determined that his drug abuse would benefit from formal treatment; because of Danny's family situation, in-patient treatment was indicated. The SAP placed him in a 45-day treatment program that accepted indigent clients.

After the treatment program ended, Danny returned to school. He attended AA meetings as aftercare (see Chapter 12) and maintained a supportive relationship with the teacher/mentor. This progress continued during the summer of his junior year and during his senior year. By taking summer school classes, Danny was able to graduate with his class. He is now gainfully employed, independent, and continuing recovery. His success has given the core team deep satisfaction and fulfillment.

A Student Assistance Program Failure Story

Juan was the proverbial star. A popular football player, he was the envy of many peers. Though he didn't really like academics, he kept his grades high enough to maintain football eligibility. His football prowess and acceptable grades led to a college football scholarship, redeemable after graduation.

However, after football season ended in his senior year, Juan's grades took a nosedive. His situation came to the attention of the school's SAP. The core team learned that he was a regular user of crack and alcohol and that his mother was an alcoholic. His response to the core team was one of manipulation and denial. This behavior was a deterrent to the intervention process, but eventually Juan completed a chemical dependency assessment. Later he attended a 30-day in-patient treatment program in another city. (Simultaneously, his mother participated in a treatment program with a different agency.)

During treatment, Juan was uncooperative and dishonest in therapy. He never relinquished denial or recognized a need to change his life. While at the treatment program he became sexually active with another client. Juan left before completing the program.

After returning to his home community, he refused to attend AA meetings or any other aftercare. He dropped out of school and lost his football scholarship. He is still abusing drugs with the same peer group.

Meanwhile the SAP program staff is dismayed at the way Juan's life is going and frustrated that the intervention was not more successful. They wonder what other steps could have helped and how Juan's scenario might have been different.

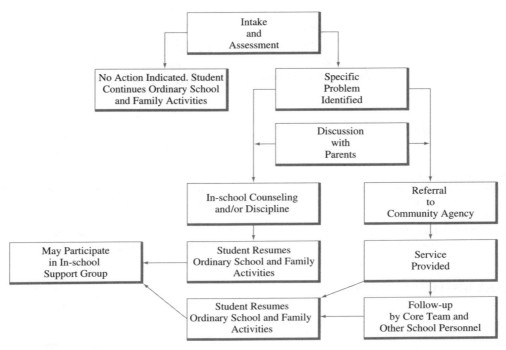

Figure 11.9 Referral Procedure

firsthand understanding of SAP services, they tend to be more supportive.

Obviously, SAPs will be more effective if students participate by making self-referrals or urging other students to seek out services. Teachers are also important in generating referrals, as are other personnel and parents.

Finally, a SAP often is called to service when a school drug policy is violated. The formation and components of a drug policy, which provides specific reasons for intervention, were discussed in Chapter 10. Although a student may be referred to a SAP without having violated a drug policy, the need for the referral will have to be established before the intervention can proceed.

Student assistance programs have been evaluated only to a limited degree. Outcome measures have included changes in use of alcohol and other drugs, improvements in academic performance and attendance, changes in the frequency of behavior problems, and **recidivism** (receiving intervention services repetitively). While there is room to be optimistic, evaluations to date indicate only modest

results.[5] The current widespread popularity of SAPs calls for much greater investment in evaluation research.

In closing this section, we must note that schools have staffs as well as students. Drug and alcohol abuse by school personnel may be just as common as it is in the general population. As student assistance programs reach out to more and more students, there is a need for schools to provide a similar intervention mechanism for troubled staff. In this regard, schools lag behind businesses and other community agencies in providing employee assistance programs.

Family Resource and Youth Service Centers

In many states, education reform is leading to the formation of centers that are designed to address a wide range of student and family problems that interfere with learning, school success, and entry into adulthood as productive members of society. Such centers are included here because the students they typically serve tend to be at high risk for alcohol and drug problems. The nature of the

HINTS & TIPS

A Student Assistance Program Preliminary Information Form

TO: _____

FROM: _____

REGARDING: Student _____

School _____ Grade _____

DATE: _____

The above student has been referred to the Student Assistance Program Core Team. In order to assist us in assessing the nature of help the program might provide, please indicate on the form below any behavior you might have noticed within the past three months or concerns you may have about the student. Please feel free to make comments where appropriate.

Please return this form to _____ as soon as possible. In order to maintain confidentiality, please return the form in an envelope or folder. After this information has been collected, it will be filed in the district's Student Assistance Program office.

Please Check Relevant Items and Comment

I. **Academic Performance**   Comments
    _____ Decline in quality of work   _____
    _____ Decline in grade earned   _____
    _____ Incomplete work   _____
    _____ Work not handed in   _____
    _____ Failing in this subject   _____

II. **Classroom Conduct**   Comments
    _____ Disruptive in class   _____
    _____ Inattentiveness   _____
    _____ Lack of concentration   _____
    _____ Lack of motivation   _____
    _____ Sleeping in class   _____
    _____ Impaired memory   _____
    _____ Extreme negativism   _____
    _____ In-school absenteeism (skipping)   _____
    _____ Tardiness to class   _____
    _____ Breaking rules   _____
    _____ Frequently needs discipline   _____
    _____ Cheating   _____
    _____ Fighting   _____
    _____ Throwing objects   _____
    _____ Defiance of authority   _____
    _____ Verbally abusive   _____
    _____ Obscene language, gestures   _____
    _____ Sudden outburst of temper   _____
    _____ Vandalism   _____
    _____ Frequent visits to counselor   _____
    _____ Frequent visits to restroom   _____
    _____ Hyperactivity, nervousness   _____

III. **Atypical Behavior**

_____ Erratic behavior day to day   _____
_____ Change in friends/peer group   _____
_____ Sudden, unexplained popularity   _____
_____ Mood swings   _____
_____ Seeks constant adult contact   _____
_____ Seeks adult advice without a specific   _____
        problem   _____
_____ Time disorientation   _____
_____ Apparent change in personal values   _____
_____ Defensiveness   _____
_____ Other students express concern about a   _____
        possible problem   _____
_____ Fantasizing; daydreaming   _____
_____ Compulsive overachievement;   _____
        preoccupied with school success   _____
_____ Perfectionism   _____
_____ Difficulty in accepting mistakes   _____
_____ Rigid obedience   _____
_____ Talks freely about drug use; bragging   _____
_____ Associates with known drug users   _____
_____ Depression   _____
_____ Sadness   _____
_____ Withdrawn from usual activities   _____
_____ Feelings of helplessness and hopelessness   _____
_____ Marked changes in sleeping patterns   _____
        and/or appetite   _____
_____ Giving away possessions or other final   _____
        arrangements   _____
_____ Impulsive   _____

IV. **Possible Alcohol/Drug-Specific Behaviors**

Witnessed	Suspected	
( )	( )	Selling, delivering
( )	( )	Possession of alcohol, drugs
( )	( )	Possession of drug paraphernalia
( )	( )	Use of alcohol, drugs
( )	( )	Intoxication
( )	( )	Physical signs, symptoms (such as weight gain or loss; appearance change; poor hygiene; red, puffy eyes; slurred speech)
( )	( )	Others

Additional Information

A. Describe the student's peer group. _____
_____

B. What role does the student play in his/her peer group? _____

C. How does the student relate to others (students, teachers, administrators) outside his/her peer group? _____
_____

D. What are the student's special interests (hobbies, clubs, sports, etc.)? _____
_____

E. What strengths does this student have?_____

F. In regard to this student's behavior, are you aware of any action that has already been taken (concern and data have been shared with student, parents have been contacted)?_____
_____

G. Additional comments _____
_____
_____
_____
_____
_____
_____
_____

Source: Warren County Schools, Warren County, Kentucky.

centers' work is intervention—addressing problems while their consequences are still limited. In some states, these centers are called family resource and youth service centers (FRYSCs); other states have other names for these centers, but their functions are similar. Some agencies that provide these services are community based, rather than located on the premises of schools. The FYI box describes Family Support America, a national organization that was established to provide support, training, advocacy, and a networking mechanism for parents and professionals working to strengthen family supports for children.

These centers are distinguished from student assistance programs because they address the unmet physical, social, and economic needs of students rather than just problematic or dysfunctional behavior. Also, these centers are not school-based clinics that concentrate on direct health services, including contraception. However, some centers may address, by referral, the unmet medical needs of students.

Political and social conservatives oppose FRYSCs for several reasons. They object to the additional government spending needed to support the centers and believe that the centers represent an unnecessary extension of government that may usurp the traditional role of parents and families. Some people believe that FRYSCs are school-based clinics in disguise, or at least a first step in their development, and they adamantly oppose education and services for sex education and birth control, especially when such services are provided without parental knowledge and consent. Those with this perspective feel that schools should be in the business of instruction, and that social and health services are inappropriate school functions.

Proponents of FRYSCs maintain that schools must do more than focus on academics that don't address the context of student lives. If it is true that education is one of the most critical ways in which children are prepared for life, and that many students labor under great impediments to learning, then a proactive approach to reducing the barriers to school success is appropriate. A compromise position is that schools and their various activities should not do anything to undermine the authority and solidarity of families, but should recognize that some families (or parents) are unable or unwilling to meet children's needs. (See Figure 11.10.)

Table 11.4 lists actual problems brought to a FRYSC located at a nonmetropolitan high school that has an enrollment of about 800 students. The list was gathered during less than half a school year.

Table 11.4

Actual Problems Served by a High School Youth Service Center in a Four-Month Period, 2000

Student abused, victim of violence

Student pregnant

Student parents needing help with parenting skills

Student and parents homeless

Student has no winter clothes

Family needs food assistance

New student has difficulty adjusting to school

Student divorcing, seeking legal assistance

Student parent needs help receiving child support

Student's family unable to buy glasses for student

Student has questions about homosexuality

Student needs help with body odor

Student needs assistance buying textbooks

Parent seeks help with problem child (student)

Student dropout seeks reenrollment assistance

Student seeks counsel on which parent he should live with after parents' divorce

Death of parent

Death of sibling

Alcoholic parent

Student needs job, doesn't know how to get one

It graphically illustrates the variety and severity of students' life problems that challenge them in reaching their full potential.

Table 11.5 lists typical generic services provided by FRYSCs. Services vary from center to center, based on unique local needs, the presence of other service programs in the school and community, and, of course, funding. In general, FRYSCs strive to be coordination and referral mechanisms rather than direct service providers. However, sometimes a lack of existing community resources reduces the feasibility of this approach; some centers are forced to be primary providers of services if the services are going to be delivered at all. Systematic documentation of the precise impact of the centers on drug abuse or related problems does not yet exist.

fyi

Family Support America

Family Support America, formerly Family Resource Coalition of America, promotes family support as the nationally recognized movement to strengthen and support families and places the principles of family support practice at the heart of every setting in which children and families are present. By identifying and connecting individuals and organizations that have contact with families; by providing technical assistance, training and education, conferences, and publications; and by promoting the voice of families, Family Support America is taking family support to scale as the national strategy for ensuring the well-being of our children today and in the years to come.

Family Support America works to bring about a completely new societal response to children, youth, and their families: one that strengthens and empowers families and communities so that they can foster the optimal development of children, youth, and adult family members—one that solves problems by preventing them. We envision a society in which all of us—families, communities, government, social service institutions, businesses—work together to provide healthy, safe environments for children and families to live and work in.

Contact Information

20 North Wacker Drive, Suite 1100, Chicago, IL 60606

Tel: 312-338-0900   Fax: 312-338-1522

http://www.familysupportamerica.org/content/home.htm

Intervention with Adults

Employee Assistance Programs

Martin Lakewood was a curriculum coordinator for Tecumseh County Schools. His 11-year career was uneventful, but mutually satisfying for him and the school system. However, his supervisor, Ms. Abbott, has noticed a change in his job performance in the past six months; he has taken more sick days and unexplained absences, missed deadlines, been complained about by other school personnel, written poor-quality reports, and has strained

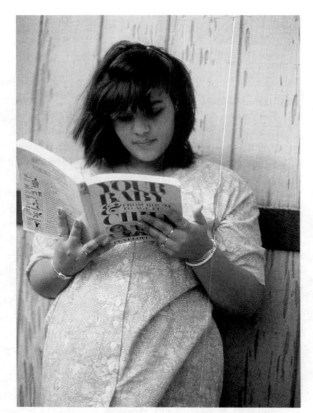

Figure 11.10 In-school Day Care Center Teen pregnancy occurs in every high school. Do you think schools should provide services to teen parents? Why or why not? (© Steve Bourgeois/Unicorn Stock Photos)

Table 11.5
Services Provided by Family Resource and Youth Service Centers
Preschool, after-school, and summer childcare
Services for pregnant students
Parenting enhancement services
Referral to health services
Referral to social services
Job development for youth
Employment counseling and related services for youth
Referral for substance abuse services
Referral for family crisis and mental health services

relationships with coworkers. When Abbott brought these observations to his attention, Lakewood was defensive and disgruntled. Abbott was calm but firm when she explained that his job performance had to improve and that, as a first step toward that end, Lakewood was expected to complete an interview with the employee assistance program (EAP) with which the school system had a contract.

The following week, Lakewood went for his first visit to the EAP. The counselor did an assessment that determined that Lakewood was using an excessive amount of prescription antianxiety drugs that he received from several physicians. This information served as a basis for recommending an outpatient counseling program financed by Tecumseh County Schools.

Meanwhile, Abbott had no knowledge of the specific nature of Lakewood's problem, but knew only that ongoing EAP services were being provided. A year later, at Lakewood's annual performance review, Abbott recognized that his work quality had improved to the high level demonstrated in earlier years.

This story is fictitious but illustrates how intervention may be done with adults. Adult intervention is an optimistic process because it rejects the notion that addiction is a downward spiral that irrevocably leads to insanity, incarceration, or death. Although this view was once conventional wisdom, we now try to reach the person at midcourse instead of waiting until he or she hits bottom.

The most strategic place for adult intervention is the workplace, but intervention can also occur in a home or community setting with the help of family members. Physicians could play an important role in intervention because a significant number of medical problems caused by alcohol or drug abuse come to their attention. So far, though, their role is minimal because they often don't associate a medical problem with drug abuse and usually are untrained in intervention skills even if they recognize a need.[6]

Many businesses and some schools have developed employee assistance programs for their workers. Business leaders recognize that alcohol and

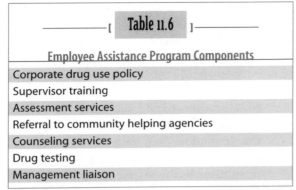

[Table 11.6]

Employee Assistance Program Components

Corporate drug use policy
Supervisor training
Assessment services
Referral to community helping agencies
Counseling services
Drug testing
Management liaison

Source: K. Dixon, "Employee Assistance Programs: A Primer for Buyer and Seller," *Hospital and Community Psychiatry*, 39, 6 (June 1988): 623–627.

drug abuse, mental health problems, serious financial difficulties, and marriage and family conflicts all interfere with job performance. Alcohol- or drug-impaired employees have inflated medical bills, make more mistakes in jobs that require physical skill, have more on-the-job accidents in industrial and other work settings, have more absences from work, and generally produce poorer-quality work.[7] Personnel are the most important component of most businesses, so there is an economic incentive to maximize workers' potential, or at least to try to remove any barriers to their work.

EAPs usually have the services listed in Table 11.6. Some companies design an EAP as an internally operated department, whereas others contract with a community EAP. An internal EAP may be less expensive for a large organization and meet its unique needs better, but a drawback is the issue of confidentiality. Employees may be reluctant to seek the EAP's services if they are unsure of the security of their EAP records. A community EAP may work better for a small organization that doesn't have enough employees to justify an internal model. External EAPs often are viewed as more confidential and not exclusively loyal to management.

EAPs depend on supervisor referrals and self-referrals. Supervisors and other managers are trained to recognize problems with their workers' job performance. When such observations are made, and a continuing problem is evident, the supervisor discusses the problem with the worker. This discussion focuses on the problem observed, not on suspicions or diagnoses. Depending on the circumstances, the supervisor may recommend or require that the employee complete an EAP assessment. The supervisor continues to monitor the worker's job performance, and after a period of time, a reassessment is made to determine if the problem has been solved or whether a different course of action is necessary.

The success of EAPs requires management to be supportive and patient as employees try to solve whatever problem is interfering with their performance. The measure of support and patience shown will vary depending on the employee's value or the ease with which he or she can be replaced. Companies with nonunion workers who labor at or near minimum wage may not provide EAP services, but instead may simply terminate troubled workers and hire nonimpaired individuals.

EAPs inform workers of their services, the procedure to access those services, and the types of problems with which the EAP can help. This strategy is intended to encourage self-referrals even before management recognizes a problem. In spite of the fact that millions of workers are provided EAP services, only a limited amount of evaluation research has been done on them; the known results are generally encouraging but not definitive.[8]

Community Intervention

Sometimes intervention takes place in a home environment. When someone is alcohol or drug impaired, family and friends observe the problematic consequences, but unfortunately may be more likely to deny the problem than an employer would be. Family members may not know what to do, may hope that the problem will get better by itself, or may be embarrassed by the problem and resolve to keep it secret. Family and friends are usually emotionally involved and find it difficult to confront the individual.

In many cases, family and friends try to compensate for the person's dysfunctional behavior by making excuses, covering up for the person's mistakes, internalizing guilt for the problem, and restructuring their lives around the person's alcohol or drug abuse. This codependency, discussed earlier in the chapter, is applied very broadly to

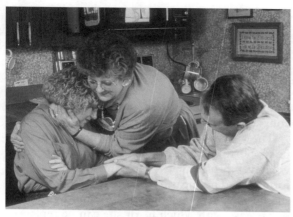

Figure 11.11 Family Intervention Often family members can be influential in getting addicted loved ones into treatment sooner rather than later, but it is very difficult. (© Skjold/PhotoEdit)

these types of behavior. Some of what has been called codependency is normal caring and concern for someone in trouble. Some of what is called codependency is inappropriately treated, sometimes fraudulently. Nevertheless, codependency is real, and it can be a barrier to intervention.

If denial can be overcome, family and friends sometimes can intervene effectively in alcohol and drug abuse by bringing the person into treatment sooner rather than later. (See **Figure 11.11.**) The process may go as follows:

1. A family member or friend talks to significant others in the drug-impaired person's life. Concerns about the person's behavior are discussed, and each tries to recall specific examples of the person's dysfunctions. A plan is established to confront the individual.

2. The group gathers to talk with the impaired person, who has no prior knowledge of the meeting. Sometimes trickery is used to get the person to come to the intervention site. One by one, friends and family recount observations and experiences when the person's behavior was dysfunctional and hurtful to them and those around them. The tone may be confrontational, but should not be condemning

or derogatory. The point is not to make the person feel guilty or to destroy any further his or her self-esteem, but rather to enable the individual to honestly face his or her problem and consider professional help. Obviously, these interventions are traumatic for all concerned and may leave some scars. The hope is that these scars will be less painful than not addressing the person's problem.

3. Family members should have a plan for treatment prior to the intervention; that is, they should have ready specific options (e.g., a mental health agency, a drug treatment facility, a 12-step program) to suggest to the individual. The group should firmly, with determination, urge the person to get help. Friends and family may not have the same power as an employer (i.e., they can't threaten the individual with being fired), but they may use other types of leverage (e.g., temporary separation, withheld financial support, confiscation of an automobile). Drastic actions may be presented in the form of ultimatums, such as, "Get help or we will _____." This strategy might be described as "tough love," and, for most people, it is hard to do.

Sometimes family interventions are guided by professional counselors. Their expertise may provide the confidence and guidance the family needs to carry out the intervention. It should also be pointed out that some people feel that family interventions as just described are coercive and manipulative and may not be an ideal way to manage human relationships. Furthermore, there may be times when the coercion is counterproductive, causing the person to resist even more. Others feel that this approach offers the most hope for early intervention.

Resources for Referral

Intervention is the first step of a two-step process. It highlights a problem and directs a person toward a solution (i.e., treatment). An intervention is not complete without referrals to specific programs or

Table 11.7
Referral Resources for Alcohol or Drug Impairment
Community mental health agencies
Clergy
Primary care physicians
School-based student assistance programs
Alcoholics Anonymous, other 12-step programs, and other support groups
Alcohol and drug dependency treatment programs
Private-practice therapists

treatment resources. Table 11.7 lists common resources for this purpose.

Summary

Successful intervention prevents the most severe consequences of alcohol and drug abuse. The chance of restoring a person to a fully functional life is greater with intervention than it is when treatment is provided at the late stages of addiction. Also, intervention may decrease the human and economic costs of treatment. While all of these results are worthwhile, the realities are that intervention often is not done, is not done successfully, or that the challenges to reducing human and organizational barriers to intervention prove too great to overcome.

Scenario | Analysis and Response

Although James Anders may have ATOD or other problems, he may not. It is not Sasha Farouk's job to determine whether James has a problem or what it is. The only step she has to take is to recognize that his appearance, demeanor, and behavior are outside the norm. It should not be very time consuming to jot down some personal notes on her observations.

Once she has done this, it is time to make a referral to the school student assistance program. The SAP director or team can then make inquiries with James's other teachers to see if there is a pattern of problem or dysfunctional behavior. If the data validate the concerns of Sasha, an appointment will be made with James and his grandparents, who are his permanent guardians.

Based on the family interview and the documentation gathered from the teachers who know James, an appointment is made for James to have an interview with a clinical counselor who is on contract with the school system. In addition, the coordinator of the school's family resources center will do an assessment to determine what types of support the family needs.

James's family and personal problems will not be solved easily or quickly, but progress will be made. James will be more successful in school than he might have been, and it all started with a small act of good will by a dedicated teacher.

Learning Activities

1. Visit local mental health or drug treatment agencies. Find out if they do assessments and, if so, how they are done. Determine how a judgment is made about a person's need for drug treatment services.

2. Go to a local school system and get a copy of its intervention and referral policy. Interview an appropriate school employee to find out how well the system works.

3. Locate a school system with a student assistance program. Discover how the SAP is organized, what services it provides, and how effective it has been.

4. Interview the director of a local employee assistance program. Obtain details on how it is organized and what types of services are provided.

Notes

1. J. D. Hawkins, D. M. Lishner, and R. F. Catalano, "Childhood Predictors and the Prevention of Adolescent Substance Abuse," in *Etiology of Drug Abuse: Implications for Prevention,* C. L. Jones and R. J. Battjes, eds., DHHS Publication No. (ADM) 87-1335 (Rockville, MD: DHHS, 1985).

2. General Accounting Office, *Health Insurance: Vulnerable Payers Lose Billions to Fraud and Abuse,* GAO/HRD-92-69 (Washington, DC: Government Printing Office, May 1992).

3. M. Klitzner et al., *Early Intervention for Adolescents* (Bethesda, MD: Pacific Institute for Research and Evaluation, 1992), 36–49.

4. J. Moskowitz, *School Drug and Alcohol Policy: A Preliminary Model Relating Policy Implementation to School Problems* (Berkeley, CA: Prevention Research Center, 1987).

5. Klitzner, *Early Intervention for Adolescents.*

6. R. Brown, W. Carter, and M. Gordon, "Diagnosis of Alcoholism in a Simulated Patient Encounter by Primary Care Physicians," *Journal of Family Practice,* 25 (1987): 259–264; S. Clement, "The Identification of Alcohol-Related Problems by General Practitioners," *British Journal of Addictions,* 81 (1986): 257–264.

7. J. Hollingsworth, "Putting a Dollar Sign on Human Life," *EAP Digest* (July/August 1989): 19, 61–62, 65.

8. C. Stanley, M. Murphy, and R. Peters, "One Organization's Experience in a Case Management/EAP Program: Implications for Monitoring and Evaluation," *Employee Assistance Quarterly,* 3, 3/4 (1988): 229–241; R. Maiden, "Employee Assistance Program Evaluation in a Federal Government Agency," *Employee Assistance Quarterly,* 3, 3/4 (1988): 191; W. Howard, "Performance-Related Outcome Measures and Participation in a Job-Based Alcoholism Counseling Program," *Dissertation Abstracts International,* 50, 7 (1990): 2244-A; J. Iutcovich, "Employee Assistance Program as Mechanism for Alleviating the Problems of Employed Alcohol Abusers," in *Preventions and Treatments of Alcohol and Drug Abuse: A Socio-epidemiological Sourcebook,* B. Forster and J. Salloway, eds. (Lewiston, NY: Edwin Mellen Press, 1991).

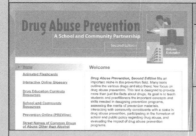

web resources

The Web site for this book offers many useful resources for educators, students, and professional counselors and is a great source for additional information. Visit the site at **http://healtheducation.jbpub.com/drugabuse/.**

Chapter Learning Objectives

Upon completion of this chapter, students will be able to:

1. Briefly define treatment.

2. Assess the need for treatment services.

3. Summarize the various formats or settings in which treatment may be provided.

4. Compare several models of addiction.

5. Compare and contrast eight approaches to drug abuse treatment.

6. Identify, briefly explain, and assess various approaches to smoking cessation.

Scenario

Jakub Green has been a middle school principal for 16 years. When he first started the job, after seven years of teaching, he was excited about the challenge and was energized by opportunities to solve problems and improve the instructional program.

Recently Jakub has found his job to be much more stressful and frustrating. He has had to manage a 10% cut in state funding and respond to significant discontent from the local board of education. Jakub has always been a social drinker, but in recent months the amount and frequency of his drinking has significantly increased. With the mounting pressures at work, he has sought refuge from it all by drinking more. Now he notices that it is harder to get through the day without a drink, but he has not shared his concerns with anyone, including his wife, who has custody of their children.

One of his best friends, Aimee Chess, is the coordinator of the school's student assistance program core team. Jakub considers confiding in her about his drinking, to get advice regarding whether he has a drinking problem or needs treatment.

Chapter 12

Treatment of Alcohol, Tobacco, and Drug Addiction

Introduction

Chapter 11 discussed early diagnosis and intervention for alcohol and drug problems. Sometimes intervention makes the need for treatment unnecessary; more times intervention prompts early treatment, which usually means more successful treatment. Sometimes early diagnosis does not occur, and the user receives no professional or other therapeutic assistance until late in the course of his or her problem. In any case, treatment is often the next step in addressing alcohol and drug problems.

The purpose of this chapter is not to teach specific skills for providing treatment for alcohol- and drug-impaired adolescents and adults; it is to familiarize the reader with the treatment system, contemporary concepts in the treatment process, and how to use treatment resources as an adjunct to drug education and abuse prevention.

For hundreds of years, efforts have been made to help people with alcohol and drug addictions. Nevertheless, the body of knowledge regarding the nature of addictions and how to treat them is still incomplete. There are many alternatives and widely divergent points of view about many treatment issues. Chapter 13 discusses the paucity of solid research and evaluation on drug abuse prevention; this deficiency is also found in evaluation of treatment programs and services. Much treatment is either not evaluated or poorly evaluated, which makes it difficult to make global recommendations. However, this chapter only occasionally makes evaluative comments about specific treatment strategies. Its main purpose is to describe what treatments are being used, not to critique them.

Some Faces of Alcoholism and Alcohol Abuse

George, age 19, is a college freshman who comes from a comfortable middle-class home in which his parents drink on occasion. He was forbidden to drink while at home, and has drunk very little in college. George recently pledged the local chapter of his father's fraternity, where heavy weekend drinking is common. Wanting to fit in, he has learned to enjoy beer, although ordinarily he does not consume large amounts. Last weekend, however, he became intoxicated and, while pursuing a dare, crashed his car and fractured his pelvis.

Ordinarily, William is a sober and well-mannered man. A loner, he lives in a rented room and rarely goes out except to work. However, from time to time, and increasingly in recent years, he suddenly starts drinking enormous quantities of alcohol, usually cheap fortified wine. Except to purchase his gallon jugs, he does not leave his room at these times, but can be heard at all hours, pacing the floor and talking loudly to himself. After a week or two (or three, in recent months), his room becomes quiet, and, looking much the worse for wear, William emerges to seek a new temporary job. When asked by his sympathetic landlady what causes him to behave in this way, he says, simply, "I don't know."

Sally has had a speech impediment since childhood. Despite considerable attention from speech therapists, she is able to speak clearly only intermittently. During her adolescence she developed the notion that she was able to speak much more clearly while under the influence of alcohol; she did not like its taste, however, so used it only sparingly. Recently she accepted a position as an assistant receptionist. When her coworker is absent, she is called upon to be the interface between the office and the outside world, something she has found difficult because of her impediment. Accordingly, she has turned increasingly to the use of alcohol, drinking vodka in the mornings before work and at lunchtime. So far her drinking has gone undetected in the workplace, but she has recognized that what was initially self-medication has become a practice that she is beginning to find gratifying in itself.

Source: Institute of Medicine, *Broadening the Base of Treatment for Alcohol Problems* (Washington, DC: National Academy Press, 1990).

Chapter 11 did not address tobacco consumption because intervention usually occurs when someone exhibits dysfunctional behavior, which generally is not present with tobacco. However, smokers are, in a physiological sense, addicts. As discussed in Chapter 3, smokers escape the despair and depravity associated with other drug addictions, but they are addicts nonetheless. Therefore, it may be appropriate to use the word *treatment* in the context of smoking and tobacco chewing cessation programs. After all, once regular smoking or chewing begins, prevention is no longer an option. On the other hand, treatment for tobacco addiction most times does not involve repairing emotional adjustment, renovating relationships, or rehabilitating skills for independent living. Tobacco addiction is more limited because treatment is restricted primarily to getting the user to quit. Recognizing both the similarities and differences between tobacco and other drug addiction, we include treatment for tobacco addiction in this chapter.

The Need for Treatment

Addiction is a mental health issue even though it has physical or organic aspects. As with all mental illness, the diagnostic criteria for addiction are not explicit or well defined, but are subjective and rely on the judgment of professionals. Of course, this is also true with physical disorders, but to a lesser degree. Experts often disagree about what is mental illness and what is not. This difficulty in diagnosing produces uncertainty about how many people are affected. The same difficulty applies to addictions. Although it is easy to obtain statistics on how many people use a drug, and how much they use, it is difficult to obtain estimates on how many people are addicted, or to know what addiction statistics mean. (See the Viewpoints box.)

Most alcohol and drug abuse treatment is funded, at least in part, by federal and state government agencies. Consequently, these agencies are the best sources of data on treatment prevalence.

			Percentage of U.S.
	Number	Percentage	Population
Gender			
Total	1,582,729	100	100
Male	1,108,452	70	48.9
Female	474,277	30	51.1
Race/Ethnicity			
White (non-Hispanic)	945,935	60.4	72.1
Black (non-Hispanic)	365,564	23.3	12.2
Hispanic	179,718	11.5	10.8
American Indian	37,327	2.4	0.7
Asian/Pacific Islander	12,940	0.8	3.8
Other	25,352	1.6	0.4
Age			
<18	134,484	8.5	25.9
18–24	245,870	15.6	9.4
25–34	451,628	28.6	13.9
35–44	508,029	32.1	16.4
45–54	190,284	12.0	13.1
55–64	40,421	2.6	8.6
65+	10,265	0.6	12.6

──────[**Table 12.1**]──────

Drug Abuse Treatment by Sex, Race/Ethnicity, and Age, 1999

Source: Substance Abuse and Mental Health Services Administration, 2001.

The U.S. Substance Abuse and Mental Health Services Administration maintains a data collection system, called the Drug and Alcohol Services Information System (DASIS), that gathers treatment data from the states. In 1999, this system identified 15,239 individual agencies that provide alcohol or drug abuse treatment or both.[1] (See Figure 12.1.) Included in this total are outpatient community programs, in-patient hospital or residential programs, and programs conducted in correctional facilities. (See Table 12.1 and Figure 12.2.) Those agencies reported about 1.6 million annual clients. The treatment agencies operated, on average, at about 84% of capacity. About 60% of treatment clients were between the ages of 25 and 44; 8.5% were under 18. About 30% were female, and 40% were nonwhite. Some clients were treated

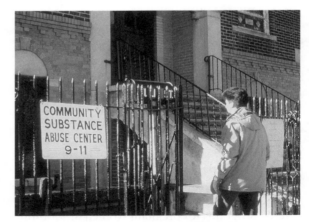

Figure 12.1 **A Drug Treatment Facility** Drug treatment facilities differ, as do their clients' treatment needs.

(© Jeff Greenberg/PhotoEdit)

The Need for Treatment　　**247**

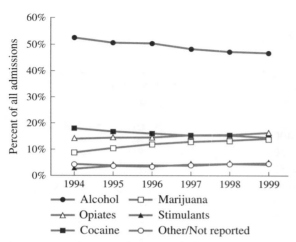

Figure 12.2 **Primary Substance of Abuse at Time of Admission, 1994–1999**

Source: Substance Abuse and Mental Health Services Administration, 2001.

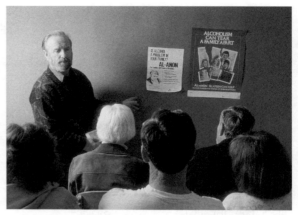

Figure 12.3 **An Alcoholics Anonymous Meeting**
Alcoholics Anonymous and similar groups are a common form of drug treatment. (© Mary Kate Denny/PhotoEdit)

for alcoholism only, others for other drug dependency only, and others for both. In 1997, about $11.9 billion was spent on drug treatment. That figure was small compared with the total social costs of $294 billion that can be attributed to substance abuse in that year.[2]

At any given time there are people in need of treatment who are not currently being served because they are unwilling to enter treatment or they lack available or accessible services. Although the 84% utilization rate cited earlier suggests a capacity greater than the need, the rate varies geographically. In some areas, utilization approaches and even exceeds 100%. Furthermore, some people in need of services are excluded because they cannot pay. Waiting lists are more common for publicly subsidized programs that are free or offered on a below-cost basis. Many programs will not accept pregnant women, adolescents, people with handicaps, or those who are HIV positive. However, data from 1999 indicate that 45% of facilities offer programs for patients with a dual diagnosis of addiction and mental illness, about 34% of programs had programs for adolescents, and 22% offered programs for pregnant women or for those with HIV/AIDS.[3] In the past it has been estimated that about 107,000 people were on waiting lists for treatment.[4]

In addition to enrollment in formal treatment programs, people participate in **mutual help** (also known as **self-help**) groups such as Alcoholics Anonymous (AA) and Narcotics Anonymous (NA). Although many of these clients also receive services from formal treatment agencies, many do not; approximately 70% of AA members are not referred from formal treatment programs.[5] Numbers from AA and similar groups are not included in the DASIS system because these groups are administratively unstructured, members are anonymous, and there is no consensus on what constitutes participation (e.g., one meeting, or five years of weekly attendance); therefore, there are not many reliable statistics on utilization of these types of groups. However, the facts that mutual support groups are found in virtually every community and that meetings are held every day suggest that the number is easily in the hundreds of thousands. (See **Figure 12.3**.)

In general, it may be said that significant numbers of people of all ages and demographic characteristics have a need for treatment of alcohol and drug abuse problems; one estimate is that each year about 5.5 million Americans need such treatment.[6] For many, the only barrier to receiving treatment is the personal recognition that help is needed. For others, there may be numerous obstacles, cost being the most significant. For service providers, the challenge is twofold: to break down denial and personal resistance to seeking treatment and to remove financial or other barriers. For counselors and therapists, a different spectrum of issues influences the recovery of drug-impaired individuals.

General Concepts of Treatment

What Is Treatment and What Is Being Treated?

Among people who use drugs, some proportion of them intensify their consumption to the point where it becomes harmful. In addition to the direct harm it causes, compulsive drug taking can take on inappropriate importance that overrides conventional aspects of life such as safety, employment, and fulfilling social responsibilities. This displacement of values can lead to significant indirect harm— broken relationships, unemployment, financial crises, and trouble with the police. Indirect harm also may be inflicted on family, coworkers, and others in the user's life. (See **Figure 12.4.**)

People whose drug or alcohol use causes them to experience these problems often can benefit from services that are called **treatment**, especially if the individual also has other emotional issues that interfere with his or her optimal functioning in society (e.g., a history of being sexually abused). The more advanced a person's addiction is, and the more extensive the related problems, the more

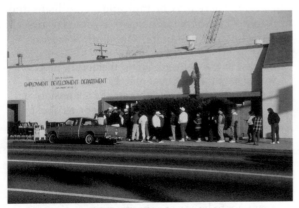

Figure 12.4 An Unemployment Line   While most unemployment is not caused by drug abuse, many who abuse drugs often experience unemployment problems.
(© Tony Freeman/PhotoEdit)

likely it is that he or she will need treatment services. The grim corollary is that the worse the person's alcohol or drug problem, the less likely it is that he or she will experience significant recovery.

The main purpose of treatment is to help the user eliminate drug use entirely or at least to adopt a use pattern that is not harmful. Hand in hand with this goal is addressing other personal and emotional problems related to the addiction. Specifically, these side issues may include reducing criminality, developing employability or vocational capabilities, restoring overall health, repairing psychological functioning, improving family life, and reducing fetal exposure to drugs.[7]

In this context the term **dual diagnosis** is often used, which refers to people with an addiction *and* a clinically diagnosable mental disorder, such as **bipolar depression** or **psychosis**. This condition presents a tremendous challenge because current drug addiction treatment methods may be far less successful in the presence of mental disorder; likewise, mental illness treatment methods may be less successful when there is a coexisting addiction. One study found that among those users seeking treatment for alcohol or drug dependency, 65% had a current mental disorder.[8] We know that many addicts have a variety of adjustment problems, but we don't know how many have a dual diagnosis significant enough to affect alcohol or drug abuse treatment effectiveness.

This chapter concentrates on treatment of the compulsive and harmful use of alcohol or other drugs. (See the FYI box.) However, there are opposing points of view in the

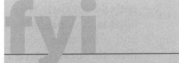

Drug Treatment Defined

Treatment refers to the broad range of services, including identification, brief intervention, assessment, diagnosis, counseling, medical services, psychiatric services, psychological services, social services, and follow-up, for persons with alcohol [or drug] problems. The overall goal of treatment is to reduce or eliminate the use of alcohol [or drugs] as a contributing factor to physical, psychological, and social dysfunction and to arrest, retard, or reverse the progress of any associated problems.

Source: Institute of Medicine, *Broadening the Base of Treatment for Alcohol Problems* (Washington, DC: National Academy Press, 1990).

treatment field about the appropriate focus of treatment. A conservative approach is to be very specific in applying treatment concepts only to alcoholism or addiction to other drugs. A more expansive approach is to advocate treatment methods for a wide variety of compulsive behaviors, including overeating, gambling, shopping, sex, anger and rage ("rage-aholism"), and so-called codependency—significant others' involvement in the dysfunctional behavior of addicts. Once these behaviors are labeled *addictions*, the next step is to apply treatment. The pros and cons of this approach are discussed later in this chapter.

Who Provides Treatment?

The question of who provides treatment implies that for a person to recover from an addiction, a treatment provider is required. There is no inherent reason why this should always be true. After all, tobacco has been described as one of the most addictive drugs, yet most quitters do so cold turkey entirely on their own. Although the cold turkey approach is probably less common with alcohol and other drug addicts, many people can recognize the destructive nature of their drug consumption and take steps to change it without any external assistance. However, the reader should recognize that many people in the drug addiction treatment field would not agree with this notion.

Nevertheless, many people either want or need some external assistance with kicking a drug habit. This assistance comes in many shapes and sizes. Treatment may be provided by private counselors and therapists who provide individual care on a fee-for-service basis. Some treatment is provided by community mental health agencies in an outpatient format. Treatment may be provided by hospitals, in which case clients may be served as in-patients, with a major focus on ridding the body of chemicals (so-called *detox*). Other in-patient programs are operated outside of hospitals. In these programs, the medical side of treatment is deemphasized while more attention is placed on personal strategies for **sobriety** and recovery. A variation of nonmedical in-patient treatment is therapeutic communities, which are residential settings that often are operated by former addicts. Professional therapists usually have a less significant role in therapeutic communities than they do in other chemical dependency treatment approaches.

Addiction as a Disease

There are many theories about the cause of alcohol and drug abuse, including sin and moral failure, nutritional deficiencies, allergies, biochemical and brain abnormalities, endocrine disorders, heredity, and social deprivation.[9] The most widespread view of addiction is that it is a disease. According to this position, people with uncontrolled drinking or other drug abuse have a disease in the same sense that one has diabetes or high blood pressure. The so-called *disease concept* or *medical model* maintains that addiction is a biological trait, probably inherited, that gets progressively worse. The affected user has no control over the condition: He or she is neither responsible for its development nor able to recover on his or her own. The reader should be clear that the disease concept is a theoretical perspective, not a statement of objective truth. In fact, most researchers in the alcoholism and addiction field disavow the disease model and counter that the supportive evidence for equating alcoholism or addiction with disease in a medical sense is unconvincing at best.

A more correct view is that alcohol and drug dependency is not a single entity, but falls into distinct subtypes with uniquely different patterns of causation. There may be multiple alcoholisms and multiple drug dependencies—a one-size-fits-all approach is not adequate. One author states:

> If at one time a major goal of the therapeutic process was to have the patient admit "I am an alcoholic," it may now be time to elaborate the confession to "I am an alcoholic who is dependent on alcohol to a certain degree (slight, moderate, severe), who is disabled to a certain degree in certain areas of functioning (physical, psychological, social), and whose problem is primarily attributable to certain vulnerabilities (physical, psychological, environmental)." The problem, and the paradox, is that there seems not to be any one specific entity conforming to our current notions of alcoholism. Rather, there appears to be a whole group of related syndromes whose only common characteristics are drinking, dependence, and damage.[10]

The disease model stands in contrast to many other perspectives.[11] The *moral model* considers the addict to be responsible for both the development of the problem and its solution or elimination. Recovery is achieved by motivation and willpower. Smoking cessation is often based on this model. In the *compensatory model*, people are not considered responsible for the development of a problem, but they can take personal responsibility to change their behavior. Treatment approaches that utilize behavior modification are based on the compensatory model. The *enlightenment model* assumes that people are responsible for the origin and development of problems, but that they cannot overcome them on their own. Alcoholics Anonymous and therapeutic communities are based on the enlightenment model. However, most proponents of AA or therapeutic communities hold to the disease model. Other models include the *public health model*, which points to interactions between the individual, the drug, and the environment, and models based on social learning theory and classical or operant conditioning.

Most of the addiction models have merits and weaknesses. For example, consider the disease model. Although alcoholism seems to run in families, many alcoholics have no family history of it, whereas some people with a strong family history of alcoholism do not develop it. This should be no surprise. Some smokers do not develop lung cancer or heart disease; it is a matter of probabilities. However, it is hard to make a case for a strong genetic link to alcoholism.[12] Many other factors are involved, some known and some not known. One strength of the disease model is that it removes the stigma of blame and guilt that may occur with the moral model. The disease model is also partially responsible for decreased criminal punishment for alcohol abuse. Although we may put drunks in jail, we also try to rehabilitate them with medical and social services. On the other hand, the disease model provides a smoke screen for alcohol promoters that claim the problem is not with alcohol but with those unfortunate drinkers who have the disease.

So far there has been little consideration of other perspectives and treatment approaches because the disease model has been so universally embraced by practitioners. The literature suggests that a more open perspective is appropriate because there is no single superior approach to treatment for all individuals.[13] Unfortunately, however, most treatment programs have a single treatment pattern: Every client is treated with identical methods and in a similar time frame. The literature demonstrates that different types of people are best served by different treatment approaches. Since at least the 1960s there have been calls to match individuals with the treatment methods best suited for their needs, but little progress has been made on this issue.[14] The treatment methods described next may be used exclusively with alcohol or drugs, or with both.

Specific Treatment Methods

Methadone Maintenance

Methadone maintenance was developed in the mid-1960s and is based on two premises. First, narcotic analgesic drugs (e.g., morphine and heroin) have similar effects: Tolerance to one drug is accompanied by tolerance to the others, and withdrawal from one drug can be blocked by administering another drug at the appropriate dose. Second, when two drugs are similar, the longest-acting drug produces the most prolonged but mildest withdrawal symptoms. Methadone, a legal prescription drug, is a long-acting narcotic analgesic. There is cross-tolerance between it and heroin; administration of methadone eliminates an addict's need for heroin, averts the dramatic highs and lows of heroin, and blocks most heroin withdrawal symptoms. Substitution of methadone for heroin enables a heroin addict to avoid street drugs and crime, and buys the addict some time to learn to cope with life without heroin. Also, because methadone is taken orally, needles can be avoided. In 1999, the DASIS system reported that there were 1,215 methadone maintenance programs with a total of 178,212 clients in the United States.[15]

Methadone programs assess the addict at the time of program entrance and determine the necessary dose of methadone. Over a period of time, the methadone dose is gradually decreased until no more of the drug is given. The typical methadone program varies in length from about 21 days to several months; duration of treatment sometimes follows a standardized timetable. In other programs, the timetable depends on the client's rate of progress toward recovery. In addition to receiving this **chemotherapy**, the client participates in counseling and rehabilitation services (such as job training). Methadone maintenance may be done in an in-patient hospital, but it is usually done on an outpatient basis. If a program is outpatient, clients are expected periodically to submit urine samples that are tested for heroin and other drugs. Some programs test weekly; others test monthly.

As methadone is reduced, the addict may experience mild withdrawal symptoms, usually about a week into the program, which may cause some patients to quit the treatment program. Others may complete the **detoxification** program successfully, but if they do not complete other dimensions of treatment, or if they return to their former residence, lifestyle, and circle of friends, they may resume heroin abuse.

Most methadone maintenance programs have the objective of eliminating use of all illicit drugs, as well as methadone. Some programs suggest that maintaining an addict on methadone for a prolonged period of time is better for the addict (and society) than returning to heroin dependency. However, many people are philosophically opposed to long-term maintenance because it appears to condone addictive drug use.

On balance, methadone maintenance program evaluations repeatedly have demonstrated their value in helping heroin addicts reduce the frequency and amount of illicit drug use, reduce criminal behavior, and become more socially responsible in employment, education, or child rearing. About one in four methadone clients is not successful with this method of treatment.[16]

Therapeutic Communities

With the opening of Synanon in 1958 came the beginning of the therapeutic community (TC) form of drug treatment. Since then, many TCs have been established, such as Daytop Village and Phoenix

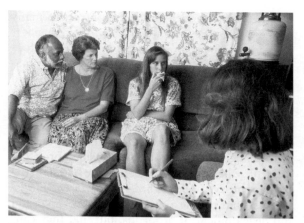

Figure 12.5 Confrontation in Group Therapy
Confrontation is a common part of group therapy that is used in therapeutic communities and many other types of drug treatment. (© Michael Newman/PhotoEdit)

House. Some TCs are operated in prisons. Therapeutic communities have several primary strategies:

1. The addict lives for an extended period (usually 2 to 24 months) in a drug-free environment with firm norms for behavior (particularly no drug use).
2. Through group and individual **psychotherapy**, there is much honest confrontation of dysfunctional feelings and behaviors such as blame, resentment, and hostility (see **Figure 12.5**).
3. Clients are expected to carry out routine responsibilities (enhanced by specific rewards and punishments) such as house cleaning, cooking, and laundry tasks. Such tasks are intended to inculcate social responsibility and normal habits and values in contrast to street hustling and other antisocial or irresponsible behavior exhibited before entering treatment.
4. Clients participate in a 12-step program such as AA or NA.
5. The longer a client resides in a TC, the more he or she assumes a staff role, with responsibility for helping newer clients to recover.

Many addicts who enter TCs leave after only a few weeks. Only about 10% "graduate" by staying for the full length of treatment as designed. However, for those who stay in TCs at least several months, one-third to two-thirds decrease their drug consumption and crime. Their posttreatment success in education or employment is about 50% greater than those who drop out or are not treated at all.[17]

Pharmacologic Treatment

Medications may be used in alcohol and drug treatment to accomplish various goals. Therapeutic drugs sometimes are helpful in minimizing the severity of withdrawal symptoms; examples are benzodiazepines (see Chapter 5) and multivitamins. Even though physical withdrawal is often mild, an addict knows that any discomfort can be relieved in minutes simply by taking a dose of the abused drug. Medications for withdrawal control can be helpful in the short run for discouraging relapse.

Medications also may be used to block the effects of a drug, effectively circumventing its **reinforcement value**. The best example is naltrexone, which is an antagonist for heroin. If someone takes a regular dose of naltrexone and then takes heroin, none of the euphoria or other wanted effects of the heroin occur. The problem with this approach is that clients usually are not compliant; they have such a strong craving for heroin that they will terminate the naltrexone therapy.

A variation of the antagonist therapy is using medication to terminate or reduce the desire for drugs or alcohol. This therapy is still in the research stage. Femeldine is an example of a drug that affects brain chemistry in such a way that the drinker's alcohol consumption decreases.[18]

Medications may be used to control drug cravings after withdrawal is completed. An example is the treatment of cocaine dependency. Some researchers and clinicians believe that cocaine addicts experience a formidable depression following cocaine use. Eventually, addicts take cocaine to avoid the depression rather than to achieve the high. Antidepressant medications may help this type of addict avoid relapse in the weeks and months following withdrawal.

Perhaps the most well-known pharmaceutical adjunct to drug treatment is Antabuse, a prescription drug first used in alcoholism treatment in 1948. Antabuse blocks the full breakdown of ingested alcohol, causing a buildup of a **metabolite** called acetaldehyde. Acetaldehyde is toxic, which causes the drinker to experience low blood pressure, nausea and vomiting, hot flashes, coughing, labored breathing, and anxiety.[19] Before Antabuse therapy begins, the drinker is forewarned about the unpleasant effects that will occur if he or she drinks alcohol; this warning is supposed to provide an external incentive for abstinence. In older, more socially stable clients, Antabuse may have some therapeutic value. However, compliance is a significant issue with most alcoholics. The effectiveness of Antabuse therapy is enhanced when the client's daily dose is monitored by a family member or by urine testing.

Finally, medications are useful in managing addicts with mental disorders. Clients with a dual diagnosis usually take psychoactive prescription drugs to enhance their recovery from addiction.

Self-Help and Mutual Support Groups

Although its roots go back to the 19th century, Alcoholics Anonymous officially began in the 1930s and has since become the prototype for many other drug abuse recovery support groups, including Narcotics Anonymous, Cocaine Anonymous, Potsmokers Anonymous, Smokers Anonymous (for tobacco addicts), Al-Anon, and Alateen. The 12-step core of AA has also been adopted by groups that address other dysfunctional behavior problems; examples include Gamblers Anonymous, Emotions Anonymous, and Overeaters Anonymous. Some drug recovery groups are not based on the 12 steps of AA, such as Women for Sobriety and Drinkwatchers.

There is considerable diversity within AA and similar support group programs, but they all are based on the 12 steps and the 12 traditions (see the FYI boxes), which provide common ground. Alcoholics Anonymous and the other 12-step groups have several standard components. The first is meetings, which are held daily at various times throughout the day. New initiates are encouraged to attend "90 meetings in 90 days." People are encouraged to attend whether they are still drinking or not; some continue affiliation for 5

The 12 Steps of Alcoholics Anonymous

1. We admitted we were powerless over alcohol—that our lives had become unmanageable;

2. Came to believe that a Power greater than ourselves could restore us to sanity;

3. Made a decision to turn our will and our lives over to the care of God as we understood Him;

4. Made a searching and fearless moral inventory of ourselves;

5. Admitted to God, to ourselves, and to another human being the exact nature of our wrongs;

6. Were entirely ready to have God remove all these defects of character;

7. Humbly asked Him to remove our shortcomings;

8. Made a list of all persons we had harmed, and became willing to make amends to them all;

9. Made direct amends to such people wherever possible, except when to do so would injure them or others;

10. Continued to take personal inventory and when we were wrong promptly admitted it;

11. Sought through prayer and meditation to improve our conscious contact with God as we understood Him, praying only for knowledge of His will for us and the power to carry that out;

12. Having had a spiritual awakening as the result of these steps, we tried to carry this message to alcoholics and to practice these principles in all our affairs.

Source: *Alcoholics Anonymous* (New York: Alcoholics Anonymous World Services, 1976), 59–60.

speaker achieve sobriety. Another meeting format is to discuss one of the 12 steps or 12 traditions. Both types of meetings provide significant fellowship and informal support.

The next component of this type of support group is studying and applying the 12 steps. Although the 12 steps were originally designed for alcohol abuse, they have been adapted to many other problems, such as narcotics and food. The steps establish three basic concepts: Users are powerless over alcohol or drugs (or food, sex, gambling, etc.), they need help from an external source (a higher power), and they can recover by making amends for the harm they have done and helping others to find sobriety. This process is called "working the steps" or "working a program." People work through the 12 steps at their own pace, with no particular expected schedule; some work the steps for the rest of their lives. This process is facilitated by reading material on the steps, published by the respective organization; the *Big Book* of AA is an example.

The third component of AA-type groups is tokens or medallions. For sobriety of various durations (one month, six months, two years, etc.), members receive a coin-like reminder of their achievement. Tokens are awarded at meetings, with fanfare and group accolade. (See **Figure 12.6.**)

A final component is that members relate to sponsors, who are group members with more time in recovery. Sponsors, essentially mentors, help the person avoid relapse, are available for support and encouragement, discuss various life problems, and guide the person through the 12 steps. Sponsors often present tokens at the appropriate times. New group members may be assigned a temporary sponsor until they choose a permanent sponsor. Members are expected eventually to take on the role of sponsor to someone else; this is considered an important part of their own recovery program.

It is conventional wisdom among treatment practitioners that AA is the most effective treatment for alcoholism, and, by implication, that other 12-step programs are most effective for treating other compulsive behavior problems. However, research does not support such an assertion. AA and other similar groups undoubtedly help many people recover from addictive behavior, but some

years, some for 10, and some for a lifetime even after they have been sober for a long time. Those people who have less success with or less attraction to the AA approach typically stop attending after only a few meetings.

Meetings are of two types: open, which anyone can attend, and closed, which are only for those who are trying to achieve sobriety. Meetings may have a speaker who tells the story of how he or she became an alcoholic and how AA helped the

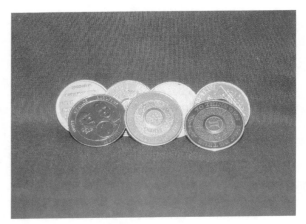

Figure 12.6 AA Medallions Alcoholics Anonymous awards tokens or medallions to commemorate periods of sobriety. (© Mindy Murray/Unicorn Stock Photos)

people are served more effectively by other approaches. There is a need for researchers to define the effectiveness of 12-step programs better, and what types of clients will respond most favorably to them.

The Minnesota Model

Besides AA and other self-help groups, the Minnesota Model is perhaps the most common approach to drug and alcohol abuse treatment and is the usual format for the typical 28-day treatment program. The name is derived from its origins in Minnesota in the 1950s. There are variations in the application of the Minnesota Model, but the most typical components include the following: (1) a one-week detoxification program to rid the client's body of the drug of abuse, (2) a three-week in-patient rehabilitation program, and (3) aftercare that is designed to last a year or more and that usually involves AA or other self-help group participation. The in-patient rehabilitation phase includes individual and group therapy, education on alcohol and the disease model, and attendance at AA or similar meetings to work the 12 steps. It may also include attention to healthful living habits and to rebuilding the client's life through assistance with employment or educational pursuits. Often there are opportunities for family therapy in the client's treatment.

The 12 Traditions of Narcotics Anonymous

1. Our common welfare should come first; personal recovery depends upon NA unity.
2. For our group purpose there is but one ultimate authority—a loving God as He may express Himself in our group conscience. Our leaders are but trusted servants, they do not govern.
3. The only requirement for membership is a desire to stop using.
4. Each group should be autonomous except in matters affecting other groups or NA as a whole.
5. Each group has but one primary purpose—to carry the message to the addict who still suffers.
6. An NA group ought never endorse, finance, or lend the NA name to any related facility or outside enterprise, lest problems of money, property, or prestige divert us from our primary purpose.
7. Every NA group ought to be fully self-supporting, declining outside contributions.
8. Narcotics Anonymous should remain forever nonprofessional, but our service centers may employ special workers.
9. NA, as such, ought never be organized, but we may create service boards or committees directly responsible to those they serve.
10. Narcotics Anonymous has no opinion on outside issues; hence the NA name ought never be drawn into public controversy.
11. Our public relations policy is based on attraction rather than promotion; we need always maintain personal anonymity at the level of press, radio, and films.
12. Anonymity is the spiritual foundation of our traditions, ever reminding us to place principles before personalities.

Source: *Narcotics Anonymous* (Van Nuys, CA: World Service Office, 1986), 7–8.

The Minnesota Model blends the self-help principles of the 12 steps with professional medical and counseling services. Personnel may include physicians and nurses (particularly during the detoxification phase), professional counselors, and nonprofessional counselors who are recovering from an addiction.

At the end of the 28-day in-patient program, clients begin an extended aftercare protocol that may include self-help groups, family therapy, Antabuse, individual and group counseling, and short-term residence in a halfway house.

Thousands of people have recovered with the help of treatment programs based on the Minnesota Model. However, it is not always successful, and it is one of the most expensive forms of treatment. Some addicts are served more effectively and efficiently with other treatment approaches.

The California Social Model

Though its theoretical roots go back to earlier decades, the California social model first was recognized as a distinct alternative treatment approach in the late 1960s and early 1970s. This treatment's perspective is that addiction is caused by social relationships and the environment as well as by individual problems and characteristics. The importance of professional services and the medical approach are discounted, and pharmacologically assisted detoxification and a passive patient role are viewed as barriers to the recovery process. The California social model puts special emphasis on participation in 12-step programs, but also may include placing clients in temporary drug-free living, such as a halfway house, and helping them form social attachments that reinforce a drug- and alcohol-free lifestyle.

Over the years the model has undergone some revisions, but as it is currently conceived, the California social model has the following conceptual characteristics:

1. The experiential knowledge of recovering addicts guides decision making (as opposed to professionals who are guided by the theory and principles of clinical practice).
2. Twelve-step programs are the foundation of recovery.
3. Recovery is lifelong and experiential in nature.
4. There is a lack of doctor-patient, therapist-client, or other power relationships.
5. Participants both receive services and give assistance.

6. Participants and staff relate in the style of an extended family.

Aversion Therapy

Aversion therapy is based on **classical conditioning** and is usually done by a counselor with an individual client. The goal is to associate alcohol or other drug use with an unpleasant sensation, such as nausea, or an undesirable consequence, such as an auto accident. The therapist assists the client in **imaging** a drinking or other drug use situation by using a "conditioning scene" (see the Hints & Tips box). Drinking or drug use is paired with something unpleasant or fear arousing. Over a period of about four weeks, the client is led in imaging escape and avoidance of drinking or drug use and its undesirable consequences. The client is led through up to 50 scenes, with each conditioning scene lasting from two to eight minutes. Evaluations of aversion therapy have shown this modality to be very effective, especially in combination with other techniques that instill problem-solving and coping strategies. (See **Figure 12.7**.)

Behavioral Self-Control Training

Alcohol problems vary in severity, from occasional problem drinking to severely dependent alcoholism. In general, it is true that the most severe problems are intractable and have a poor **prognosis**

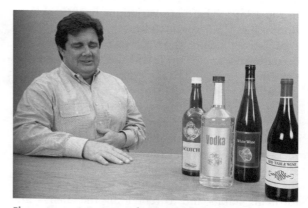

Figure 12.7 A Person Who Is Conditioned to Be Repulsed by Alcohol Aversion therapy conditions people to be repulsed by alcoholic beverages.

for recovery. However, some therapies are more suitable for drinking problems that are less entrenched and serious. Behavioral self-control training (BSCT) is just such an approach. It is used most often with a goal of moderation, but the same techniques can be directed toward abstinence.

BSCT can be directed by a therapist with individual clients or in a group. It can also be done individually through a self-help approach, with minimal professional intervention. The therapist-directed version typically is done in weekly 90-minute sessions over a period of eight weeks. Between sessions, clients complete homework designed to help them gain skills to control drinking and cope with problems in ways other than alcohol abuse. Specific BSCT strategies include the following:

1. Setting limits on the number of drinks per day
2. Self-monitoring of drinking behavior
3. Changing the rate of drinking
4. Practicing assertiveness in refusing drinks (see **Figure 12.8**)
5. Setting up a reward system for achievement of goals
6. Learning which **antecedents** result in overdrinking
7. Learning other coping skills instead of drinking

Evaluations of BSCT show that many people respond successfully to this treatment approach and can continue to drink moderately or remain abstinent for long periods of time.[20]

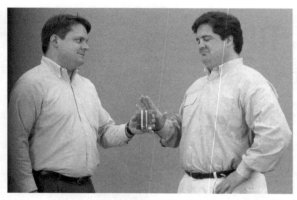

Figure 12.8 Learning How to Say "No" Adults with less severe drinking problems can learn many skills to manage their drinking, including saying "no" to alcohol in social situations.

Conflicting Perspectives on Treatment

The most widely held belief among treatment professionals is that once someone has had a drug or drinking problem, he or she must strive for lifelong abstinence in order to maintain sobriety and avoid relapse. This view reflects the dominance of the disease concept of alcohol and drug addiction.

Some researchers and clinicians have suggested that moderate use is also a feasible goal, at least for legal substances, but their assertions have been criticized as being unrealistic, unprofessional, dangerous, and unethical. However, there is evidence to support the notion that some alcoholics can safely include moderate drinking in posttreatment recovery.[21] For those people with the most advanced addictions, moderation probably won't be effective, but a trial with moderation may be a first step in convincing them of the need for abstinence.

Every form of treatment has proponents who may be zealous about the value of their particular approach. The truth is that many treatment modalities can achieve success, and treatment professionals must be open to all of the strategies in order to find the most suitable approach for each client. This practice is not being followed very often for several reasons. Various options may not be available in a given community, the entity that recommends treatment may be tied to a specific approach (insurance companies, for example, favor a medical or professional approach as a general policy, even though other strategies may be more effective and less expensive), and the techniques to match patients with specific treatment approaches are not well developed and are not widely understood by practitioners. The practice of matching clients to particular treatment strategies will certainly increase in the future.

As mentioned at the beginning of this chapter, many people view addicts as victims; that is, addicts are seen as casualties of forces beyond their control who require intensive external help and lifelong immersion in a recovery process. A minority of researchers and treatment professionals think that this attitude becomes a self-fulfilling prophecy that leads to defeat or at least to less than optimal recovery.[22] They attribute much value to self-efficacy instead of the idea that addicts are powerless over their addiction. The self-efficacy approach has the following general components:

1. The individual must want to change.
2. The things that are important in life can provide important motivation for change. These things must be identified and highlighted in contrast to the addictive behavior.
3. Individuals with addictions can and must improve personal skills and self-confidence.
4. Investing time, energy, and money in family, job, community, hobbies, and so forth can promote success in overcoming addiction.
5. Community and social support for wholesome and productive activity in all aspects of life can be a powerful force for maintaining an addiction-free lifestyle.

Recovery services based on these premises seem to have much to offer and might be a refreshing alternative to some of the more limited or traditional approaches. However, drug addiction is such a prevalent and worrisome problem that we should be open to researching every strategy that offers promise.

Smoking and Chewing Cessation

For more than 40 years, efforts have been made to help people quit using tobacco. During that time, many approaches have been tried; some have been discarded and others have been modified. Although still not 100% successful, the state of the art has advanced considerably. Most tobacco users who have quit have done so entirely on their own; users who are less motivated or have severe addiction often can be helped by various kinds of external assistance.[23] The resources and technology for smoking cessation are much more developed than those for chewing cessation. It is assumed that what works for smoking will also work for chewing, including counseling, behavioral strategies, and nicotine replacement therapy,[24] but more research and development is needed to clarify this issue further. Likewise, most of what is known about smoking cessation is based on work with adults. There is a great need to help adolescents quit smoking and chewing, but the knowledge base in this area is minimal.

Help may include self-help materials that are published by governmental agencies and many private-sector organizations. The best of these publications include information about the consequences of smoking, specific strategies and exercises for successful quitting, information targeted to special audiences, specific strategies and exercises for avoiding relapse, and strategies for trying again in case of initial failure or relapse. (See **Figure 12.9**.) Self-help guides can be printed manuals and brochures, audiotapes, or videotapes.[25] Numerous Internet-based guides to smoking cessation also exist.

In many communities, private counselors offer **hypnosis** as an aid to smoking cessation; such services are widely advertised. Hypnosis may be done on an individual or group basis, in a single session or in multiple sessions, and as a single strategy or as part of a combination of several strategies. Undoubtedly, some people quit smoking with this approach, but it is not considered the most promising method by itself. Many people are unwilling or unable to be hypnotized, so this approach is not suitable for them. It is clear that success with hypnosis is contingent upon the client's motivation to quit; without such motivation, success is very unlikely. Also, the training of the hypnotist is critical; let the buyer beware!

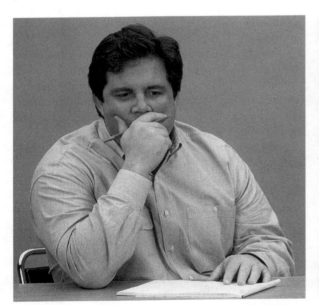 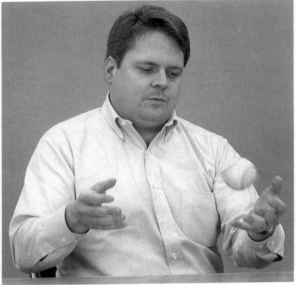

Figure 12.9 Techniques Used to Stop Smoking (Left: Invention/Reasons to Quit; Right: Keeping Hands Busy)
Many quit-smoking skills can be learned from self-help material or in smoking cessation classes.

There has been some interest in **acupuncture** as a cessation procedure. Evaluations show that acupuncture alone is not very effective, but its value might be improved if it is combined with other strategies. As with all cessation methods, the tobacco user's desire to quit is the most important variable.

Another cessation technique is nicotine replacement therapy. Nicotine gum and nicotine skin patches were once available only by prescription from a physician, but are now available over the counter. (See **Figure 12.10**.) A nicotine inhaler and nicotine nasal spray are available by prescription. These devices give the user a controlled source of nicotine that is reduced over a period of time. In the meantime, smoking behavior can terminate, as well as the hazards of inhaling carbon monoxide and tar. To be most valuable, gum or patches should be used in combination with a self-help program or a group cessation program. Most people attempting to quit will not succeed with nicotine supplements alone.

Another medication shown to be helpful in tobacco cessation is bupropion (brand name Zyban). This prescription medication, used in combination with nicotine replacement therapy and behavioral support programs, has been shown to promote tobacco abstinence.[26]

Aversion therapy, available from private practitioners and agencies, is sometimes effective. It is based on the same concepts described for aversion therapy in the treatment of alcohol and other drug abuse. The tobacco user is taught to associate tobacco use with an unpleasant experience or sensation. This may be done by imaging unpleasant stimuli, with electric shock, or with rapid smoking. In rapid smoking, the client is directed to inhale from a cigarette every six seconds until he or she becomes nauseated or cannot tolerate any more cigarettes. Over a period of time, smoking becomes aversive and unwanted, at least in theory.

In general, aversion therapy has not proven to be effective, but it is still available in some places. When it is combined with other complementary strategies that promote long-term maintenance, aversion can have good results. These programs tend to be expensive. Consumers should carefully review the components and success rates of specific programs.

Another well-known resource for tobacco cessation is a group quitting program. These programs are available in most communities and may be sponsored by governmental agencies, hospitals, voluntary agencies, churches, and for-profit businesses. They are typically structured to last from four to eight weeks; most programs are outpatient, but there are some residential quit-smoking group programs.

Group programs typically include education on the benefits of quitting and pay significant

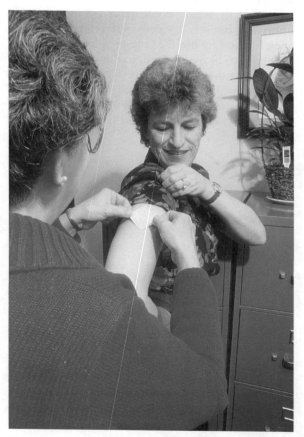

Figure 12.10 Nicotine Skin Patch Nicotine gum or skin patches can help many people successfully quit smoking. (© Tony Freeman/PhotoEdit)

Tobacco Cessation Resources

American Cancer Society
1599 Clifton Road NE
Atlanta, GA 30329
(800) ACS-2345
www.cancer.org/

American Heart Association
National Center,
7272 Greenville Ave.
Dallas, TX 75231
(800) AHA-8721
www.americanheart.org

National Cancer Institute
NCI Public Inquiries Office
Suite 3036A
6116 Executive Boulevard, MSC8322
Bethesda, MD 20892-8322
(800) 4-CANCER
www.nci.nih.gov

American Dental Association
211 East Chicago Ave.
Chicago, IL 60611
(312) 440-2500
www.ada.org/

American Lung Association
61 Broadway, 6th Floor
New York, NY 10006
(212) 315-8700
www.lungusa.org/

Tobacco Information and Prevention Source (TIPS)
U.S. Department of Health and Human Services
Parklawn Building, Room 110
5600 Fishers Lane
Rockville, MD 20857
(301) 443-1575
www.cdc.gov/tobacco/

Tobacco Cessation Guideline
Office of the U.S. Surgeon General
www.surgeongeneral.gov/tobacco/

QuitNet
www.quitnet.com/
Consult your phone directory for your local health department or hospital.

attention to **quitting skills**. They also address topics of special concern, such as weight gain and stress. In addition to conventional instruction in concepts and skills, these programs have the benefit of group support. Participants share and discuss issues that can help them avoid relapse, pressure each other to keep trying, and reinforce each other for short-term quitting success. The proprietary programs tend to be quite expensive, and there is no evidence to show that they are more effective than programs offered by nonprofit

agencies. Evaluation studies of group programs yield an average one-year success rate of 33%.[27] This benchmark is useful for judging specific programs.

Like all drug treatment, some quitting methods work better than others, depending on the individual. If a user is unsuccessful with one method, it is worthwhile to try different approaches until one is found that works. The FYI box lists tobacco cessation resources that are available to most communities.

Summary

This book is intended for personnel interested in ATOD prevention. The authors believe prevention is the best way to address problems of drug abuse. However, a comprehensive approach calls for cooperation and coordination between prevention, intervention, and treatment. Educators and prevention specialists should know the various alternatives for the treatment of drug problems, including those for the cessation of smoking. They must be prepared to ask questions about why someone needs treatment and what sort of treatment will be provided, and be able to assess the merits of the answers. Educators and specialists should know when to refer someone for treatment. Understanding the treatment process will help provide support for ongoing recovery. This chapter has been included to expand the prevention specialist's ability to work on a comprehensive team, cooperating with treatment personnel to more effectively respond to drug problems that occur in our communities.

Scenario | Analysis and Response

Jakub hesitates to talk to Aimee Chess because she is an employee of the school, and he worries about rumors spreading that he has a drinking problem. However, he is worried about his drinking, and decides he has to trust his friend.

Aimee decides that since Jakub's personal relationships are still intact, and he has not had severe work problems, he does not need anything as intensive as a 28-day treatment program. Instead, she advises him to go to a local community mental health agency that offers behavioral self-control training. In addition, she makes suggestions on ways Jakub could relieve stress and lead a more balanced life.

Learning Activities

1. Obtain statistics on the client capacity of drug abuse treatment programs in your state. Determine how many clients are actually served each year, and what provisions are made for addicts who can't pay for treatment services.

2. Visit local drug abuse treatment agencies in your community and determine how their programs are organized and implemented. Categorize each program according to the treatment approaches described in this chapter.

3. Interview a chemical dependency counselor and discuss his or her views on the causes of addiction. In your own mind, try to classify the counselor's view by the models described in this chapter.

4. Do an inventory of the local smoking cessation resources and programs.

5. Do a library and Internet search on evaluation studies of adolescent smoking cessation programs or methods.

Notes

1. Office of Applied Studies, Substance Abuse and Mental Health Services Administration, "New and Repeat Admissions to Substance Abuse Treatment," *The DASIS Report,* April 26, 2002.

2. R. M. Coffey, T. Mark, E. King, et al., "National Estimates of Expenditures for Substance Abuse Treatment, 1997," SAMHSA Publication No. SMA-01-3511 (Rockville, MD: Center for Substance Abuse Treatment and Center for Mental Health Services, Substance Abuse and Mental Health Services Administration, February 2001).

3. Office of Applied Studies, "New and Repeat Admissions."

4. H. L. Batten, C. M. Horgan, and J. M. Prottas, *Drug Services Research Survey Provisional Report: Phase I* (Rockville, MD: National Institute on Drug Abuse, November 1990).

5. J. Wallace, "The Attack of the 'Anti-Traditionalist' Lobby," *Professional Counselor,* (January/February 1987): 21–39.

6. D. R. Gerstein and H. J. Harwood, eds., *Treating Drug Problems,* Vol. I (Washington, DC: National Academy Press, 1990).

7. Ibid.

8. H. Ross, F. Glaser, and T. Germanson, "The Prevalence of Psychiatric Disorders in Patients with Alcohol and Other Drug Problems," *Archives of General Psychiatry,* 45 (1988): 1023–1031.

9. R. K. Hester and W. R. Miller, eds., *Handbook of Alcoholism Treatment Approaches: Effective Alternatives* (New York: Pergamon Press, 1989).

10. T. Babor, "Evaluating the Evaluation Process," in *Evaluation of the Alcoholic: Implications for Research, Theory, and Treatment,* R. Meyer et al., eds., Research

Monograph No. 5 (Rockville, MD: National Institute on Alcohol Abuse and Alcoholism, 1981), xiii.

11. Hester and Miller, *Handbook of Alcoholism Treatment Approaches*; P. Brickman et al., "Models of Helping and Coping," *American Psychologist*, 37 (1982): 368–384.

12. A. M. Bolos et al., "Population and Pedigree Studies Reveal a Lack of Association Between the Dopamine D_2 Receptor Gene and Alcoholism," *Journal of the American Medical Association*, 264 (1990): 3156–3160.

13. Hester and Miller, *Handbook of Alcoholism Treatment Approaches*.

14. R. M. Glasscote et al., *The Treatment of Alcohol Problems: A Study of Programs and Problems* (Washington, DC: Joint Information Service of the American Psychiatric Association and the National Association of Mental Health, 1967).

15. Office of Applied Statistics, Substance Abuse and Mental Health Administration, *National Survey of Substance Abuse Treatment Services,* October 1, 2000.

16. Gerstein and Harwood, *Treating Drug Problems,* Vol. I, 147.

17. Substance Abuse and Mental Health Services Administrations, *National Drug and Alcohol Treatment Unit Survey (NDATUS): 1992 Main Findings Report,* DHHS Publication No. (SMA) 93-2007 (Rockville, MD: DHHS, 1993).

18. Ross, Glaser, and Germanson, "Prevalence of Psychiatric Disorders."

19. Ibid.

20. Hester and Miller, *Handbook of Alcoholism Treatment Approaches*.

21. Ibid.

22. S. Peele and A. Brodsky, *The Truth About Addiction and Recovery* (New York: Simon & Schuster, 1991).

23. J. L. Schwartz, *Review and Evaluation of Smoking Cessation Methods: The United States and Canada, 1978–1985,* NIH Publication No. 87-2940 (Bethesda, MD: National Cancer Institute, 1987).

24. M. C. Fiore, W. C. Bailey, S. J. Cohen, et al., *Treating Tobacco Use and Dependence: Clinical Practice Guideline* (Rockville, MD: U.S. Department of Health and Human Services, 2000).

25. T. J. Glynn, G. M. Boyd, and J. C. Gruman, *Self-Guided Strategies for Smoking Cessation: A Program Planner's Guide,* NIH Publication No. 91-3104 (Bethesda, MD: National Cancer Institute, 1990).

26. Fiore et al., *Treating Tobacco Use and Dependence.*

27. Schwartz, *Review and Evaluation of Smoking Cessation Methods.*

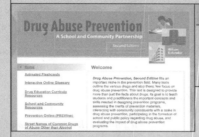
Chapter Learning Objectives

Upon completion of this chapter, students will be able to:

1. Compare and contrast six different needs assessment strategies.

2. Assess the strengths and weaknesses of several survey designs.

3. Suggest appropriate needs assessment strategies for their own school or community.

4. Write examples of several types of objectives.

5. Compare the differences between three different levels of evaluation.

6. Suggest appropriate evaluation strategies for various objectives.

Scenario

The Big Sandy Regional Drug Coalition has been in operation for many years. The coalition's budget comes from the United Way, allocations from city and county governments in the region, state grants, and local fundraising.

For the last six years, the coalition has set aside 40% of its annual budget for minigrants to constituent groups. If a school or church or civic group wanted to do a drug abuse prevention project, it could apply to the Big Sandy Coalition for funds. The only requirement was that the group had to provide a project description, tell how the funds would be used, and submit a report at the end of the project describing the project's results.

Recently, some of the coalition's leadership has been attending training programs, conducted by the state mental health agency, regarding science-based concepts, accountability, and evaluation. They have been convinced that the minigrant program has to be strengthened by requiring that projects be based on an assessment, be guided by measurable objectives, and have a careful evaluation plan.

When the new minigrant guidelines are released, many of the previous grantees are bewildered. They don't understand the reason for the change in the minigrant program, and don't know how to address the stipulations of the new guidelines. Some are wondering if the minigrant program will survive for long.

Chapter 13

Needs Assessment and Program Evaluation

Introduction

One of the ironies of drug education is that we have spent a lot of time doing something that is ineffective—disseminating drug facts—and almost no time doing what could improve effectiveness significantly—**evaluation**. This failure is worth exploring. Why are so much energy and so many resources expended on programs without serious consideration of their impact? We can gain some comfort from realizing that this issue transcends drug education and is an ongoing problem in all health education and promotion and human services in general.

The list of barriers to evaluation is a long one. Institutions of higher education have neither impressed on educators-in-training the importance of evaluation nor expected them to learn evaluation skills. Professionals who provide education and prevention often feel inadequate to tackle evaluation because they don't know how to go about it or may be intimidated by statistics. They just want to work with students or clients, and they think the work must be doing some good because it is personally rewarding. Often no time or budget support is provided for evaluation.

The results of evaluations that have been done often are not disseminated effectively. If evaluations of ineffective programs consistently were made known to practitioners, these programs might not be used and the importance of evaluation would be even more recognized.

Unsuccessful evaluations are ignored for two primary reasons: (1) A profit motive may drive some entrepreneurs who are not constrained by ethics to continue selling ineffective materials, and (2) practitioners deny the results because they have invested energy in and are committed to the program. To discover that the program doesn't work threatens their egos and self-esteem.

Needless to say, some blame can be placed on all concerned, but it doesn't have to be this way. Drug educators' work can be made progressively and consistently better, and resources can be used more conservatively to bring to students and others who are served programs that work rather than yesterday's mistakes.

Needs Assessment

One way that drug education can be made more effective is to identify and prioritize problems and needs at the very beginning. To do this, practitioners first should make efforts to carefully determine what is required and what should be done before they launch headlong into programming. Second, they should plan the evaluation process at the beginning rather than after the program is completed.

The social services and public health sectors have long practiced needs assessment. In drug education, however, much of school-based education is guided by K–12 scope and sequence schemes, and students are expected to conform to the schemes rather than the other way around. Consequently, most teachers are unaccustomed to doing any formal assessing of needs. Perhaps this strategy doesn't need to be changed. However, the prevention approach advocated in this text is a comprehensive, public health approach, and in order for prevention efforts to be most effective, needs assessment must be done. Everyone who provides drug education should at least understand the concept and importance of needs assessment, and drug education leaders should have some skills in this area.

The general purpose of needs assessment is to gain a fuller understanding of the **target group** to be addressed: characteristics that are relevant to an education or prevention program, what the main problems are, and what might be an appropriate way to intervene. In this case, a needs assessment seeks to determine the nature and extent of drug problems; drug use knowledge, attitudes, and behavior; patterns of risk and protective factors; relevant available resources; and prevailing per-

Table 13.1
Relevant Considerations for a Drug Education Needs Assessment
Demographic traits
Police records of illegal drug activity
Drug use levels and trends
Drug knowledge and attitudes
Available curricula
Available instructional materials
Current prevention activities
Cohesiveness of a community coalition
Student opinions
School drug policies
Prevalence of drug policy violations
Relevant public opinions
Felt needs

ceptions about drug problems and potential program activities. (See Table 13.1.)

Needs assessment sometimes seeks to determine *felt needs*, that is, what people feel about community problems and how they should be addressed. Felt needs may be quite different from the clinical conclusions of professionals. This discrepancy presents a challenge to educators to find common ground between quantified, objective assessment findings and the subjective views of target group representatives.

Besides giving prevention specialists more complete understanding of the target group and what needs to be done for them, needs assessment determines a specific basis for program objectives. Once the most important problems are identified and the context is understood, the next step is to develop objectives. These objectives are built on the rationale provided by the needs assessment findings.

This step is a very important concept. Despite the billions of dollars that are poured into drug education and prevention programs, there is never enough money to do all that we would like to do. Needs assessment can curtail squandering of resources on programs and activities for which there is no documented need and promote interventions for

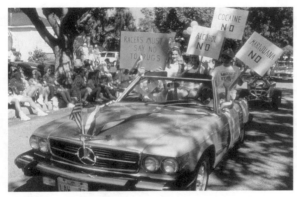

Figure 13.1 Just Say "No" to Drugs Rally How do we know if this type of prevention effort is worthwhile?

(© Joe Sohm/Unicorn Stock Photos)

those problems shown to be most significant. (See **Figure 13.1.**) Furthermore, needs assessment is not just about efficiency; it is also a matter of stewardship. Most drug education (school based or otherwise) is funded with public dollars. Prevention specialists have a responsibility to invest those funds in the most appropriate way, as identified by needs assessment.

Needs Assessment Strategies

Program planners may conduct needs assessment using various techniques. Some techniques are quite simple and easy to use, whereas others are more involved and complicated. There is no single ideal way for a needs assessment to be conducted; the approach depends on available resources, the nature of the community or target group, and, certainly, the skills of the planner. The following sections review the more common needs assessment strategies.

Existing Data Sources

Planners' first impulse at this stage of program planning often is to do a survey or take other steps to gather original data. However, a wealth of data may already exist. Schools and the rainbow of community agencies gather and maintain data that may be relevant for assessing the need for drug abuse prevention. For example, the police have records on drunk driving and other drug law violations, schools maintain records on drug-related disciplinary incidents,

mental health agencies maintain records on the numbers of addiction clients and statistics on the drugs most often encountered, and social welfare agencies maintain records on the alcohol-related domestic violence or other family problems.

Obviously, these data do not paint a totally accurate picture, but each bit of information can contribute to a greater understanding of the needs that exist. The process of gathering data presents an opportunity for planners to network with diverse segments of the helping community; these contacts can be advantageous in other aspects of the prevention program. Contacts are especially important for school-based educators who are accustomed to working in a self-contained environment. As discussed in Chapter 7, the most effective prevention is community oriented and not limited to in-school strategies.

Literature

There is a large volume of published literature on the drug problem. Practitioners, researchers, government personnel, advocates, educators, and many others have been prolific in writing about various dimensions of this issue. Although not much may have been written specifically for a local community, much of the general literature sheds light on the needs of a given community. Examples include the nature of and differences between various drug problems and the unique needs of a community's ethnic groups.

These materials can be obtained from a public or university library. Electronic search technology is also available at libraries. State agencies and the National Clearinghouse for Alcohol and Drug Information can help locate appropriate literature. And, of course, the Web makes this material available in ways never before possible.

Selected Interviews

The selected interview is one of the least rigorous needs assessment strategies, but it can yield good information to guide programming. There are two steps to this strategy. First, construct a set of questions that you want answered. Typically, they are **open-ended**, subjective questions such as "What do you think is the worst drug problem in this community?" or "What do you think needs to be done?" The development of these questions should be guided by a planning or advisory committee.

The second step is to identify a group of people who represent various segments of the school or community population, including students, teachers, parents, medical professionals, clergy, police, social service workers, mental health workers, minority groups, and any others deemed appropriate.

A balance must be achieved between interviewing a sufficient number of people to obtain adequate input and not including so many people that the process gets bogged down in the "paralysis of analysis." The planner should take careful notes as each interviewee responds to the standardized questions. Then the planner must summarize all of the responses to make conclusions and identify a precise direction for the program. If resources are available, there are sophisticated computer techniques that can be used to analyze these data.

Focus Groups

Focus groups are similar to selected interviews except that data are gathered from group discussions. The planner brings together a small number of people (five to ten) with common interests. Examples include groups of students, groups of parents, groups of teachers, groups of police officers, groups of clergy, and so forth. Before the group meets, the planner develops a standardized set of open-ended questions. During group discussions, the planner should listen and note comments carefully, particularly areas of consensus. A tape recorder or video camera can facilitate the recording process, but may change the dynamics of discussion if group members have reservations about being taped.

Focus groups have two advantages over selected interviews. First, they are more efficient because they obtain input from several people at a time rather than just one. Second, **group dynamics** may generate ideas that would never come out in individual interviews. Focus groups also have some disadvantages. They may be difficult to organize; scheduling an interview time with many people may be challenging. In addition, some group members may be reluctant to express their feelings and ideas in front of others.

After the focus group meets, the planner should summarize the notes and draw conclusions.

Nominal Group Process

Nominal group process (NGP) is similar to focus groups in that the planner brings together a group of individuals with some common characteristics to discuss some problem or issue. However, NGP systematically promotes equal participation by all group members, and the group identifies the precise conclusions of the discussion. NGP is done in seven steps.

Step 1 identifies an open-ended question to which the group will respond. The question should not be categorical (i.e., a yes/no or multiple-choice response) because participants must discuss and brainstorm. (Categorical answers can be obtained from surveys.) The following are examples of appropriate questions: What is the most important drug problem in this community? What can we do to help parents be more effective in helping their children avoid drug problems? What can be done in the church community to help prevent alcohol, tobacco, and other drug problems? What can be done to decrease alcohol abuse by college students?

Step 2 brings together the group. Groups may be small (five to ten participants), like focus groups, or a larger number of members may be sorted into smaller units that assemble in different areas of a large room or in separate meeting rooms. NGP requires one to two hours to complete. Participants need paper and pens, and each group needs either a flip chart, blackboard, or marker board. Groups can be oriented and directed by one facilitator, or a facilitator can be assigned to each small group.

In step 3, participants are given the question and asked to independently write down a list of possible ideas, solutions, strategies, and reasons. This step requires five to ten minutes. Participants should not discuss their responses with others, nor should they try to summarize, streamline, or prioritize.

The object of step 4 is to consolidate the individual lists that were generated in step 3. One by one, group members state one response on their list, which a recorder writes down on a flip chart or blackboard. This reporting continues in a round-robin fashion until all responses are recorded on the master list. While reporting and recording are in progress, there should be no concern for duplication, nor should members explain or debate the responses. All responses are accepted and given equal credibility.

In step 5, the group scrutinizes the master list. Participants may ask for clarification on specific items, but they should not debate or critique. If some responses seem to be duplicates, inquiries can be made to determine if the items have the same intent or whether they are unique; redundant items can be merged into one. The facilitator should be nondirective and avoid asserting his or her own values or point of view.

In step 6, group members individually review the semifinal master list and individually select the best five items. After the selection, they are instructed to rank the five responses by assigning five points to the top choice, four points to the next highest, and so on. Then participants mark their choices and the corresponding point values on the master list. The facilitator eliminates all items not selected in this last round, and ranks the selected items according to the total points each received. If the NGP has more than one group, all groups can be brought together and their priority lists posted for all to examine. Then one more vote can be taken to come up with a final priority list.

Step 7, the last step, is a chance for the group to reflect on and discuss their decisions. What does the priority list mean, and what are its implications? What is the appropriate course of action? Who needs to be involved, and what are their roles? Will the list have to be approved by a decision maker or board or discussed in another arena? How can the group's ideas be implemented?

NGP's value is equal participation from all participants; it is very democratic. It solicits precise conclusions rather than vague impressions gleaned from conversations. The downside of NGP is the difficulty of finding people who are willing to commit the time required. Also, it sometimes requires participants to take a leap of faith to accept equally, in a democratic way, all points of view.

Surveys

Surveying can be done with specific groups, such as restaurant owners, employees of a specific company, clients of a medical practice, and, of course, students. All of these would call for specific and unique procedures.

Fortunately for educators and prevention specialists, there is an abundance of survey data on the use of alcohol, tobacco, and other drugs. Federal, state, and local agencies (especially schools) have been very aggressive in gathering this kind of data. (See Figure 13.2.) Valuable information can be gleaned by comparing data from the three levels. For example, a finding that a state or local community has a higher rate of Ecstasy use than the national average indicates that Ecstasy abuse prevention should be made a priority in programming. On the other hand, if a state or local community has drug use rates that are lower than the national average, these fortunate communities may be instructive to the communities with higher rates.

Unfortunately, the proliferation of surveys has been accompanied by a proliferation of survey instruments. Data collected are not comparable because of the way questions are phrased. As illustrated in the FYI box, differences in survey construction make it difficult for prevention specialists to draw conclusions; that is, they are trying to compare grapes and cherries, which are close but not identical. Ideally, a local agency would identify an instrument used at the state or federal level that measures items of common interest. Then the local survey can be patterned after the larger survey. This would permit direct cross-reference of one survey to another. This situation is illustrated in Table 13.2, which shows that the local community has a higher marijuana use rate than the state or the nation.

The main sources of national data are Monitoring the Future, Parents Resource Institute for Drug Education (the PRIDE survey), the National Household Survey on Drug Abuse, the Drug Abuse Warning Network (DAWN), the Youth Risk Behavior Surveillance System, and the Drug and Alcohol Services Information System. These sources provide valid and reliable data on various dimensions of drug use and related issues.

Binge drinking on campus hurts sober students: survey

CHICAGO (AP) — Binge drinking is rampant on almost a third of the nation's campuses — and where it prevails, sober students suffer, a survey found.

"Students on campuses where there's a lot of binge drinking are affected in a number of ways — including physical assault, sexual harassment, property damage and interrupted sleep or study time," said Henry Wechsler, director of the Alcohol Studies Program at the Harvard School of Public Health.

His team surveyed 17,592 students on 140 campuses last year. Findings appear in today's Journal of the American Medical Association.

Forty-four percent of students reported binging, defined as downing five drinks or beers in a row for men or four in a row for women at least once in the two weeks before the survey.

Nineteen percent of all students were frequent bingers — having at least three binges in the period. The five or four drinks did not have to be consumed within a specific time period to qualify as binging.

Bingers tend to drink for the express purpose of getting drunk, Wechsler said.

Jacob Talbott knows the type. The freshman at Southern Illinois University in Carbondale said off-campus bars that lure students with discounted pitchers of beer only make matters worse.

"They've got all those specials at the bars on weekdays, so that's when everybody goes," Talbott said.

"They'll come in (the dorm) at 2 or 3 in the morning, and maybe I'm actually trying to get to bed early that night," he said. "They'll be running up and down the halls and stuff. Then I can't get to sleep. If I've got a 9 or 10 o'clock class the next day, I'm not very happy."

Bingers were seven times as likely to have unprotected sex as non-binge drinkers, 10 times as likely to drive after drinking and 11 times as likely to fall behind in their studies, the survey said.

At about one-third of the schools, more than 50 percent of students surveyed were bingers. At another third, fewer than 35 percent were

bingers. The survey did not identify particular schools.

Sober students at the heavy-drinking schools were much more likely to endure abuse from drinking students than teetotalers at the lowest-level drinking schools.

At the heavy-drinking schools, sober students were more than twice as likely to be insulted, hit, assaulted or experience unwanted sexual advances from drinking students.

They were also about 2½ times as likely to have their study or sleep interrupted or their property damaged by drinkers, the survey said.

Katharine C. Lyall, president of University of Wisconsin System and chair of the advisory board for the Harvard study, said orientation and counseling programs aimed at binge drinkers at her schools have been largely unsuccessful.

"I increasingly encounter students who comment they have a roommate whose drinking interferes with their study time," Lyall said. "Or that they were out on Saturday ... with a friend who got so drunk they got sick and ruined everybody's evening."

Figure 13.2 **A Newspaper Headline Reflects Survey Findings** Surveys of drug use in local communities, states, and the nation as a whole are done frequently.

Survey data also can be used to make self-comparisons over time. Data from several consecutive years may show trends such as increased, decreased, or unchanged drug use. These data can alert planners that a change in priorities, emphasis, or strategies is needed. An example of such a trend analysis is illustrated in Table 13.3.

This kind of comparison is possible only if survey instruments remain constant. Once a local school system selects or develops a questionnaire, it should stick with that questionnaire for at least several years. Otherwise, self-comparison is precluded.

Whenever surveying is done, important technical issues must be considered. The national data sources mentioned earlier are all credible and generally accepted. However, no matter how scientifically rigorous a survey instrument or its administration and analysis is, there is always a question

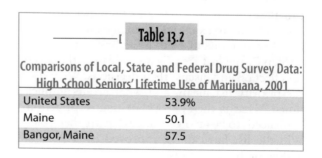

[Table 13.2]	
Comparisons of Local, State, and Federal Drug Survey Data: High School Seniors' Lifetime Use of Marijuana, 2001	
United States	53.9%
Maine	50.1
Bangor, Maine	57.5

about validity. Do people underreport or overreport their personal drug use? Undoubtedly, they do both. (See **Figure 13.3**.) The percentage of students who use a specific drug may be higher or lower than survey results indicate. Research suggests that underreporting is a greater problem than overreporting.[1] Underreporting or overreporting occur for a variety of causes, such as rebellious dishonesty, denial, and survey administration procedures.

| Table 13.3 |

Percentage of High School Seniors Reporting Any Lifetime Use of Selected Drugs, Mahoning County, Ohio

	1998	1999	2000	2001
Alcohol	81.4	80.0	80.3	79.7
Cigarettes	65.3	64.6	62.5	61.0
Cocaine	9.3	9.8	8.6	8.2
Marijuana	49.1	49.7	48.8	49.0

However, the rate of inaccuracy is usually consistent from year to year, so even though a figure for one year could be disputed, the trend over a period of years is probably valid.

Programmers should be sure to understand the meaning of the national data sources. It is important that they know the methods used to form the sample and collect the data. For example, data from the medical examiner portion of DAWN are gathered from a set of cities across the country and show the number of drug-related deaths in those cities. National averages cannot be calculated, or even rates, because neither the total number of deaths nor the total population served by the medical examiners in those cities is reported. Such limitations must be taken into account when programmers attempt to make meaningful comparisons at the local level. Another example is the PRIDE survey. The national composite data reported from this survey do not evenly represent the U.S. school population as a whole, but only those school systems that use the survey. Comparisons should be made with caution.

At the state level, drug surveys are typically done by one or more of the following: a department of education, a drug abuse agency, or a health and human services department. When survey data from one of those sources are obtained, the local educator or prevention specialist should always inquire about the validity and reliability of the questionnaire and the representativeness of the sample included in the survey. These issues need to be clarified.

Validity refers to the degree to which an instrument measures what it claims to measure. This

Incompatible Data from Parallel Surveys

Item from Monitoring the Future survey:

On how many occasions have you had alcoholic beverages to drink in your lifetime?

_____ 0 occasions   _____ 10–19 occasions

_____ 1–2 occasions   _____ 20–39 occasions

_____ 3–5 occasions   _____ 40 or more occasions

_____ 6–9 occasions

Item from Kentucky Department of Education alcohol and drug survey:

I have used alcohol

_____ never in my life

_____ 1–5 times in my life

_____ In the past week

_____ 2–10 times in the past month

_____ 11–30 times in the past month

Item from Warren County, Kentucky, student drug survey:

How many times, if any, have you had alcohol to drink in your lifetime (more than a few sips)?

_____ Never

_____ 1–2 times

_____ 3–10 times

_____ 11–20 times

_____ 21 or more times

process becomes very complex if the instrument is trying to measure psychological traits (e.g., the Minnesota Multiphasic Personality Inventory) or personality types to produce a score to be contrasted with group means. Fortunately, this issue is fairly simple for a straightforward drug survey. Do the questions cover the important issues? Are questions clear and unambiguous? Are the response options clear and not overlapping? To improve the validity of a questionnaire being developed, a variety of people, including students, should critique the instrument prior to large-scale administration of it.

Reliability means that questionnaire respondents answer questions the same way if they are

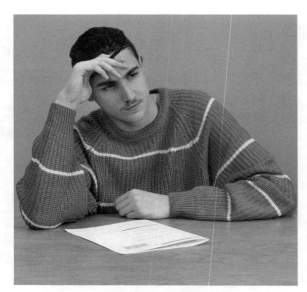

Figure 13.3 **Student Fills out Questionnaire** Do students tell the truth when they fill out drug surveys? Why or why not?

asked the same questions more than once, or if they answer a set of questions that measure the same object of interest (e.g., use of alcohol). Response consistency across two or more time intervals is known as *test-retest reliability*. Reliability in a set of items that measure the same construct is known as *internal consistency*.

If a student answers one time that he has not used LSD in the past month but then later answers a similar question and indicates that he used LSD four times in the past month, reliability of the data is questionable. It is understood that people are not always consistent; the reasons for their fabrications may be complex. However, reliability is also a function of the instrument: the phrasing and sequence of questions and the format and layout of the questionnaire.

Reliability can be measured in many ways, but for a typical drug survey, two techniques usually suffice. First, a single questionnaire includes the same question more than once or elicits the same information in more than one way. This technique provides an internal check of respondent consistency. Another approach is to use a *test-retest method*. With this method, the questionnaire is administered to a group and then given again to the same group several days later, without any drug education or program activities in the interim. The mathematical correspondence between the test and the retest responses is the level of test-retest reliability. Common statistics used to assess internal consistency are Kuder-Richardson-20 and Cronbach's alpha.

Sampling involves forming a group that is representative of the larger population. State and national surveys usually only sample the total population (that is, they select a small group to represent the whole). Efforts must be made to ensure that a sample closely reflects the gender, race, ethnicity, urbanicity, and so forth, of the total population so that meaningful inferences can be drawn. At the local level, school system surveys typically include all students in attendance on the day of the survey. The drug use rates of absentee students typically are greater than those of the student population as a whole, so even a schoolwide survey may not reflect accurately the exact level of ATOD use in a particular school. (See **Figure 13.4**.)

Another surveying issue is *anonymity*. Survey developers have an ethical responsibility to protect respondents' anonymity, especially if the questionnaire asks personal questions about drug use. Beyond the ethical issue, ensuring anonymity leads to more accurate self-reports. Anonymity can be established by including a verbal or written statement before the survey is administered, by proscribing any identification on instruments or answer sheets, and by administering the questionnaire in such a way that respondents feel their identity is protected. Further, students should be assured that answer sheets will not be examined by their teachers. It has been observed that the drug use estimates from the Monitoring the Future survey are higher than those from a parallel age group in the National Household Survey. This discrepancy is thought to be due to adolescents feeling more anonymous when they answer questions at school rather than at home.

At the local level, educators can choose to adopt a questionnaire developed by a surveying agency (e.g., state agency, PRIDE) or develop their own. If they adopt an instrument, they should discuss

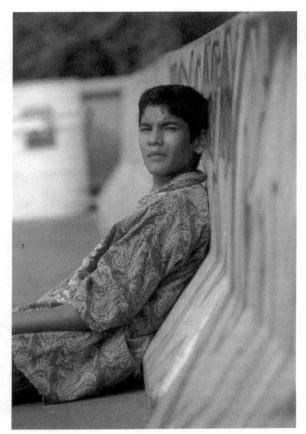

Figure 13.4 **A Student Absent from School** School dropouts may use drugs more than adolescents who graduate. (© AbleStock)

its validity and reliability with the sponsoring agency. If they develop their own, they should consult a local statistician or professional evaluator to address validity and reliability. In general, the authors recommend that local-level educators who want to conduct a drug survey seek the counsel and assistance of an appropriate agency in state government, such as a department of education or a department of health. Even if consultants are used to carry out a survey, educators should be familiar with the basic issues of survey administration and design.

In the future, more surveying will be done using the Web, but in most communities it is not yet a feasible design for the general public.

Survey Designs

Group Survey Administration

A group survey is the most convenient approach because many people can be surveyed all at once, and, at least in school, you have a captive audience. Respondents' trust in anonymity is less than with a mailed instrument, but greater than with a household interview. One concern about this type of survey is that of missing group members. For example, students who are absent when a school questionnaire is administered might be assumed to be more frequent drug users. This issue is a concern for other survey approaches as well; respondents who fail to return mailed questionnaires or cannot be reached by phone may be different from respondents who participate in the survey. A second issue with group surveys is to ensure that when multiple groups are surveyed, instructions and administration conditions are uniform.

Mailed Questionnaires

Sometimes mailed questionnaires are the most feasible method, such as when target group members don't normally assemble together. For example, if a program's goal is to promote more effective parenting, needs assessment data probably wouldn't be gathered at school. Both mail and telephone surveys would be used to reach respondents. Mailed questionnaires are efficient because they can all be mailed at the same time with one mass mailing. With this method, however, there is less control over who responds to the questionnaire and whether respondents comply with directions.

Another problem is nonresponses. An ideal response rate is at least 50%; of course, the goal is 100%, but this rate is rarely reached. Response rates can be improved by designing easy-to-answer questions; keeping the instrument short; providing a self-addressed, stamped return envelope; providing an incentive such as a small gift or a redeemable coupon for returning the questionnaire; and sending out reminders and follow-up questionnaires to nonresponders. For obvious reasons, mailed questionnaires are not appropriate for gathering data on transient or homeless persons.

Goal

The purpose of the program is to promote the healthy development of adolescents and to facilitate their successful entrance into a productive and satisfying adult life.

Program Objectives

- The incidence of alcohol-related highway crashes among California drivers in the 16 to 24 age group will decrease 25% by the year 2008.

- The incidence of smoking-related birth defects and perinatal health problems will decrease in Texas by 20% by the year 2008.
- The annual U.S. incidence of drug-abuse-related hospital emergency department visits will be reduced by 20% by the year 2010.
- The annual rate of liver cirrhosis deaths among African American men will be no more than 12 per 100,000 by the year 2010.
- The annual incidence of fetal alcohol syndrome among Native Americans will be no more than 2 per 1,000 live births by the year 2010.

Telephone Surveys

Telephone surveys also are used to reach target group members who don't assemble together. Although several callbacks may be required to reach some people, the response rate is usually higher than with mailed surveys. Telephone surveys afford less anonymity, and some respondents may object. Also, telephone surveys are very labor intensive—callers have to be recruited, uniformly trained, and supervised—and they don't reach people with unlisted numbers, cell phones only, or no phones at all. This limitation may indicate that another survey method should be used.

The proliferation of telemarketing has made people less tolerant and patient with phone calls from people they don't know. In addition, the movement away from land-based phones to cell phones may make it harder to reach people since cell phone numbers are generally not published or publically available.

Household Surveys

A household survey is the most time-consuming and labor-intensive approach. However, an advantage is a respondent's willingness to answer lengthy questionnaires in person. Another advantage is that more than one family member in the same household can be surveyed. Household surveys are

perhaps the least frequently used method of gathering behavioral data.

In summary, needs assessment is designed to provide a greater understanding of the target group and the priority issues for drug education. Needs assessment is successful when it provides a clear basis and rationale for writing objectives to guide the program.

Writing Objectives

The task of writing objectives is usually the responsibility of program planners, whether they are developing units and lesson plans or designing a broad-based initiative for the school or general community at large. Objectives, and how to write them, are discussed here because they logically flow from needs assessment and because they provide a key focus for some aspects of evaluation.

During program planning, planners first focus attention on long-term, broad issues and systematically narrow them down to the most immediate, short-term issues. To be specific, the needs assessment suggests a **goal** that is a statement of overall hope and intent, written in general terms. An example of a goal is given in the Hints & Tips box. Once the goal is conceived, it is accomplished by targeting efforts toward a set of objectives, some

Example Behavioral Objectives

- Over the next five years, Pennsylvania State University students' practice of driving after having five or more drinks will decrease by 40%.
- The annual use of marijuana by 12- to 17-year-olds in Hennepin County, Minnesota, will decline by 40% by the year 2010.
- By 2008, the initiation of tobacco smoking by 12- to 17-year-olds in Dade County, Florida, will decline by 20%.

- Among pregnant women in the United States, regular cigarette smoking will be reduced to no more than 10% by the year 2010.
- Use of anabolic steroids by high school seniors in Shelby County, Tennessee, will be reduced to no more than 2% by the year 2010.

of which are short term and some of which are long term.

Whether their training was classroom or community oriented, education students have been taught for a long time that objectives should be measurable and specifically stated. Mager's *Preparing Instructional Objectives* may be the classic text for teachers on how to write precise objectives.[2] In the public health education field, Green, in his work with the PRECEDE-PROCEED model (see Chapter 8), was one of the early proponents of articulating objectives with explicit dimensions.[3]

One type of objective, called a **program objective**, addresses the health and social consequences of drug use (see the Hints & Tips box for examples). School-based educators typically do not articulate program objectives because they seem to be beyond the traditional focus of schools. However, we promote a comprehensive, community-based approach to drug abuse prevention, and this broader perspective described by program objectives must become more recognized. Program objectives should specify (1) the health or social problem to be influenced, (2) the identity of the target group, (3) the time frame for completion of the objective, and (4) the magnitude of the influence (e.g., percent increase or decrease).

Once program objectives are stated explicitly, it is necessary to determine related **behavioral objectives**. The needs assessment should help the planner become familiar with the behavioral causes of drug-related problems. For example, if a program objective addresses HIV infection, the behavioral objective might address IV drug use. Behavioral objectives, like program objectives, should be precise in their language and include all but one of the four components of program objectives. The exception is that instead of specifying a health or social problem, the objectives specify a behavior. The accompanying Hints & Tips box gives examples of behavioral objectives.

In conventional practice, school-based drug education aims to reduce drug use of all types, and this is usually a starting point. Strategies are then developed to reach that objective. However, planners should be familiar with the more comprehensive approach discussed earlier. Sometimes just focusing on drug use will have only limited impact. For example, most schools have programs and activities to discourage drunk driving. A better approach is to look at the consequences: highway accidents that lead to injury or death. We know that highway accidents can be caused by alcohol use prior to driving, but those accidents are also caused by excessive speed and other poor driving practices. Therefore, it is appropriate to address the other causes of highway accidents as well as drunk driving. This comprehensive approach could significantly boost schools' effectiveness in promoting the health and social well-being of children and adolescents.

Once behavioral objectives are defined, the next step is to write instructional and resource objectives. This step will be guided by theory and actual

Example Instructional and Resource Objectives

Instructional Objectives

- By the year 2010, the proportion of high school seniors in Suffolk County, New York, who associate risk of physical or psychological harm with the heavy use of alcohol will increase to 70%.
- By the year 2010, the proportion of high school seniors in Bannock County, Idaho, who perceive social disapproval associated with the occasional use of marijuana will increase to 85%.
- Eighty-five percent of sixth graders in Bowling Green Junior High will satisfactorily demonstrate drug refusal skills by the end of the 2005–2006 school year.

- By 2007, 200 parents in Osage County, Oklahoma, will successfully complete a parent education program.
- Fifty percent of the smoking employees at Electric Motors, Inc., will master a set of smoking cessation skills during 2006.

Resource Objectives

- Economic and transportation barriers to Greenwood High School students' participation in extracurricular activities will be eliminated by the beginning of the 2006–2007 school year.
- By January 1, 2007, ten persons will be trained as coordinators/facilitators of group smoking cessation programs to be conducted in Greene County, Ohio.

---

information regarding the causes of behavior. **Instructional objectives,** which are most familiar to classroom teachers, focus on student **cognitive, affective,** and skill learning. **Resource objectives** address system barriers to be breached or specific resource deficits that must be supplied in order for the behavioral objectives to be accomplished. This third type of objective must be stated clearly, but may not require all four components needed to establish program and behavioral objectives. Examples of instructional and resource objectives are found in the Hints & Tips box.

In summary, objectives drive the evaluation process. The more carefully objectives are written, the easier the job of evaluation.

Evaluation

We asserted at the beginning of the chapter that evaluation must be formulated in the early stages of program planning rather than after the program is completed. There are at least two reasons for this. First, the discipline of evaluation forces programmers to write clear, coherent, and measurable objectives, which has a constructive impact on

program implementation. In other words, if an exact destination is known, it is easier to select routes to get there.

The second reason for designing evaluation at the beginning is that mechanisms for gathering evaluation data must be in place as the program unfolds. Otherwise, it may be impossible to gather these data after the program is completed.

The evaluation process is often organized in three levels. The first level is process evaluation, sometimes called *formative evaluation*.

Process Evaluation

Process evaluation should tell what a program did and how it was done. It assesses the quantity of activities, the number of people served, and the quality of program elements. Process evaluation can help programmers fine-tune the program in progress, thus enabling midcourse adjustments. (See Figure 13.5.) It also can identify ways in which program implementation can be improved if it is repeated in the future. Examples of process evaluation strategies are provided in Table 13.4. Process evaluation often is overlooked, but it is helpful in improving drug education.

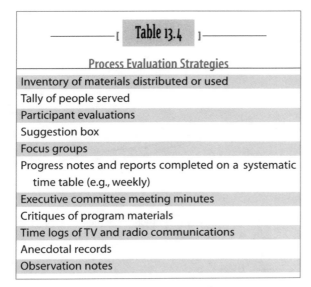

Table 13.4
Process Evaluation Strategies
Inventory of materials distributed or used
Tally of people served
Participant evaluations
Suggestion box
Focus groups
Progress notes and reports completed on a systematic time table (e.g., weekly)
Executive committee meeting minutes
Critiques of program materials
Time logs of TV and radio communications
Anecdotal records
Observation notes

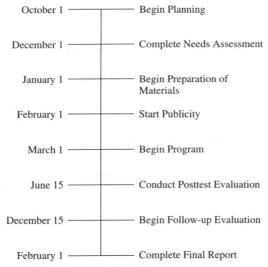

October 1	——	Begin Planning
December 1	——	Complete Needs Assessment
January 1	——	Begin Preparation of Materials
February 1	——	Start Publicity
March 1	——	Begin Program
June 15	——	Conduct Posttest Evaluation
December 15	——	Begin Follow-up Evaluation
February 1	——	Complete Final Report

Figure 13.5 A Project Time Line   Process evaluation may include a project time line.

Impact Evaluation

Far more important than process evaluation is *impact evaluation,* which determines whether the instructional objectives, resource objectives, and behavioral objectives have been achieved. In other words, this level documents whether participants mastered knowledge and skills and adopted desirable attitudes, whether required resource supports were provided, and whether the targeted behavior change was accomplished.

Knowledge and skills testing is familiar to most people because it occurs so frequently in school. Skills usually are evaluated by standardized observation. Knowledge and attitudes may be assessed with a variety of test question formats, by reviewing journal writing, and by assessing art, creative writing, or other types of projects. Testing methods must closely reference the learning objectives, and questions should be phrased precisely enough to produce reliable results. Evaluation of resource objectives is accomplished by asking the team members on site whether the necessary resources were provided.

Evaluating behavioral objectives is a bit more challenging. The most logical approach is to refer to the needs assessment; if the needs assessment produced a baseline measure for some behavior, the method used to determine that baseline should be repeated, noting what change has occurred. Generally, there are two primary ways to obtain behavioral data. The first method is with some type of survey—questionnaires completed in classes or other groups, mailed questionnaires, telephone surveys, or household surveys. All of these alternatives have advantages and disadvantages, including differences in cost, time, and personnel required, expected response rates, and respondents' willingness to be forthright. (See **Figure 13.6**.)

The second way to gather behavioral data is by tracking data from existing sources. For example, imagine that an objective is to increase the number of drug-impaired students who seek services from the student assistance program (SAP). It would have been determined at baseline that some number of such students contacted the SAP during an average month in the past year. SAP intake statistics could then be monitored into the future to ascertain whether the average monthly service load increased according to the objective. The underlying assumption is that the absolute number of drug-impaired students remains constant. This assumption could be verified by survey.

In many cases, both methods can be used. For example, in a community drunk-driving prevention program, the behavior to be assessed is driving under

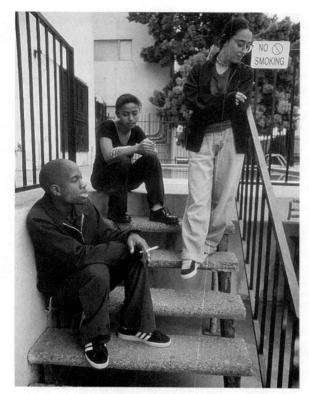

Figure 13.6 **Evaluating Student Behavior**   How do we know if a program has resulted in postponed drug use by teens? (© Michael Newman/PhotoEdit)

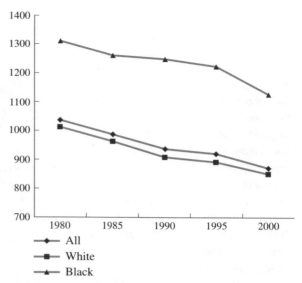

Figure 13.7 **Death Rates for African Americans and Whites**   Health status of a target group changes slowly.

Source: National Center for Health Statistics.

the influence of alcohol. To measure progress toward this objective, a sample of the population could be surveyed, police records on the number of drunk-driving arrests could be monitored, and the number of persons for whom bars and taverns helped find alternative transportation could be tracked. These statistics are meaningful only if needs assessment baseline measures exist.

Outcome Evaluation

The third level of evaluation, *outcome evaluation*, measures the achievement of the program objectives: whether or not the targeted change in drug-use-related health status occurred. Another outcome measure may be economic costs associated with drug abuse. For example, a company may be interested in reducing the cost of alcohol-related illness and absenteeism among its workforce. In some instances,

outcome evaluation has a short time frame, such as in the case of drunk-driving crash fatalities. In other cases, it covers the long term, such as illness caused by smoking. (See Figure 13.7.)

If the needs assessment was done thoroughly, there should be an unequivocal relationship between the health problem identified in the program objective and the behaviors targeted by the behavioral objectives. If this is the case, then evaluation of the program objectives may be less important. If the behavioral objectives are met, there should be no doubt that the program objective and health problem have been affected. An example may be taken from antitobacco education. The object of such education is to prevent the use of cigarettes and smokeless tobacco, and because the impact of tobacco use on various health problems already has been so thoroughly demonstrated, it is not necessary to test it again in a specific local community.

This is also a practical problem in undertaking outcome evaluation. For example, 15 to 20 years' follow-up is required to evaluate the health status of students who didn't initiate smoking versus those who did.

The point here is that there is extensive harmful drug use worth preventing, more than we can

HINTS & TIPS

A Workshop Participant Rating Form

Please rate the following items by placing an X in the appropriate blank.

	Strongly Agree 1	Agree 2	Undecided 3	Disagree 4	Strongly Disagree 5
1. My knowledge of drug information was increased by the workshop.	_____	_____	_____	_____	_____
2. Drug information presented will be useful to me professionally or personally.	_____	_____	_____	_____	_____
3. My knowledge of prevention techniques was increased by the workshop.	_____	_____	_____	_____	_____
4. I will be able to apply the prevention techniques presented in the workshop.	_____	_____	_____	_____	_____
5. The workshop presenter was well organized.	_____	_____	_____	_____	_____
6. Comfort and physical facilities were satisfactory.	_____	_____	_____	_____	_____
7. My objective for attending this workshop was achieved.	_____	_____	_____	_____	_____

address all at once. Little can be gained from targeting drug use behavior that is not well documented to cause undesirable social or health consequences.

Analyzing Data

Data analysis may be quite simple or profoundly arcane, depending on the level of evaluation and the needs of the evaluator. This section begins with a discussion of the process evaluation level and progresses to the impact and outcome levels. Emphasis is on more common evaluation needs as opposed to evaluation research.

Data that are gathered in process evaluation often are simple counts of things or people, or written documentation of various aspects of program implementation. These data usually do not require complex statistical analysis. The Hints & Tips box provides an example of a participant rating form for a drug abuse prevention workshop. Process evaluation data gathered with such a form will be fairly simple to tabulate and analyze.

The items on the form in the box are designed as Likert scales (ranked from Strongly Agree to Strongly Disagree). For each item, the evaluator adds all of the numbers marked on completed questionnaires and divides the total by the number of respondents. This number gives the group's average assessment for each item. Another approach is to calculate the percentage of all responses captured by each response option (e.g., 40% marked response 1, 25% marked response 2, etc.). These data are analyzed by comparing the evaluation findings for the same workshop or program presented on different occasions or by different presenters.

Analysis of data gathered in impact evaluation usually starts with students' grasp of factual information. Instructors typically calculate the percentage of correct answers out of the total possible correct answers. Scores for a group then are summed

Table 13.5

Comparison of Group Means

Group A Scores (%)	Group B Scores (%)
87	70
75	82
77	74
80	69
96	55
68	53
84	83
75	65
88	62
92	58
Mean for Group A: 82.2	Mean for Group B: 67.1

$t = 3.18, df = 9, p < 0.05.$

and divided by the number of scores to obtain an average or mean. A mean for one group may be compared with another group's mean (e.g., two groups take a test; one group has completed a drug education unit, one group has not). The statistical tool used to analyze the mean is either a **t-test** or an **analysis of variance (ANOVA)**, which indicates whether one mean is significantly greater and whether any observed difference could be due to chance. A comparison of group means is shown in Table 13.5. When used in the context of prevention, means are also a matter for professional judgment. Statistical significance is a mathematical concept; the difference between two means may be statistically significant (i.e., the means are not equal, the difference is not due to chance) but not different enough to have meaningful implications for prevention programs.

It is also a common practice to gather data before a program begins in order to rule out some extraneous variables. Let's say we want to implement a fifth-grade tobacco information program, and decide it is worthwhile to test the instructional value of the adopted curriculum. Before the program begins, a knowledge test is administered to two groups of students. One group will receive the program (a treatment group) and one group will not (a control group). After the treatment group

receives the program, the knowledge test is administered again to both groups. Pretest and posttest scores for the two groups then are analyzed with the analysis of covariance (ANCOVA) tool. ANCOVA takes into account the difference in scores before the program was offered to determine the real significance of any difference in posttest scores. By including both the pretest and posttest scores in the analysis, we can determine more definitively the program's effect as opposed to factors such as family influences, mass media communications, and coincidental educational experiences.

Sometimes education objectives target attitudes, which usually are assessed with a Likert-type scale. The most conventional way to analyze data of this sort is to create a cross-tabulation and apply a **chi-square test,** shown in Table 13.6. The example in the table shows that a stronger attitude that personal use of marijuana is "bad" is associated with Group A, presumably because this group was exposed to a drug education strategy.

Data on drug use that was targeted by behavioral objectives usually indicate whether a target has been reached, for example, what percentage of students are currently using marijuana and whether that percentage has changed by the targeted decrement since baseline. No other calculated statistics are required for this evaluation. However, sometimes an effort is made to rule out the influence of other variables. For example, suppose a smoking cessation program is conducted. A behavioral objective is stated: There will be a 5% decrease in adult smoking over the next two years. A **social marketing campaign** is mounted to accomplish the objective. As the two years draw to an end, smoking data are gathered in the same way they were gathered in the needs assessment. Let's say the data show a gratifying 5% decrease in smoking. However, the decrease may have occurred without the social marketing campaign, and may be due to other influences in society.

One simple solution is to compare smoking rates in the local community with those for the state and nation. Table 13.7 shows that smoking declined in Maricopa County, Arizona, by 5%, whereas it only changed by 1% in the state and nation. This comparison indicates that the social marketing

---[**Table 13.6**]---

Analysis of a Drug-Related Attitude

Questionnaire item: My use of marijuana would be bad

	Strongly Agree 1	Agree 2	Undecided 3	Disagree 4	Strongly Disagree 5
Group A	40 (52%)	20 (26%)	11 (14.2%)	5 (6.4%)	1 (1.2%)
Group B	25 (31.2%)	15 (18.7%)	25 (31.2%)	9 (11.2%)	6 (7.5%)

Chi-square = 14.28, df = 4, $p < 0.01$.

---[**Table 13.7**]---

Comparison of Adult Smoking at Local, State, and National Levels for a Three-Year Period

	2000	2001	2002	Percent Change
Maricopa County	37.0%	36.0%	35.0%	5.4%
Arizona	35.0	35.0	34.6	1.1
United States	29.0	28.9	28.7	1.0

---[**Table 13.8**]---

Adult Smoking as Influenced by a Social Marketing Campaign: Comparison of a Study Community with a Control Community

	2000	2001	2002	Percent Change
Maricopa County	37.0%	36.0%	35.0%	5.4%
Madison County	38.4	38.1	37.8	1.6

campaign had an impact on smoking cessation in the local community.

A more rigorous approach is to find a similar community in terms of demographics and social indicators but which was not exposed to the social marketing campaign. This comparison is shown in Table 13.8. Comparisons become more complex if we select some communities to receive all of the social marketing campaign, some to receive parts of it, and some to receive none of it. All of these comparisons on smoking probably would be analyzed with cross-tabulations and the chi-square test.

Finally, program objectives typically are evaluated by gathering data on the incidence or prevalence of the targeted health or social problem. These rates are calculated at the end of the objectives' time frame and compared with the targeted change.

Drug education data analysis may be very complicated and challenging. Educators and prevention specialists without advanced training in statistics and evaluation should consult an expert at a local university, planning agency, or government body. Consultation always should be done prior to the program. Planning and implementation have to proceed in certain ways to make more sophisticated evaluation designs possible. However, the most common evaluation needs can be satisfied without such expert consultation.

Disseminating Evaluation Findings

After evaluation is completed, or at least as various phases are completed, it is important to communicate the findings to appropriate individuals and agencies. Every person on the program team should have a chance to review and discuss the end results of the program, noting in particular the strengths and weaknesses of implementation and whether the educational, resource, behavioral, and outcome objectives were achieved. These individuals' participation in this process is critical for programming excellence in the future. It may be required, but also desirable, to share findings with administrative superiors. Good news (program success) is well received and promotes future support. Bad news (limited or no success) is more difficult to share, but being forthright with administrators builds trust and may provide an opportunity to discuss reasons for this failure and generate suggestions for improvement.

A note of caution: Some administrators may take a cue from program success, particularly declining student drug use, and redirect funds away from prevention programs in the mistaken belief that the problem is solved. They must be persuaded that long-term success requires continuing effort and investment. Other administrators may deny increasing levels of student drug use and choose to believe that drug problems are bad in other places but not in their system. Sometimes corroboration with student focus groups or a comparison with nearby school districts helps break through this denial.

Some evaluation results may be communicated to the local community: parents, community leaders, and citizens at large. Usually only changes in drug use or the consequences of drug use are of interest to this audience. If these measures show that problems are getting worse, this news may generate increased support for prevention programs in the future. If evaluation results show that progress has been made, the community may have increased confidence in the need for and value of the programs. However, there is a risk that too much good news fosters apathy because people believe that the problems require no further concern. Educators should deliver good news with a note of caution that some problems remain. Likewise, bad news brings the risk that schools will be blamed for the problems. Communities sometimes find schools to be an easy target, and don't consider the responsibility of families, churches, the business community, and the media.

Educators also should recognize the ethical issue of overemphasizing bad news for self-serving reasons. An example is characterizing the drug problem as much worse than it really is in order to protect program budgets or secure additional funding.

A related ethical issue is overstating the positive benefits of a program or prevention activity. For self-serving reasons, prevention workers sometimes characterize their programs or efforts as very successful, with little or no objective evidence. Not only is this unethical, but it blocks a culling of ineffective programs and prevents more rapid progress in achieving health goals.

Finally, it is often valuable to share evaluation results with other professionals who are involved in similar pursuits. Sharing may be done in a variety of ways, including presentations at local or regional coalitions, state or national conferences, newsletters, and journal articles. Computer technology also may come into play; for example, e-mail list serves, specialized electronic bulletin boards, and websites increasingly are being used to share information.

The Role of the Evaluator

Evaluation may be done by an external consultant or a permanent staff member. External consultants may be a better choice; they have more objectivity because they have not invested their own time and effort into the program's planning and implementation. If the evaluation is done by a staff member, it may be important to arrange for a well-chosen advisory group, one with the tenacity and expertise to review and oversee the evaluation.

It is also important for the evaluator to communicate the evaluation findings with clarity and coherence. Good verbal and writing skills are critical, but charts and diagrams may be tremendously useful. Ubiquitous computer technology makes graphic techniques readily available.

Summary

The need for more continuous and rigorous evaluation of drug education activities is immense, and findings must be shared and applied more consistently. While some aspects of evaluation require the skills of evaluation experts, much can be done by local-level educators and prevention specialists.

Big Sandy Coalition has astute leadership, and they are right to try to institute higher standards of accountability for scarce prevention dollars. Following a national trend, they recognize that it is no longer tenable to invest program funds in activities that may be enjoyable, well received, and seem reasonable, but that have no solid evidence of effectiveness.

At the same time, they have to work with the groups and communities that are their constituents. They decide to reserve part of the minigrant budget for programs that can show evidence of effectiveness. The other portion of the budget is set aside for programs that may not have an established record of effectiveness; however, the projects must have a stronger evaluation plan in order to be funded.

Their next step will be to conduct workshops for potential grantees, establishing greater expertise in evaluation and assessment. The process will be long, but rewarding in the long run.

Learning Activities

1. Find journal articles about the evaluation of a drug education or prevention program or activity. Identify the evaluation methods used, the levels of evaluation considered, and the statistics used in data analysis.

2. Obtain examples of drug use survey instruments. Try to determine, from the source, the validity and reliability of the instruments.

3. Try to secure results of drug use surveys conducted by local school systems. Compare the results with state and national statistics.

4. Using the guidelines presented in this chapter, conduct a focus group and a nominal group process on a drug abuse prevention topic.

5. Select a drug education curriculum or a generic prevention strategy, such as Project Prom or antidrug media campaigns. Search a library and the Internet to learn about the evaluation findings regarding that curriculum or strategy.

Notes

1. L. D. Johnston and P. M. O'Malley, "Issues of Validity and Population Coverage in Student Surveys of Drug Use," in *Self-Report Methods of Estimating Drug Use: Meeting Current Challenges of Validity,* B. A. Rouse, N. J. Dozel, and L. G. Richards, eds., DHHS Publication No. ADM 85–1402 (Washington, DC: U.S. Government Printing Office, 1985).

2. R. F. Mager, *Preparing Instructional Objectives* (Palo Alto, CA: Fearon, 1962).

3. L. W. Green et al., *Health Education Planning: A Diagnostic Approach* (Palo Alto, CA: Mayfield, 1980).

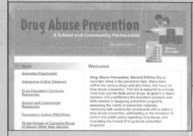

web resources

The Web site for this book offers many useful resources for educators, students, and professional counselors and is a great source for additional information. Visit the site at **http://healtheducation.jbpub.com/drugabuse/.**

Chapter Learning Objectives

Upon completion of this chapter, students will be able to:

1. Propose a compromise position on the drug legalization debate, considering all of the major points of view.

2. Compare the way public policy has addressed tobacco promotion and alcohol promotion, and predict what further actions might be taken in the future.

3. Contrast the relative merits of advertising restrictions versus taxation as a prevention policy.

4. Suggest ways to implement needle distribution programs that are sensitive to community needs and concerns.

5. Recall several of the Healthy People 2010 objectives related to alcohol, tobacco, and other drug abuse.

Scenario

In your state, the AIDS advocacy group has mounted a statewide ballot initiative for legislation to make it legal for AIDS patients and others with serious illnesses to legally purchase marijuana for their own use. The rationale for the initiative is that the marijuana will help control the nausea and weight loss associated with the illness and some drug treatment. Support by medical groups in the state is mixed: Some support the proposal, while others do not. The state attorney general is publically opposing this step to legalize marijuana. The U.S. Justice Department has made it known that it will take legal action to block such legislation if it were to pass.

The drug abuse coalition in your community has been approached by leaders of the ballot initiative for a public endorsement supporting the legalization of marijuana in circumstances of serious illness. As the coordinator of the coalition, you are considering your position on the issue and how to approach the membership about it.

Chapter 14

Public Policy and Drug Abuse Prevention

Introduction

The attention span of the American public is measured in nanoseconds. Public opinion polls are released seemingly every day, and they are as volatile as a thermometer. Interest in various public issues fluctuates wildly as our attention quickly shifts from one issue to another. Politicians both exploit and are victimized by this phenomenon. They can be on center stage by taking a bold stand on an issue to which the public is riveted, promising to lead us to the brave new world. When the public is distracted by the next issue that comes along, the politician no longer has a constituency.

No issue has been touched more by the fickle finger of fashion fate than alcohol and drug abuse. In the 1960s and early 1970s, America was shocked by the strange, new phenomenon of drugs in schools, on campuses, at concerts, and in neighborhoods; this shock was exacerbated by a deluge of headlines and TV soundbites. The frenzy eventually subsided, though it never disappeared. With the advent of crack cocaine and the link between IV drugs and AIDS, drug abuse again grabbed the nation's attention. This attention climaxed in 1987 when Len Bias, a University of Maryland basketball player, and Don Rogers, an NFL football player, died from cocaine overdoses. In the same year, Douglas Ginsberg was eliminated from consideration for appointment to the U.S. Supreme Court when it became known that he had used drugs earlier in his life. During the second half of the 1980s, drugs consistently were cited as the greatest domestic concern of Americans.

It became widely recognized in America late in the 1980s that the use of tobacco, alcohol, and illicit drugs was consistently and convincingly declining, both for adolescents

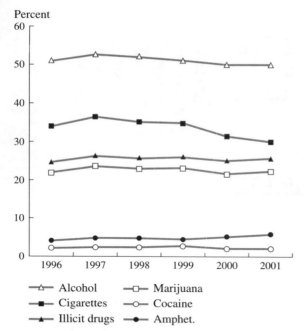

Percent

—△— Alcohol   —□— Marijuana
—■— Cigarettes   —○— Cocaine
—▲— Illicit drugs   —●— Amphet.

Figure 14.1 Past-Month Use of Drugs, 12th Graders, 1996–2001.

Source: Monitoring the Future.

and adults. Paradoxically, the success of the prevention efforts led to public apathy. Politicians and other leaders took the cue and put drug abuse prevention on the back burner of policy formation and executive action. At the same time, violence, health care reform, welfare reform, and economic issues generated consternation and contentious debate. It is ironic that ATOD abuse has ties to all of those issues, but somehow apathy remains widespread. Since the early 1990s, drug use generally has declined very little; in many cases it has remained unchanged or even increased. (See **Figure 14.1**.)

In the 21st century, drug abuse has received inconsistent attention in the public eye. The National Office of Drug Control Policy identified a link between terrorism and illegal drug use. In the context of the war on terrorism, this caused a bit of a stir, but not for long. Illegal sales of oxycontin, trafficking in methamphetamines, and club drugs get occasional attention, but the media usually cover these stories like other crime stories. A white-hot

public spotlight rarely targets these issues, unlike what was common in the 1980s. Drug abuse is just barely on the radar screen of most politicians.

A national public opinion poll conducted in 2001 found that the drug abuse problem was seen by 90% of 1,513 respondents as either a crisis or a serious problem. However, in the same survey, 74% of respondents said we were losing the drug war.[1]

It remains to be seen how society will respond in the future. Will there be changes in patterns of public funding that will support school-based prevention more generously? Will there be a competing push to put more funds into law enforcement and supply reduction, consonant with our current focus on violence? Will we at last reject single-strategy efforts and embrace a more comprehensive approach to prevention? Only time will tell.

The waxing and waning of support for prevention is perhaps unavoidable in our free and open society of diversity and pluralism. However, long-term success would be more assured if society's responses to drug problems were not so characterized by faltering support and vacillating interest. The lesson to be learned is that prevention professionals must work harder to frame the issues, and not abdicate this role to the media. We must bring the nature and extent of drug abuse problems to the attention of communities in more creative ways. Without preaching gloom and doom, we must find means to kindle consistent support for and commitment to comprehensive prevention programs.

In addition to managing the public agenda better, we will have to come to grips with a variety of troubling issues. Solving some issues will require a buildup of public support to combat forces that are opposed to prevention (e.g., the alcohol and tobacco industries and their allies). Solving other issues will require serious application of evaluation research and rejection of familiar and comfortable strategies in favor of strategies that show more promise for success. Still other issues demand research and development of new technology and more effective prevention strategies.

This chapter addresses a variety of issues that school personnel and others on the front line of prevention need to understand. As their understanding increases, they can become more involved in public debate and more confident and assertive in policy formation. Their influence can provide a more consistent base for comprehensive community prevention.

Public Policy Issues in Prevention

Legalization of Drugs

In the past the American public was generally opposed to legalizing drugs. Elected officials have rarely been willing to question the war on drugs or to suggest that strict and broad prohibition is not good public policy. However, the fact that legalization has been entertained seriously and continuously for more than 30 years indicates that its proponents have some very sound arguments.

Perhaps as a bellwether of shifting public opinion, the Hollywood movie *Traffic* portrayed the futility of the drug war. In addition, there has been much debate about the legalization of marijuana for those who have AIDS or who are undergoing cancer treatment. When the drug warriors stand opposed to drug use by these patients, they don't get much sympathy from the public.

Legalization is not an issue that polarizes people; instead, views fall on a continuum. There are variations in the degree to which people think the law enforcement approach has failed and how much retrenchment is appropriate. Some people propose **decriminalization** of possession of small quantities for personal use. Others believe that drugs should be legalized but highly regulated. Some people would establish degrees of legalization, based on the threat posed by specific drugs. Still others would make it possible for physicians to prescribe cocaine and heroin to established addicts, or marijuana to those suffering from AIDS or cancer. A few libertarians advocate total legalization, thereby allowing consumers to decide whether or not they want to use drugs. These complexities will not be addressed here, but the simple dichotomy of legalization versus prohibition will be discussed.

The basic premise of the call for legalization of drugs is that governments have tried to suppress drug use since the 1914 Harrison Act that put restrictions on the use of opiates and cocaine (see Chapter 2) and the 18th Amendment that in 1920 instituted national prohibition of alcohol. Since the Harrison Act was passed, there has been a long list of ever-tougher and more comprehensive efforts to use the power of government to stop the sale and use of illicit drugs.

What has been learned from all of this legislation is that it is impossible to stop completely the supply of alcohol and drugs from reaching consumers who are willing to buy them. Alcohol prohibition did decrease alcohol consumption, but the social costs outweighed the benefits realized from less drinking.[2] It is difficult to say whether the laws that regulate illicit drugs have affected their supply or consumption. What is known is that drugs seem to be abundantly available, particularly in cities. Whether the supply would be even greater without legal restrictions and criminal penalties is impossible to determine. Nevertheless, proponents make several points for reversing our reliance on law enforcement to fight the war on drugs.

Arguments in Favor of Legalization

The first point made by proponents is that legal control and prohibition have failed in the past, and there is no reason to believe that they will succeed in the future. It is true that staggering sums of money (tens of billions of dollars) have been spent on the war on drugs; the federal government alone will spend $19.2 billion in 2003; states spend about an equal amount.[3] This combined amount is about $133 for every man, woman, and child, and about $104 million every day. About 79% of state and local and 67% of federal drug control spending went for supply reduction, law enforcement, and criminal justice system expenses. Funds have been allocated for more police officers, undercover operations, confiscation of drugs that enter the country illegally (**interdiction**), more prisons, aerial reconnaissance of marijuana and cocaine fields, border patrols, and police-type operations in foreign countries. There has been virtually no accountability for all of this spending; that is, specific expenditures have not been linked to objective results.[4]

One could posit that the decline in illicit drug use during the 1980s was partly due to law enforcement efforts, but there is no clear evidence that supports that conclusion, nor estimates of the magnitude of law enforcement's impact. Some of the objectives of prohibition-type efforts are to decrease the supply, decrease the purity, and increase the price of drugs. These objectives have not been met. The cost of heroin at the retail level declined from an estimated $3,295 per gram in 1981 at 4% purity to $2,087 per gram at 25% purity in 2000; the cost of cocaine at the retail level declined from an estimated $423 per gram in 1981 at 36% purity to $212 per gram at 61% purity in 2000.[5]

Michael Massing, writing in the *New York Review of Books*, presents a typical scenario:

> [Prosecutor] Giuliani's office spent five years gathering evidence in the [Pizza Connection] case. His associates videotaped meetings, gathered airline passenger seat lists, recovered ticket stubs, pored over hotel registers, kept surveillance logs, and retrieved immigration records. Teams of six agents listened to 47 telephones around the clock, taping a total of 55,000 conversations; the 900 most important were transcribed and collated in nine bound volumes. So vast was the evidence that it took a full year to be presented in court.
>
> In the end, the government was rewarded for its pains. All but two of the defendants were convicted, and most were sentenced to long terms. Still, as [author Shana] Alexander observes, the case "did not make the slightest dent in the nation's desperate drug problem. More heroin and more cocaine is on the streets today than before [the trial began]. The trial severely overtaxed every branch of our legal system—law enforcement, bench and bar—and taxed the unfortunate jurors most of all."[6]

An international comparison shows that many Western countries are much less invested in law enforcement drug control efforts, yet the size of their drug problems is much smaller. "In some Western European nations, including Italy, the Netherlands, Spain, and Switzerland, much more emphasis has been given to the health consequences of drug addiction, and there has been a reluctance to use the criminal law against users at all. [See Figure 14.2.] Other Western European nations, notably Germany, Norway, and Sweden, have viewed drug use as a moral issue. They have also used criminal law against users, but not nearly as

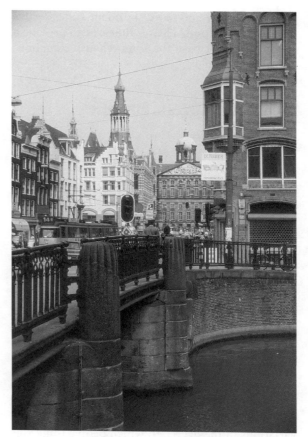

Figure 14.2 **Amsterdam** Some European countries are more permissive regarding drugs than the United States. (© Charles E. Schmidt/Unicorn Stock Photos)

aggressively as has the United States."[7] International comparisons must be made with caution because there are many social and cultural differences that are hard to assess. Policy that is effective in Europe may not be successful in the United States or Canada.

The second point made by proponents of legalization is that prohibition contributes to crime, victimizing all of society. A lot of money can be made from drugs, so there is constant violence among drug dealers and with the police; many of the casualties are innocent bystanders. Heroin and cocaine addicts often resort to prostitution and theft to support their drug habits because the cost of their habit is far too great to be financed by conventional employment. Alcohol or tobacco

A Latin American Perspective on Drug Trafficking

The government of Colombia and its law-abiding citizens will continue to wage all-out war on drugs and drug trafficking. But it is a war we cannot win by ourselves. We must form an alliance with the governments, and the citizens, of the drug-consuming nations of the world. And this means first and foremost the United States. If there is one central element in the drug trade, it is demand in the U.S., which consumes 50 percent of the world's illicit cocaine.

Until this demand is forced down, the illegal profit incentive will eclipse the efforts made on all other fronts and violence and corruption in both our countries will continue to spiral up.

Source: Victor Mosquera Chaux, Colombian Ambassador to the United States, letter to the editor, *New York Review of Books*, March 2, 1989.

addiction are different because those products are legally available and in ample supply.

The rejoinder to this point is that law enforcement officials consider it one of their goals to make the price of drugs so expensive that potential users will be discouraged and current addicts will be motivated to seek treatment. As mentioned previously, this goal has not been achieved. Drug use is **price sensitive**, and higher prices drive some addicts into treatment. However, some addicts who enter treatment are not rehabilitated, and other addicts resolve to steal more when the price of drugs goes up. If drugs were legalized, their prices would naturally go down. Governments could keep prices artificially high with tariffs, but if the official prices were too high, a black market would develop to undercut legitimate sales.

The third main point for legalization is that our aggressive law enforcement efforts disrupt and distort foreign policy. Latin American countries in particular have experienced intensive U.S. pressure to take action against their own citizens to stop the production and export of cocaine, marijuana, and heroin. These actions include sanctioning growers, destroying laboratories and seizing production chemicals, and prosecuting the so-called drug lords. These actions have caused significant political unrest, shocking assassinations, and government corruption. It is estimated that Columbian narcotics cartels spend $100 million on bribes to Colombian officials each year.[8]

Some officials in these countries are ambivalent about drug control efforts because the drug business provides employment and an economic stimulus to communities that are deprived and desperate. For example, in 1993, 98% of Bolivia's foreign exchange earnings from goods and services came from the coca market.[9] Other officials are supportive in principle because they are opposed to their countries aiding and abetting the illicit drug trade, but they are resentful of the damage done to their countries by an insatiable U.S. demand for drugs. (See the Viewpoints box.) They object to strong-arm U.S. pressure and think we should do more to cut U.S. demand for drugs. Incidentally, there is no evidence that U.S. drug control operatives are effective in foreign countries.[10]

A fourth argument of legalization forces is that legal controls and the war on drugs violate citizens' civil rights. This position argues that the currently illegal drugs are no more hazardous than alcohol and tobacco—400,000 deaths per year are attributable to tobacco, 100,000 to alcohol, and 18,000 to illicit drug use, including about 11,600 deaths associated with AIDS transmitted by IV drug use.[11] Although proponents recognize the potential harm that can be done by cocaine, amphetamines, heroin, and the like, they claim that illegal drugs can be used moderately in the same way as alcohol is used. Furthermore, they say that aggressive police action—violent intrusion of suspects' residences and seizure of assets—is an abuse

On Freedom, Parenting, and Social Responsibility

At some point between Lamaze and PTA, it becomes clear that one of your main jobs as a parent is to counter the culture. What the media deliver to children by the masses, you are expected to rebut one at a time. But it occurs to me now that the call for "parental responsibility" is increasing in direct proportion to the irresponsibility of the marketplace. Parents are expected to protect their children from an increasingly hostile environment. Are the kids being sold junk food? Just say no. Is TV bad? Turn it off. Are there messages about sex, drugs, violence all around? Counter the culture. Without wallowing in false nostalgia, there has been a fundamental shift. Americans once expected parents to raise their children in accordance with the dominant cultural messages. Today they are expected to raise their children in opposition. Once the chorus of cultural values was full of ministers, teachers, neighbors, leaders. They demanded more conformity, but offered more support. Now the messengers are Ninja Turtles, Madonna, rap groups, and celebrities pushing sneakers. Parents are considered "responsible" only if they are successful in their resistance.

Source: Ellen Goodman, "Battling Our Culture Is Parents' Task," *Chicago Tribune*, August 18, 1993.

---

of power and a violation of privacy and property rights. While these points may have some validity, opponents feel that our society needs to be less concerned with rights and more concerned with responsibility and family and community welfare.

Finally, some proponents of legalization refer to concepts of cost-benefit analysis. Public policies to control drug use have benefits and costs.[12] By some accounting, the costs of current drug control policies (e.g., overcrowded prisons and criminal justice systems) outweigh their benefits. Public policies should be such that the expense of addressing a problem is equal to or less than the cost incurred by the problem itself. The war on drugs does not seem to meet this standard, particularly for marijuana.[13] However, many of the values (e.g., responsibility, delay of gratification) protected by the drug warriors are not readily quantified or assessed in monetary terms.

Arguments Against Legalization

Most people are against legalizing drugs because "drugs are bad" and, therefore, it is in society's best interest to stop people from using them. Similar logic is used in support of helmet laws. There is no question that drug abuse inflicts extensive personal and social harm; however, legal drugs do more harm. Antilegalization spokespersons recognize this fact, but say that just because some harmful things are legal is no reason to make all harmful things legal.

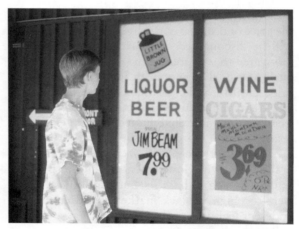

Figure 14.3 **Advertising of Legal Drugs May Confuse Children** Children may wonder "Who's right, the ads or my parents and school?" (© Rod Furason/Unicorn Stock Photos)

Second, many people assert that legalization would send mixed messages to young people. (See Figure 14.3.) Legal use of drugs in society makes prevention more difficult, because schools and parents teach youth to say "no" while other forces in the community teach them to say "yes." (See the Viewpoints box "On Freedom, Parenting, and Social Responsibility.")

There is some validity to this issue of mixed messages, as illustrated by the tug of war experienced in preventing alcohol and tobacco use. The decline in drug use during the 1980s was much more pronounced for illegal drugs than it was for alcohol and tobacco: Between 1980 and 1990, high school seniors' lifetime reported use dropped 27% for illicit drugs, 9% for tobacco, and 4% for alcohol. These numbers might suggest that the presence of mixed messages is potentially significant. However, for the last five years, use of alcohol and tobacco has decreased slightly, while the use of illicit drugs has slightly increased. (See Figure 14.1.)

A third antilegalization argument is for a return to traditional moral values. Those people opposed to legalization believe that antidrug laws reinforce moral standards, declaring society's definitions of right and wrong. They point to the decay of the family, high rates of teen sexual activity and pregnancy, the AIDS epidemic, abortions, child abuse, and other violence as indicators of America's moral decline.

> Our society now places less value than before on what we owe others as a matter of moral obligation; less value on sacrifice as a moral good; less value on social conformity, respectability, and observing the rules; and less value on correctness and restraint in matters of physical pleasure and sexuality. Higher value is now placed on things like self-expression, individualism, self-realization, and personal choice."[14]

From this point of view, legalizing drugs would drive yet one more nail into the national coffin.

A fourth antilegalization argument is one of history, best articulated by David Musto, a psychiatrist and medical historian from Yale University. He cites the fact that the drug epidemic that occurred in the late 1800s and early 1900s ended largely because mainstream society began to view drug use as a threat and rejected drug-using lifestyles, and argues that this development will recur as history repeats itself. A fundamental shift in public attitudes toward drug use was apparent in the 1980s as the current drug epidemic declined; sanctions were necessary to support this shift. Legalization would disrupt the trend, and block or reverse continuing progress.[15] In the 1990s, however, use of illicit drugs changed very little, in spite of strong sanctions; this fact tends to refute this argument.

Opponents of legalization also say that drugs certainly should not be legally available to youth, any more than alcohol or tobacco should be. As long as drugs are partly illegal (e.g., for youth), there will still be efforts to make illegal sales, and law enforcement efforts will still be required.

It is difficult to pin down the position of the American public with respect to legalization of drugs. About two-thirds of people believe it is very or somewhat effective to arrest drug users. Only 49% of people believe that possession of small amounts of marijuana should be treated as a criminal offense. About 75% of people believe that we will never be able to stop drugs from coming into this country and that we are losing the drug war.[16] These opinions probably are not informed by the issues just discussed. When former Surgeon General Jocelyn Elders suggested publicly in December 1993 that the issue of legalization should be studied, she was loudly criticized by leaders in Congress and received no support from the White House. Nevertheless, the country is moving away from the war on drugs as it was fought in the recent past. In the late 1980s and early 1990s, about 70% of federal drug spending was allocated to law enforcement; about 30% was split between prevention and treatment. In the drug control plan unveiled by President Bush in 2002, about two-thirds of spending was to go for law enforcement and about one-third was earmarked for prevention and treatment. (See Table 14.1.) The challenge is to spend dollars in all categories in a cost-effective way and to address some of the serious social problems that contribute to the abuse of drugs. Also needed is more prevention work focusing on alcohol and tobacco. Heretofore, efforts have been deficient in these areas.

Drug Abuse and the First Amendment

One of the great paradoxes of society is that while we go to great lengths to stamp out illicit drugs, we allow persuasive messages about alcohol and tobacco to be shouted from the rooftops. Alcohol and tobacco account for a huge segment of the advertising industry, which has not gone unnoticed by prevention advocates. (See the Viewpoints box "A Public Health Perspective on Tobacco Advertising.") In 1965, a new federal law required

A Public Health Perspective on Tobacco Advertising

While this Institute spent $47 million last year to develop and disseminate effective smoking intervention technologies, the major cigarette manufacturers spent $3.6 billion in an effort to convince people that smoking is necessary for social acceptance, that it makes one attractive to the opposite sex, and that it enhances self-image. Over the past four years alone, expenditures for all cigarette advertising and promotional activities have increased nearly 50 percent and, increasingly, they appear to be targeting youth.

Perhaps the most criticized campaign of recent years was the introduction, in 1988, of the "smooth character" cartoon Joe the Camel. In 1989, RJR Nabisco ran a particularly outrageous four-page ad in youth-oriented *Rolling Stone* magazine, in which dating advice was offered for young men. On the first page of the ad is a cartoon of a beautiful woman asking if the male teen is "bored? lonely? restless?" Inside, the "smooth character" gives "foolproof dating advice" for impressing someone on the beach:

> Run into the water, grab someone and drag her back to the shore, as if you've saved her from drowning. *The more she kicks and screams, the better* [emphasis added].

While the tone and slant of this advice constitute an insulting provocation to the women of our country, perhaps equally troubling is the information on the back page of the ad: "How to get a FREE pack even if you don't like to redeem coupons." The suggestion: Just ask "your best friend" or "a kind-looking stranger" to redeem the coupon for you.

Who is really the target of such an advertisement? Certainly, the camel cartoon character could not have much appeal for an adult. And how many people would feel compelled to ask "a kind-looking stranger" to redeem a coupon for free merchandise—unless, of course, they were underage?

No doubt the success of the "smooth character" campaign is one reason that RJR Nabisco more than tripled its advertising expenditures for Camel cigarettes. In the wake of Joe the Camel's popularity, Brown & Williamson Tobacco Corp. has begun test marketing of a penguin cartoon character to promote Kool cigarettes in billboards, magazines, and store displays. It is not difficult to imagine what impact such large-scale, youth-oriented promotions may have on the sale of these brands to teenagers. Unfortunately, by the time we resolve this question, millions of our young people already will have become addicted to cigarettes. While the economic costs to our future program of health care delivery will be staggering, the future human costs are beyond reckoning.

As public health officials, we must devise effective strategies to counter such seductive promotions, and we will not shy away from this mission. Yet, for every $1 that NCI spends on research to combat smoking, the tobacco industry spends $80 to promote the addiction. Where the cigarette manufacturers can offer free packs of cigarettes, cigarette lighters, and premiums such as attractive clothing, we can offer only warnings about the dangers of smoking and advice about how to quit.

As health professionals, we need to understand that smoking is not only an individual's problem, but also a societal problem—"a social carcinogen," as one prominent researcher characterized it.

Source: National Cancer Institute, 1991.

Table 14.1

U.S. Federal Drug Control Spending (in millions), 2001–2003

	2001	2002	2003	Percent Change
Prevention	2,578.7	2,548.6	2,473.4	−4.0
Treatment	3,335.0	3,587.5	3,811.7	14.3
Law enforcement	12,182.0	12,686.7	12,894.6	5.8
Total	18,095.7	18,822.8	19,179.7	5.9

Source: Office of National Drug Control Policy.

warning labels on tobacco packages; later, warnings were required on all tobacco advertising. In the 1960s, the Fairness Doctrine was invoked to provide free air time for antitobacco spots to counterbalance tobacco ads on television; in 1971, cigarette advertising on television was completely banned. The Alcoholic Beverage Labeling Act was passed in 1988, which required warning messages on alcoholic beverage containers. In 1992, the Sensible Advertising and Family Education Act was brought before Congress. The law would have required warning messages on all alcohol advertising, including TV, radio, billboards, and print media, but it was not passed. (See the FYI box.) Some advocates are encouraging a total ban on alcohol promotion on TV and radio, or at least a restriction of such advertising during hours when minors are likely to be tuned in.

As advertising is targeted more aggressively by prevention advocates, several issues are ever more hotly debated: Do advertising appeals influence smoking or drinking behavior? Are alcohol and tobacco warning labels necessary? Are warning labels effective in altering smoking and drinking behavior? To what extent are alcohol and tobacco ads protected by freedom of speech provisions of the First Amendment to the U.S. Constitution? (See **Figure 14.4**.)

That advertising causes smoking and drinking is, of course, denied by industry spokespersons. Their standard claim is that advertising influences brand selection but does not persuade someone to purchase and use a product. In fact, there is little evidence from experimental research to show that advertising *causes* smoking or drinking.[17] However, many studies demonstrate associations between advertising and behavior and the precursors of behavior.[18]

Numerous surveys of adolescents have asked them what influenced them to smoke or drink. Advertising is among the factors they identify, but it is far less significant than family and peer influences. There is evidence that children pay attention to advertising and that ads do affect their brand selection. In spite of their denials, the alcohol and tobacco industries are adamantly opposed to advertising restrictions or regulations; apparently they believe advertising has an impact. In countries

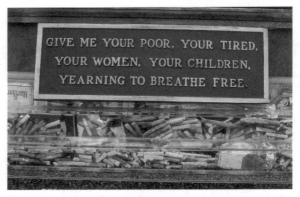

Figure 14.4 Antitobacco Speech Freedom of speech may protect drug advertising, but it also ensures the right to criticize the alcohol and tobacco industries.

(© Aneal Vohra/Unicorn Stock Photos)

where alcohol and tobacco are less regulated, advertising and promotion are even more aggressive.

Prevention advocates recognize that the influence of advertising on behavior may be small, but that even a small impact on a big problem is worth achieving. Advertising as a prevention target should not be disregarded, because it can be a significant influence on some youth. Furthermore, it is much easier to control marketing campaigns than to alter family or peer influences. It is hoped that future research will better explain the role of advertising in the initiation of smoking and drinking.

Some people maintain that warning labels are unnecessary because everyone knows about the hazards of tobacco and alcohol, and people who are prone to drug abuse are unlikely to be influenced by a printed warning.[19] Although it is true that public knowledge about the risks of alcohol and tobacco use is widespread, it is limited in some population subgroups, including children, youth, and people with limited education. A 1991 study of 956 junior and senior high school students in eight states found widespread misinformation about alcoholic beverages.[20] These information gaps could be filled in other ways, but the alcohol industry should be expected to play a role in educating youth honestly about the products it sells.

Both tobacco and alcohol companies have mounted campaigns that they claim are designed to discourage young people from using their products. However, these campaigns never mention the hazards of smoking or drinking, but tell young people that smoking and drinking are for adults only. It is hard to believe that those campaigns are really what the industries say they are. Prevention specialists also should recognize that warning labels are merely information; they have value only when they are supported by comprehensive prevention strategies.

After we ask whether warning labels are needed, we must ask whether they have an impact on smoking or drinking. This question is awkward for the prevention field, because the evidence that warning labels are effective is inconclusive. Some researchers report that warning labels can influence consumers;[21] others seem less certain.[22] In countries where warning labels are not required, the alcohol and tobacco companies do not use them. One conclusion that can be drawn from this is that the companies are afraid that the warning labels will discourage people from buying their products. It is fair to say that warning labels can influence

awareness and attitudes and may have a small impact on behavior. However, when warning labels are combined with other education and prevention activities, they can serve a more useful purpose.

The push for greater controls on advertising has prompted the alcohol and tobacco industries to frame their position in constitutional terms. Their position is built on two principal points: (1) Alcohol and tobacco are legal products, and (2) the First Amendment to the U.S. Constitution guarantees them the right to speak freely, in the form of advertising, about their products. They further maintain that freedom of speech includes the right not to speak. In other words, they claim the right not to say things in their ads that might be harmful to their business. (See **Figure 14.5.**)

When cigarette ads were banned from the airwaves, industries did not challenge the ban because they believed that the antitobacco public service ads required by the Fairness Doctrine were more detrimental to them than the loss of TV and radio exposure. To compensate, they shifted cigarette marketing to other media, such as magazines and sponsorship of auto racing events. In the three years prior to the ban, per capita cigarette consumption declined; after the ban, it increased for each of the next three years.[23]

When warning labels first were proposed for all cigarette packages and alcoholic beverage containers, the alcohol and tobacco industries' constitutional argument was rejected by Congress and

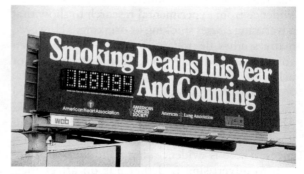

Figure 14.5 **A Public Statement About Tobacco**
Tobacco companies have cast smoking as a constitutionally guaranteed freedom. Freedom and addiction are not easily linked. (© A. Rodham/Unicorn Stock Photos)

the courts. The Sensible Advertising and Family Education Act (S.674/H.R. 1823) would have required warning labels on all alcohol advertising. The alcohol industry's stance was that marketplace information is critical for the effective operation of a capitalist economy, and that therefore commercial speech is just as important as political and civil speech. It also claims that while tobacco is harmful with normal use, alcohol is harmful only when it is abused, and that all products (e.g., automobiles) are potentially harmful if they are abused. The industry concedes that container warning labels may be appropriate, much like information on food labels, but that advertising targets everyone, consumers and nonconsumers alike.

If the proposed legislation had passed, it undoubtedly would have been challenged in the court system. Only then would the constitutionality of required warning labels on alcohol advertising be definitively determined. However, judicial precedent provides some benchmarks for the decision. Commercial speech has some protection under the First Amendment, but much less so than civic or political speech. The degree of protection is not standardized, but depends on the value of the commercial information to consumers.

There is, of course, full legal precedent for barring false or deceptive commercial speech. Court decisions have determined that "nondeceptive commercial speech can be banned if a substantial State interest is furthered" and that "nonmisleading commercial speech for a legal product may be regulated if the Government directly and materially advances a substantial Government interest by means no more extensive than necessary."[24] "Regulation" could be interpreted to include required warning labels. If the courts continue to agree that such a requirement can be constitutional, perhaps the decision will then rest on whether or not the labels are effective. As discussed earlier, this case will be hard to prove unequivocally.

Incidentally, the alcohol industry claims that labels are ineffective and therefore should not be required. However, it has used devious methods to make beverage container warning labels difficult to read and easy to overlook, such as by printing them in very small type, printing them with noncontrasting backgrounds, printing them so that they are partially covered by overlapping labels, or otherwise positioning them to be hidden within label graphics and layout.[25]

Taxation as a Prevention Policy

Alcohol and tobacco are consumer goods, and prevention workers have made efforts to make them more expensive as a way to discourage consumption. Conventional wisdom is that people, especially if they are addicted, will buy these products regardless of what they cost. However, research has conclusively demonstrated that both alcohol and tobacco purchases are price sensitive: As price increases relative to the cost of living, consumption declines.[26] The National Academy of Sciences studied this issue with respect to alcohol and concluded that

> even relatively small changes in prices may influence not only the quantity of consumption but also the most serious health effects as well. Taxes affect prices, prices affect the quantity of consumption, and the quantity of consumption affects the health and safety of drinkers. An increased tax on alcoholic beverages has the particular effect of improving the chronic health picture (as indexed by liver failure) of the heavier drinkers—who are, it can be added, paying most of the tax increase. Therefore, we see good grounds for incorporating an interest in the prevention of alcohol problems into the setting of tax rates on alcohol.[27]

That price affects consumption is particularly true for youth and the lower social classes.[28] It has even been demonstrated that alcoholics are sensitive to prices and drink less when the beverage price increases.[29] Taxes on tobacco and alcohol are quite popular with the general public, as verified by public opinion polls. They are a relatively painless way (especially for nonsmokers or moderate drinkers) to pay for government programs, and they can reduce the health and economic damage done by these products.

By international standards, U.S. tobacco taxes are among the lowest of those levied by industrialized nations, and as a proportion of the retail price, those taxes declined from 47% in 1970 to 30% in 1993.[30] Since that time, numerous states

Table 14.2

Tobacco Tax Increases in Selected States

State	Date of Increase	Tax Increase ($)	State's New Tax ($)	Smoking Decline (%)	New Revenue (millions)
Alaska	10/97	0.71	1.00	13.5	28.7
California	1/99	0.50	0.87	18.9	555.4
Hawaii	7/98	0.20	1.00	8.1	6.4
Illinois	12/97	0.14	0.58	8.9	77.4
Maine	11/97	0.37	0.74	15.5	30.8
Maryland	7/99	0.30	0.66	16.3	68.0
Massachusetts	10/96	0.25	0.76	14.3	64.1
Michigan	5/94	0.50	0.75	20.8	341.0
New Hampshire	7/99	0.15	0.52	10.4	19.6
New Jersey	1/98	0.40	0.80	16.8	166.6
New York	3/00	0.55	1.11	20.2	365.4
Oregon	2/97	0.30	0.78	8.3	79.8
Rhode Island	7/97	0.10	0.71	1.5	8.6
South Dakota	7/95	0.10	0.33	5.6	6.1
Utah	7/97	0.25	0.515	25.7	17.6
Vermont	7/95	0.24	0.44	16.3	11.7
Wisconsin	11/97	0.15	0.59	6.5	52.9

Source: National Campaign for Tobacco Free Kids.

Table 14.3

Federal Alcohol Excise Taxes, 2002

Product	Tax	Tax per Container
Beer	$18/barrel	$0.05/12-oz can
Wine, ≤14% alcohol	$1.07/gallon	$0.21/750-ml bottle
Wine, >14% to 21%	$1.57/gallon	$0.31/750-ml bottle
Hard cider	$0.226/gallon	$0.04/750-ml bottle
Distilled spirits	$13.50/gallon	$2.14/750-ml bottle

Source: U.S. Bureau of Alcohol, Tobacco, and Firearms.

have increased their tobacco excise taxes; without exception, the result has been a decline in smoking and increased revenues. As of 2002, the average state excise tax was $0.60 per pack,[31] but many other states were expected to raise their taxes. (See Table 14.2.) Federal tobacco taxes amounted to $7.2 billion in 2000. State governments collect many more billions in excise and sales taxes.

Alcohol taxes have not been adjusted to keep up with the consumer price index; federal beer and wine taxes remained the same from 1951 to 1991. Liquor taxes remained the same from 1951 to 1985, being raised once again in 1991. In 1951, the federal excise tax on distilled spirits was $10.50 per gallon, increasing to $13.50 in 1991. Meanwhile, inflation made a dollar in 1951 equal to $5.24 in 1991.[32] Federal alcohol taxes amounted to $8.1 billion in 2000. As with tobacco, state governments also levy alcohol excise taxes. To the great disappointment of drug abuse prevention and treatment advocates, there has been serious consideration in Congress of lowering federal alcohol taxes.[33] (See Table 14.3.)

Until recently, cigarette and alcohol excise taxes have been less than the social cost of these products' use.[34] Taxes on tobacco have been increasing lately, so the balance of cost versus tax revenue has been becoming more equal. It has been predicted that a 10% increase in the price of tobacco products will lead to a 4% decrease in adult consumption and a 7% decrease in youth consumption.[35] According to that formula, a $0.75 tax increase on a $3.00 pack of cigarettes should result in a 17.5% decrease in youth consumption.

Americans support cigarette tax increases, partly because only about 25% of the population would pay the tax. On the other hand, the tobacco industry and agricultural groups in tobacco-growing states are opposed. It remains to be seen who has the most power, the majority or special interests. The political reality is that an alcohol tax increase would be much more difficult to enact, even though it would be even more appropriate than a cigarette tax increase. Given the current political climate in Washington and most state capitals, it is unlikely that any alcohol taxes will be raised in the near future, no matter how justified.

As an effective prevention strategy, taxation has one principal pitfall. If purchase price becomes too high, consumers will find ways to circumvent paying the tax, such as by crossing state lines to buy cigarettes or alcohol in neighboring states that have lower state taxes. In Canada, tobacco taxes were about $3 per pack in the early 1990s, compared with about $0.50 in the United States; this high Canadian tax contributed to a 40% decline in smoking among Canadian adults and a two-thirds decline among teens.[36] The Canadian government has since reduced its tobacco tax because of widespread cigarette smuggling from the United States. This problem will be ameliorated when U.S. taxes are raised to the Canadian level.

Drugs and AIDS

When the AIDS epidemic was recognized in the early 1980s, it was quickly determined that IV drug use was a principal risk factor. As of December 2001, approximately 467,910 people had died from the disease since the first cases were diagnosed in 1981.[37] In comparison with the number of ATOD-related

[**Table 14.4**]

The Proportion of Adolescent and Adult AIDS Cases Attributed to IV Drug Use Among Different Population Subgroups, 2001

White males	17%
African American males	40%
Hispanic males	20%
White females	41%
African American females	39%
All adolescents/adults	31%

Source: Centers for Disease Control and Prevention, 2002.

deaths (518,000 per year), this number is relatively small, although AIDS deaths could become much more numerous in the future. Nevertheless, AIDS is a serious threat to our health and the economic welfare of the health care system. People who primarily are concerned with drug abuse or AIDS have begun to mount cooperative efforts.

There are as many as 2.4 million IV drug users in the United States,[38] and about one-third of AIDS cases are caused by IV drug use exposure alone or in combination with other risk behaviors. However, the percentage of cases attributed to dirty needles varies markedly among different population groups. (See Table 14.4.) In major metropolitan areas where there is a greater number of IV drug users, the significance of needle-transmitted AIDS is staggering in terms of the drain on the medical care system and the toll of human lives. Although only 3% to 4% of the U.S. population live in New York City, about 15% of the cumulative U.S. AIDS cases since 1981 have been among IV drug users who live in that city.[39]

In about 113 U.S. cities and others in Canada, Europe, and Australia, public health officials have initiated distribution and exchange of IV needles and syringes as a way to limit HIV infection.[40] (See Figure 14.6.) While recognizing the hazards of drug addiction, leaders view AIDS as a more urgent and serious matter, and the distribution of needles a lesser evil than the spread of the AIDS virus.

Opponents of these programs say that spending tax dollars to subsidize destructive and illegal

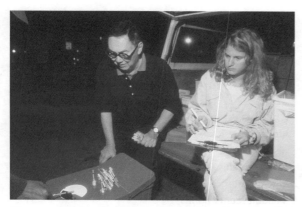

Figure 14.6 Needle Distribution on an Urban Street
Needle distribution has been promoted as a way to limit the spread of AIDS, but it conflicts with mainstream social values. (© Ramey/Unicorn Stock Photos)

activity is bad policy and may facilitate or even increase IV drug use. Opponents further assert that the threat of AIDS may give junkies an incentive to seek out treatment. Although it might be ideal for addicts to enter treatment and quit their drug habit, many of the cities that operate needle distribution programs have a shortage of treatment resources, and people are placed on waiting lists.

Evidence shows that (1) addicts seek out clean needles if they are available,[41] (2) needle sharing declines among participants of needle distribution programs,[42] and (3) people do not become IV drug abusers because clean needles are available.[43] An additional benefit is that needle exchange programs promise to save health care dollars because the cost of providing needles is much less than the cost of providing lifetime medical care to an HIV-infected individual, which is about $200,000.[44] Furthermore, IV drug users are socially isolated and hard to reach with social and public health programs, so when they exchange their needles it may be a good opportunity to give them information on risk reduction, condoms, and referral into treatment programs.

The End of the Beginning

Many teachers and researchers in the drug abuse prevention field have spent the better part of their adult lives wrestling with understanding the nature and extent of drug abuse problems and how they

could be reduced. Given the presence of free will and the limitations of social engineering, the best we can hope for is **harm reduction**, diminishing the proportion of people involved in drug abuse and the magnitude of the damage.

The drug problem will never disappear, though it may shrink or expand in historical trends. Consequently, whenever and wherever one practices prevention, it is simply at the beginning of the next 10 years, regardless of whether the current trend is ascending or descending. We now have a considerable body of knowledge about what works and doesn't work in prevention, much more than existed two decades ago. From the micro perspective, it will be necessary to ensure that only effective strategies are implemented and that prevention strategies are carried out in a way that maximizes their impact. From the macro perspective, efforts must be comprehensive, and all agencies (or systems) must collaborate. The authors believe that a 1994 agreement between the U.S. Department of Education and the U.S. Department of Health and Human Services is a step in the right direction (See the FYI box). Although the statement is dated, the principles are still valid and worthwhile.

Healthy People 2010 Objectives for the Nation for Alcohol, Tobacco, and Other Drugs

In 2000, the federal government released an extensive list of health promotion objectives to be achieved by the year 2010. The overall label for the objectives and the effort they represent is Healthy People 2010. While the objectives cover all health issues, the concern here is with alcohol, tobacco, and other drugs. What follows are a few examples of the national objectives to diminish the harm done by ATOD abuse.

- By the year 2010, reduce deaths caused by alcohol-related motor vehicle crashes to no greater than 4 per 100,000 population.
- By the year 2010, reduce drug-induced deaths to no greater than 1 per 100,000 population.
- By the year 2010, reduce to no greater than 30% the proportion of adolescents who

Joint Statement on School Health: The Secretaries of Education and Health and Human Services

Health and education are joined in fundamental ways with each other and with the destinies of the Nation's children. Because of our national leadership responsibilities for education and health, we have initiated unprecedented cooperative efforts between our Departments. In support of comprehensive school health programs, we affirm the following:

America's children face many compelling educational and health and developmental challenges that affect their lives and their futures.

These challenges include poor levels of achievement, unacceptably high drop-out rates, low literacy, violence, drug abuse, preventable injuries, physical and mental illness, developmental disabilities, and sexual activity resulting in sexually transmitted diseases, including HIV, and unintended pregnancy. These facts demand a reassessment of the contributions of education and health programs in safeguarding our children's present lives and preparing them for productive, responsible, and fulfilling futures.

To help children meet these challenges, education and health must be linked in partnership.

Schools are the only public institutions that touch nearly every young person in this country. Schools have a unique opportunity to affect the lives of children and their families, but they cannot address all of our children's needs alone. Health, education, and human service programs must be integrated, and schools must have the support of public and private health care providers, communities, and families.

School health programs support the education process, integrate services for disadvantaged and disabled children, and improve children's health prospects.

Through school health programs, children and their families can develop the knowledge, attitudes, beliefs, and behaviors necessary to remain healthy and perform well in school. These learning environments enhance safety, nutrition, and disease prevention; encourage exercise and fitness; support healthy physical, mental, and emotional development; promote abstinence and prevent sexual behaviors that result in HIV infection, other sexually transmitted diseases, and unintended teenage pregnancy; discourage use of illegal drugs, alcohol, and tobacco; and help young people develop problem-solving and decision-making skills.

Reforms in health care and in education offer opportunities to forge the partnerships needed for our children in the 1990s.

The benefits of integrated health and education services can be achieved by working together to create a "seamless" network of service, both through the school setting and through linkages with other community resources.

Goals 2000 and Healthy People 2000 provide complementary visions that, together, can support our joint efforts in pursuit of a healthier, better educated Nation for the next century.

Goals 2000 challenges us to ensure that all children arrive at school ready to learn; to increase the high school graduation rate; to achieve basic subject matter competencies; to achieve universal adult literacy; and to ensure that school environments are safe, disciplined, and drug free. Healthy People 2000 challenges us to increase the span of healthy life for the American people, to reduce and finally to eliminate health disparities among population groups, and to ensure access to services for all Americans.

In support of Goals 2000 and Healthy People 2000, we have established the Interagency Committee on School Health, co-chaired by the Assistant Secretary for Elementary and Secondary Education and the Assistant Secretary for Health, and we have convened the National Coordinating Committee on School Health to bring together representatives of major national education and health organizations to work with us.

We call upon professionals in the fields of education and health and concerned citizens across the Nation to join with us in a renewed effort and a reaffirmation of our mutual responsibility to our Nation's children.

Richard W. Riley
Secretary of Education

Donna E. Shalala
Secretary of Health
and Human Services

report that they rode, during the previous 30 days, with a driver who had been drinking alcohol.

- By the year 2010, reduce to no greater than 20% the proportion of college students engaging in binge drinking of alcoholic beverages.
- By the year 2010, increase to at least 80% the proportion of adolescents who perceive great risk associated with using cocaine once per month.
- By the year 2010, extend legal requirements for maximum blood alcohol concentration levels of 0.08% for motor vehicle drivers aged 21 years and older to all states and the District of Columbia.
- Reduce cigarette smoking to no greater than 12% of adults by the year 2010.
- Reduce past-month cigarette smoking to no greater than 16% of adolescents by the year 2010.
- Increase the average age of first use of tobacco products by adolescents to 14 by the year 2010.
- By the year 2010, at least 30% of pregnant smokers will quit during their pregnancy.
- By the year 2010, reduce to no greater than 10% the proportion of children who are regularly exposed to tobacco smoke at home.

The accomplishment of all 46 of the ATOD objectives will require partnerships between all levels of government and between the public and private sectors. The objectives provide benchmarks for local prevention programs, validating the importance of recognized needs. The objectives also represent the comprehensive prevention approach advocated throughout this text.

Summary

Our future challenge is to build on the lessons of the history of prevention that are documented in prevention literature and discussed in this text. In addition to school-based curricula and policy, community supports need to be addressed. We must examine the way law enforcement and the criminal justice system have been used to prevent drug abuse. We must consider the public presentation and advertising of alcohol and tobacco. We should be open to using price manipulation and taxes as a way to discourage drug abuse, and we should intervene collaboratively to diminish the related problems of drug abuse, AIDS, and violence. Perhaps the trials and errors of past efforts will not be forgotten when we are on high alert for the next rise in drug abuse.

Scenario | Analysis and Response

The issue of the legalization of marijuana is a delicate one for a community antidrug coalition. On the one hand, many people sympathize with AIDS and cancer victims and the suffering they experience. Many people, even if they have not personally used marijuana, feel that those patients should be able to have access to any remedy that will improve the quality of their lives. Strongly opposing marijuana legalization in this instance seems very cold and insensitive.

On the other hand, the public is also expecting your coalition to unilaterally oppose drug abuse, and many are unable to distinguish the difference between irresponsible drug abuse and the use of marijuana by certain patients. There is some concern about the mixed messages that would ensue from endorsing legalization.

In addition, the coalition is dependent on funding from the state and federal governments. At least some segments of those governments are opposed to the legalization of marijuana for patients. Will support by the coalition jeopardize future funding? Will it lead to a loss of support from constituents in the local community?

As the coalition's coordinator, you must approach this issue with caution. There should be full and open debate about whether to issue an endorsement of the initiative. The full membership should be included in deliberations, not just officers or the executive committee. It is essential that all views be aired and all consequences considered.

Learning Activities

1. Obtain copies of state laws that mandate age restrictions on the purchase and use of alcohol and tobacco. Also acquire copies of legislation that regulates drunk driving.

2. Examine magazine ads for alcohol and tobacco products. Summarize the theme of each ad, and try to identify the target audience. Make comparisons between different types of magazines (e.g., news magazines, women's magazines, sports magazines) and different points in time (e.g., December 1980, 1985, 1990, 1995, 2000).

3. Discover the current taxes levied on alcohol and tobacco products in your community. Trace the history of those taxes: how long they have been in place, for what the funds are used, and whether any effort has been made to raise or lower the taxes.

4. Determine the location of the nearest needle distribution program. Find out how the program is operated and funded, how many people participate, how the program has been received in the local community, and if there are any indications of the program's impact. A source for this information might be an AIDS outreach program or agency.

5. Read the *Healthy People 2010* chapters on tobacco (www. health.gov/healthypeople/ Document/HTML/Volume2/ 27Tobacco.htm) and substance abuse (www.health.gov/ healthypeople/Document/HTML/Volume2/26 Substance.htm). Identify several objectives, and outline the strategies proposed to achieve the objectives.

Notes

1. Princeton Survey Research Associates, Pew Research Center for the People & the Press Survey, February 2001.

2. A. Goldstein and H. Kalant, "Drug Policy: Striking the Right Balance," *Science,* 249 (September 1990): 1513–1521.

3. Office of National Drug Control Policy, *State and Local Spending on Drug Control Activities* (Washington, DC: The White House, October 1993); Gary E. Johnson, "Bad Investment," Mother Jones.Com, July 10, 2001.

4. P. Reuter and J. Caulkins, "ONDCP's First Four Years as a Policy Agency," testimony before the House Committee on Government Operations, October 5, 1993.

5. Abt Associates, *The Price of Illicit Drugs: 1981 Through the Second Quarter of 2000* (Washington, DC: Office of National Drug Control Policy, October 2001), 43.

6. M. Massing, "Desperate over Drugs," *New York Review of Books,* March 30, 1989, 22.

7. P. Reuter, M. Falco, and R. MacCoun, *Comparing Western European and North American Drug Policies: An International Conference Report* (Santa Monica, CA: RAND, 1993), viii.

8. Trade and Environmental Database (TED), *TED Case Studies: Columbia Coca Trade* (Washington, DC: American University, 1997), 4.

9. U.S. Congress, Office of Technology Assessment, *Alternative Coca Reduction Strategies in the Andean Region* (Washington, DC: U.S. Government Printing Office, July 1993).

10. National Narcotics Intelligence Consumers Committee, *The NNICC Report, 1992: The Supply of Illicit Drugs to the United States* (Arlington, VA: Drug Enforcement Administration, September 1993); Institute for Health Policy, Brandeis University, *Substance Abuse: The Nation's Number One Health Problem. Key Indicators for Policy* (Princeton, NJ: Robert Wood Johnson Foundation, 1993), 50.

11. National Center for HIV, STD, and TB Prevention, Divisions of HIV/AIDS Prevention, "Drug-Associated HIV Transmission Continues in the United States," Centers for Disease Control and Prevention, March 11, 2002.

12. M. Kleiman, "Neither Prohibition nor Legalization: Grudging Toleration in Drug Control Policy," *Daedalus,* 121, 3 (1992): 53–83.

13. H. Saffer, and F. Chaloupka, "State Drug Control and Illicit Drug Participation," National Bureau of Economic Research, working paper No. w7114, May 1999.

14. W. Bennett, *The Index of Leading Cultural Indicators* (Washington, DC: The Heritage Foundation, 1993).

15. D. Musto, testimony presented to the U.S. House of Representatives, Select Committee on Narcotics Abuse and Control, September 29, 1988.

16. Princeton Survey Research Associates.

17. R. Smart, "Does Alcohol Advertising Affect Overall Consumption? A Review of Empirical Studies," *Journal of Studies on Alcohol,* 49, 4 (1988): 413–423.

18. C. Atkin, "Effects of Televised Alcohol Messages on Teenage Drinking Patterns," *Journal of Adolescent Health Care,* 11, 1 (1990): 10–24; L. Wallack, D. Cassady, and J. Grube, *TV Beer Commercials and Children: Exposure, Attention, Beliefs, and Expectations About Drinking as an Adult* (Washington, DC: AAA Foundation for Traffic Safety, 1990); H. Saffer, *Alcohol Advertising Bans and Alcohol Abuse: An International Perspective* (Cambridge, MA: National Bureau of Economic Research, July 1989); J. Grube and L. Wallack, "Television Beer Advertising and Drinking Knowledge, Beliefs, and Intentions Among School Children," *American Journal of Public Health,* 84, 2 (1994): 254–259; J. Pierce, L. Lee, and E. Gilpin, "Smoking Initiation by Adolescent Girls, 1944 Through 1988: An Association with Targeted Advertising," *Journal*

of the American Medical Association, 271, 8 (February 23, 1994): 608–611.

19. B. Neuborne, testimony presented to the United States Senate, Committee on Commerce, Science, and Transportation, May 13, 1993.

20. Office of the Inspector General, *Youth and Alcohol: A National Survey* (Washington, DC: DHHS, June 1991).

21. L. Kaskutas and T. Greenfield, "First Effects of Warning Labels on Alcoholic Beverage Containers," *Drug and Alcohol Dependence,* 31 (1992): 1–14; R. Smart, "Health Warning Labels for Alcoholic Beverages in Canada," *Canadian Journal of Public Health,* 81, 4 (1990): 280–283; D. Polowchena, "Right to Know," in *Controversies in the Addiction Field: Volume One,* R. C. Engs, ed. (Dubuque, IA: Kendall/Hunt, 1990).

22. R. Engs, "Do Warning Labels on Alcoholic Beverages Deter Alcohol Abuse?" *Journal of School Health,* 59, 3 (1989): 116–118; P. Richardson et al., *Review of the Research Literature on the Effects of Health Warning Labels: A Report to the United States Congress* (Washington, DC: DHHS, June 1987); D. Pittman, "Health Warning Labels on Alcoholic Beverages," in *Controversies in the Addiction Field: Volume One*; D. Scammon, R. Mayer, and K. Smith, "Alcohol Warnings: How Do You Know When You Have Had One Too Many?" *Journal of Public Policy and Marketing,* 10, 1 (1991): 214–228.

23. T. MacKenzie, C. Bartecchi, and R. Schrier, "The Human Costs of Tobacco Use," *New England Journal of Medicine,* 330, 14 (April 7, 1994): 975–980.

24. S. Shiffrin, testimony presented to the United States Senate, Committee on Commerce, Science, and Transportation, May 13, 1993.

25. Center for Science in the Public Interest, "BATF Cites Warning Label Problems," *Booze News,* 6, 1 (Winter 1994): 3.

26. P. Cook, "The Economics of Alcohol Consumption and Abuse," in *Alcoholism and Related Problems: Issues for the American Public,* L. West, ed. (Englewood Cliffs, NJ: Prentice-Hall, 1984), 56–77; U.S. Department of Health and Human Services, *Reducing the Health Consequences of Smoking: 25 Years of Progress. A Report of the Surgeon General,* DHHS Publication No. (CDC) 89-8411 (Washington, DC: Government Printing Office, 1989); J. Harris, "The 1983 Increase in the Federal Cigarette Excise Tax," in *Tax Policy and the Economy,* Vol. 1, L. Summers, ed. (Cambridge, MA: Massachusetts Institute of Technology Press, 1987), 87–111.

27. M. Moore and D. Gerstein, eds., *Alcohol and Public Policy: Beyond the Shadow of Prohibition* (Washington, DC: National Academy Press, 1981).

28. U.S. General Accounting Office, *Teenage Smoking: Higher Excise Tax Should Significantly Reduce the Number of Smokers* (Washington, DC: General Accounting Office, June 1989); J. Townsend, "Cigarette Tax, Economic Welfare and Social Class Patterns of Smoking," *Applied Economics,* 19 (1987): 355–365.

29. Goldstein and Kalant, "Drug Policy."

30. Institute for Health Policy, *Substance Abuse,* 54.

31. Campaign for Tobacco-Free Kids, "State Cigarette Excise Tax Rates and Rankings," fact sheet, September 19, 2002.

32. U.S. Bureau of Labor Statistics, Consumer Price Index.

33. Associated Press, "Some in Congress Support Cutting Alcohol Tax," August 27, 2002.

34. M. Grossman et al., "Alcohol and Cigarette Taxes," *Journal of Economic Perspectives,* 7, 2 (Fall 1993): 211–222; W. Manning et al., "The Taxes of Sin: Do Smokers and Drinkers Pay Their Own Way?" *Journal of the American Medical Association,* 261 (1989): 1604–1609.

35. Centers for Disease Control and Prevention, "Reducing Tobacco Use: A Report of the Surgeon General [Executive Summary]," *Morbidity and Mortality Weekly Reports,* 49, RR16 (December 22, 2000): 1–27.

36. D. Sweanor, "Tobacco Taxes: How to Raise Billions of Dollars While Saving Millions of Lives," *Prevention File* (Summer 1993): 13–15.

37. Centers for Disease Control and Prevention, National Center for HIV, STD, and TB Prevention, Division of HIV/AIDS Prevention, September 27, 2002.

38. AIDS Action, "Needle Exchange Facts," *Policy Facts,* June 2001.

39. Centers for Disease Control and Prevention.

40. AIDS Action. "Needle Exchange Facts."

41. J. Watters et al., "Syringe and Needle Exchange as HIV/AIDS Prevention for Injection Drug Users," *Journal of the American Medical Association,* 271, 2 (January 12, 1994): 115–120.

42. Institute for Health Policy Studies, *The Public Health Impact of Needle Exchange Programs in the United States and Abroad: Summary, Conclusions, and Recommendations* (San Francisco: University of California and Berkeley: School of Public Health, University of California, September 1993).

43. Watters, "Syringe and Needle Exchange"; Institute for Health Policy Studies, *The Public Health Impact of Needle Exchange Programs*; J. Guydish et al., "Evaluating Needle Exchange: Are There Negative Effects?" *AIDS,* 7 (1993): 871–876.

44. AIDS Action, "Needle Exchange Facts."

Criteria for the Development or Selection of Drug Prevention Curricula

Curriculum Information Sheet

Title: _____

Ordering Information: _____

Telephone: _____

Contact Person: _____

Cost: _____

Materials: _____

Teacher Edition: _____

Student Edition: _____

Workbooks: _____

Videos: _____

Consumables: _____

Training: _____

   (Initial): _____

   (Subsequent): _____

   (Location): _____

Consulting: _____

Assessment Costs: _____

Time Needed to Implement: _____

   Training of Teachers: _____

   The Curriculum: _____

Curriculum Assessment Instrument

The most important part of the curriculum is its content. Using the checklist provided below, evaluate each criterion using a numerical value up to and including the possible total points designated in the parenthesis preceding each criterion. If you do not assign at least 1 point to the first two criteria, do not proceed.

General (15 Points)
_____ (2)   Contains a clearly stated no-use philosophy.
_____ (2)   Supports a total abstinence approach to alcohol, tobacco, and other drugs for school-age children.
_____ (3)   Demonstrates respect for the laws and values of society.
_____ (3)   Promotes healthy, safe, and responsible attitudes and behavior both in and out of the school environment.
_____ (4)   Includes strategies to involve parents, family members, and the community in the effort to prevent the use of tobacco, alcohol, and other drugs.
_____ (1)   Contains differential programming for targeted or diverse populations.

Drug Information (30 Points)
_____ (9)   Stresses the unhealthy and harmful effects of tobacco, alcohol, and other drugs.
_____ (9)   Contains alcohol, tobacco, and other drug-specific factual and accurate information.
_____ (7)   Contains appropriate intervention and resource information, such as referral sources within the school and the community.
_____ (5)   Contains appropriate information concerning legal consequences to self and others.

Personal/Social Responsibility (25 Points)
_____ (6)   Demonstrates that each individual is unique and valued and has an important role in society.
_____ (6)   Focuses on the social consequences of drug use and the effect drug use has on self-esteem.
_____ (7)   Disarms the sense of personal invulnerability.
_____ (6)   Builds in awareness and resistance to influences (family, peer, community, and media) that encourage alcohol and other drug use.

Skill Building (35 Points)
Contains skill-building exercises in the following areas:
_____ (6)   Self-concept/self-empowerment
_____ (6)   Healthy relationships
_____ (7)   Communication and refusal
_____ (5)   Team building/group dynamics
_____ (6)   Decision making/critical thinking
_____ (5)   Personal responsibility

Organization (15 Points)
_____ (3)   Contains learning objectives which are well defined, behavioral, and measurable, and includes both long-term and short-term outcomes as identified by the district.
_____ (2)   Includes both cognitive and affective objectives.
_____ (2)   Is grade and age appropriate.
_____ (3)   Is capable of being integrated into and/or reinforced in a variety of subject areas.
_____ (5)   Promotes a comprehensive approach to health education.

Instructional Strategies and Methodologies

Research findings show that a variety of instructional methods to accommodate different learning styles provides a more effective curriculum. Using the checklist provided below, determine the types of instructional methods used in the curriculum that match specified objectives. (25 Points)

The program includes a variety of instructional methods:
_____ (2)   Simulation exercises
_____ (1)   Socratic instruction (questioning)
_____ (1)   Student-centered learning
_____ (2)   Applied learning activities
_____ (2)   Small-group discussion
_____ (1)   Opportunities to learn and practice skills related to the objectives of the program
_____ (2)   Sample tests or other assessment methods
_____ (1)   Uses "healthy" peers as role models— not recovering alcoholics or addicts
The program includes activities that focus on developing:
_____ (2)   Decision-making skills
_____ (2)   Refusal skills
_____ (2)   Critical thinking skills
_____ (2)   Goal-setting skills
_____ (2)   Self-responsible behavior
_____ (2)   Self-esteem/self-empowerment

Curriculum Materials

Curriculum materials are an important element in the overall effectiveness of the curriculum. The following is a list of basic criteria which should be met. (10 Points)

The curriculum materials should be:

_____ (2) Current (published or revised within the last four years)
_____ (1) Grade appropriate
_____ (1) Relevant to the program objective
_____ (1) Free from culture, ethnic, and sex bias
_____ (1) Teacher friendly
_____ (1) Durable and safe (no jagged edges or loose parts)
_____ (1) Capable of being easily updated
_____ (1) Referenced
_____ (1) Transportable

Commitment to Time

The amount of time that a school district can devote to drug prevention is limited; therefore, time is an important element. (10 Points)

Does the curriculum package include:

_____ (3) Sufficient time for the objectives to be met?
_____ (2) Time frames for implementation which fit the scheduling needs of the district?
_____ (3) Time frames and conditions for teacher training?
_____ (2) Time frames and conditions for teacher re-training?

Community-Specific Criteria

Identifying and matching district-specific criteria with the curriculum allows for a greater likelihood of success. This list is not comprehensive; it is a starting point for the curriculum assessment team. There are undoubtedly many other factors that can and should be identified. Use the blank space provided below to include any additional criteria that have been identified as needs in your community. (25 Points)

_____ (3) Does the curriculum include materials that are relevant to ethnic groups represented in the district?
_____ (3) Does the cost of the curriculum fit within the funds available?
_____ (1) Does the program provide for annual content assessment?
_____ (2) Does the program match the time frame available for development and implementation?
_____ (3) Is there availability of trainer and/or technical assistance to implement the program?
_____ (3) Is there availability of trainer and/or technical assistance to update the program?

_____ (2) Does the curriculum respond to the drug(s) of choice identified in the district?
_____ (1) Has the curriculum been evaluated on a readability scale and is it grade appropriate?
_____ (3) Does the curriculum have a parental involvement component?
_____ (2) Does the curriculum address the identification and utilization of community resources?
_____ (2) Does the curriculum provide an avenue for student involvement which encourages bonding with the community through service?

Additional community-specific criteria:

Assessment

Validation of curricula that deal with drug education/prevention is becoming the most demanding area in drug education. The U.S. Department of Education, along with many other organizations, is requiring that programs be evaluated for effectiveness in preventing and/or reducing drug use in the community. The following is a list of criteria that should be made available to the consumer prior to the purchase of any curriculum. Even though the curriculum may be accompanied by evaluating data, it is best to have an independent resource examine and verify the information. If your organization does not have an in-house resource, your state department of education, a university, or a college may be of assistance in locating an expert in your area to help with this component. Check assessment components present in the curriculum. (10 Points)

_____ (2) The program was thoroughly evaluated for both validity and reliability prior to dissemination.
_____ (1) The assessment was clearly linked to program objectives.
_____ (3) The assessment shows evidence of changes in attitudes, behaviors, and beliefs toward drug use.
_____ (1) The assessment shows evidence of reduction of drug use.
_____ (1) The program provides for an ongoing assessment by program implementors.
_____ (1) The program provides an analysis model for the implementers to follow.
_____ (1) The statistical method used to evaluate the studies was appropriate.

Grade-Specific Criteria: Prekindergarten Through Second Grade

The most important part of the curriculum is its content. Using the checklist provided below, evaluate each criteria using a numerical value up to and including the possible total points designated in the parentheses preceding each criterion. These will be weighted and added on the summary sheet at the end of this instrument.

General (5 Points)
_____ (3) Meets district-specific objectives.
_____ (2) Contains clearly stated no-use philosophy and supports a total abstinence approach to alcohol, tobacco, and other drugs.

Drug Information (15 Points)
_____ (1) Includes definition of drugs and teaches children to distinguish between foods, poisons, medicines, and drugs.
_____ (1) Provides age-appropriate information on alcohol, tobacco, and other drugs.
_____ (1) Provides information that medicines can be misused and harmful.
_____ (1) Stresses the avoidance of unknown and possibly poisonous and dangerous objects.
_____ (2) Emphasizes the importance of having good health habits—nutrition, hygiene, sleep, and exercise.
_____ (1) Helps child to identify "safe," responsible adults both in and out of school.
_____ (2) Discusses the dangers of harmful substances.
_____ (2) Discusses issue that a child is not responsible for another person's use of alcohol and other drugs.
_____ (2) Addresses how a problem with drugs affects everyone in the family.

Personal/Social Responsibility (15 Points)
_____ (3) Stresses that every individual is unique and valuable.
_____ (1) Emphasizes that the child is an important member of the family.
_____ (3) Stresses that the individual is responsible for his/her well-being and that the parent and the child share this responsibility.
_____ (1) Teaches concepts of sharing and relationship building.
_____ (1) Facilitates understanding of how one person's action affects others.
_____ (1) Demonstrates ways to protect children from strangers.

_____ (2) Builds assertiveness skills to assist children in saying "no" to things they have been taught are wrong.
_____ (1) Teaches children responsibility to tell appropriate adults about strangers, episodes, and problems.

Skill Building (15 Points)
_____ (4) Self-esteem
_____ (4) Developing healthy relationships
_____ (3) Assertiveness skills/peer refusal
_____ (4) Decision making/critical thinking

Grade-Specific Criteria: Third Through Fifth Grade

The content of the curriculum and its learning objectives should focus on the developmental issues that children face during this period. Although family is still an important influence, peers take on a greater role and exert a significant influence. Often risk-taking behaviors such as experimentation with tobacco, alcohol, and other drugs may begin during this developmental period.

Using the checklist provided below, evaluate each criterion using a numerical value up to and including the possible total points designated in the parentheses preceding each criterion.

General (5 Points)
_____ (2) Meets district-specific objectives.
_____ (1) Contains a clearly stated no-use philosophy and supports an abstinence approach to tobacco, alcohol, marijuana, crack, and other drugs.
_____ (1) Includes strategies to involve parents, family members, and the community in the effort to prevent the use of tobacco, alcohol, and other drugs.
_____ (1) Promotes healthy, safe, and responsible attitudes and behavior both in and out of the school environment.

Drug Information (15 Points)
_____ (2) Contains alcohol, tobacco, marijuana, and other drug-specific factual information.
_____ (2) Stresses the unhealthy and harmful effects of drugs.
_____ (1) Demonstrates ways to identify specific drugs (e.g., alcohol, tobacco, crack, inhalants, wine coolers, and other drugs).
_____ (3) Educates why various drugs should not be used and the consequences of their use.
_____ (2) Stresses the fact that alcohol, tobacco, and other drugs are illegal, either for minors

or all persons, and that they are against state law and/or school policy.

_____ (1) Teaches specifically that tobacco, alcohol, and other drugs are illegal for minors to possess, use, and/or distribute.

_____ (2) Promotes healthy, safe, and responsible attitudes and behavior.

_____ (2) Helps students to identify persons and institutions who can assist them in time of trouble.

Skill Building (15 Points)
_____ (3) Self-esteem/self-concept
_____ (3) Healthy relationship building
_____ (3) Assertiveness/refusal
_____ (3) Decision making/critical thinking
_____ (3) Cooperative team processes

Personal/Social Responsibility (15 Points)
_____ (3) Stresses the importance of obeying laws and the consequences of breaking them, especially those governing onset of legal use of alcohol.

_____ (2) Supports and emphasizes the value of positive role models.

_____ (3) Teaches students how to recognize and respond to social influences, such as peer pressure, advertising, and other environmental messages, that promote drug use.

_____ (2) Educates about the concept of addiction, what it is, and how it affects others, including family members.

_____ (2) Teaches the importance of getting help for someone (family, friends, self) who has a drug problem.

_____ (2) Demonstrates and teaches good citizenship practices.

_____ (1) Stresses the need for maintaining good health practices and the consequences of bad habits.

Grade-Specific Criteria: Sixth Through Eighth Grade

The content of the prevention curriculum and its learning objectives should address the developmental issues facing children who are in this age range. Their rapid physical development often leaves them feeling uncomfortable, unattractive, and uncoordinated. These factors, coupled with the changes that are occurring cognitively and socially, often place the child in situations that are conducive to risk-taking and experimenting behaviors.

Using the checklist provided below, evaluate each criterion using a numerical value up to and including the possible total points designated in the parentheses preceding each criterion. These numbers will be transferred to the last page of this instrument in the grade-specific category.

General (5 Points)
_____ (3) Meets district-specific objectives.
_____ (2) Contains a clearly stated no-use philosophy and supports an abstinence approach to alcohol (including wine coolers), tobacco, marijuana, and other drugs.

Drug Information (15 Points)
_____ (2) Includes knowledge of the characteristics and chemical nature of specific drugs and drug interactions, including, but not limited to, alcohol, marijuana, tobacco, cocaine, crack, and other drugs.

_____ (2) Describes the physiology of drug effects on the circulatory, respiratory, nervous, reproductive, and immune systems.

_____ (2) Creates an awareness of the stages of drug addiction and the lack of predictability from one person to another.

_____ (2) Discusses how heredity and other factors impact a person's susceptibility to addiction.

_____ (1) Incorporates an awareness of the short-term and long-term effects of drugs on appearance and physical, mental, and social functioning.

_____ (1) Creates an understanding of how using drugs affects activities requiring motor coordination, such as operating vehicles or playing sports.

_____ (1) Examines the issues of the drug problem faced by society, the tactics society has adopted to fight the problem, and the responsibilities individual citizens have in overcoming this problem on the local level.

_____ (1) Identifies the relationship between drug use and HIV and acquired immuno-deficiency syndrome (AIDS).

_____ (1) Includes knowledge of local, state, and federal laws and policies regarding drug use, including school policy.

_____ (1) Identifies local resources that assist the community in eliminating drug problems.

Personal/Social Responsibility (15 Points)
_____ (3) Fosters a developing sense of self-worth and appreciation of the positive aspects of growing up.

_____ (3) Encourages youth to think and behave as valued members of school, family, and community.

_____ (3) Fosters drug-free living.

_____ (3) Encourages youth to become involved in school and community-related activities such as sports, service clubs, and other activities that promote drug-free lifestyles.

_____ (3) Develops awareness and resistance to messages that promote drug use, especially music, peers, and media.

Skill Building (15 Points)

_____ (3) Self-esteem/self-concept

_____ (3) Assertiveness/peer resistance

_____ (3) Decision making/critical thinking

_____ (3) Healthy relationships

_____ (3) Personal responsibility

_____ (1) Healthy alternatives

Grade-Specific Criteria: Ninth Through Twelfth Grade

The focus of the prevention curriculum at this age level should encompass the idea that these youth quickly are becoming adult citizens. They are primarily concerned with individual identity, financial independence, deepening relationships, independence from family, and self-rule.

Using the checklist provided below, evaluate each criterion using a numerical value up to and including the possible total points designated in the parentheses preceding each criterion. At the conclusion of this section, transfer the numbers to the summary page.

General (5 Points)

_____ (3) Meets district-specific objectives.

_____ (2) Contains a clearly stated no-use philosophy and supports a total abstinence approach to alcohol, tobacco, and other drugs.

Drug Information (15 Points)

_____ (3) Incorporates an understanding of both the long-term and short-term physical, mental, and social effects of drugs.

_____ (3) Explores the relationship of drug use to related diseases and disabilities, including HIV/AIDS, learning disorders, handicapping conditions, birth defects, and heart, lung, and liver diseases.

_____ (3) Demonstrates an understanding of how alcohol, tobacco, and other drugs can affect the mother and fetus before, during, and after pregnancy (including lactation).

_____ (2) Provides information regarding legal, social, and economic consequences of drug use, both for self and others.

_____ (2) Discusses international, economic, political, and social implications of drug use (including tobacco).

_____ (2) Provides information on role expectations as consumers, role models, and partners in relationships.

Personal/Social Responsibility (15 Points)

_____ (15) Focuses on the fact that students are maturing young adults and that, as such, they have a responsibility to be drug-free, well-educated, healthy, productive citizens.

Skill Building (15 Points)

_____ (3) Self-concept

_____ (2) Peer leadership

_____ (3) Communication/assertiveness

_____ (2) Healthy relationships

_____ (2) Decision making/critical thinking

_____ (2) Personal responsibility

_____ (1) Healthy alternatives

Curriculum Assessment Summary

To use the assessment instrument to assess the curriculum you are examining quantitatively, use this page to add the points assigned to each section and divide the total by 250 (possible points). If you did not evaluate the curriculum using one of the grade-specific components, divide the total points by 200 instead of 250. The resulting score will give you a percentage to use in comparing one curriculum with another.

Content

General (15) _____

Drug Information (30) _____

Personal/Social Responsibility (25) _____

Skill Building (35) _____

Organization (15) _____

• Instructional Strategies (25) _____

• Curriculum Materials (10) _____

• Commitment to Time (10) _____

• Community-Specific (25) _____

• Assessment (10) _____

• Grade-Specific (50) _____

• Total_____

• Divide Total by 250 (or 200) _____

Source: U.S. Department of Health and Human Services. Prevention Plus III, 1991.

Selected Evaluation Instruments

Alcohol, Tobacco, and Other Drugs: Knowledge, Attitudes, and Behavior

We are interested in what you know about alcohol, tobacco, and other drugs and how you feel about using ATOD. Your answers to these questions will be kept confidential.

Please circle the number or fill out the blank space that most closely corresponds to your answer. You are to circle one number only for each item or question asked.

Thank you for your participation.

I. Knowledge About the Effects of Alcohol, Tobacco, and Other Drugs

1. How much do you think people risk harming themselves physically, mentally, or in other ways if they:

	No Risk	Little Risk	Some Risk	Great Risk	Can't Say
a. Smoke one or more packs of cigarettes every day	1	2	3	4	5
b. Chew smokeless tobacco every day	1	2	3	4	5
c. Take four or five drinks of an alcoholic beverage (beer, wine, liquor) every day	1	2	3	4	5
d. Use marijuana regularly	1	2	3	4	5
e. Use heroin regularly	1	2	3	4	5
f. Use cocaine regularly	1	2	3	4	5
g. Use other drugs (uppers, downers, LSD) regularly	1	2	3	4	5

II. Attitude Toward Alcohol, Tobacco, and Other Drugs

2. How do you feel about people 18 or older who do each of the following?

	Strongly Disapprove	Disapprove	No Opinion	Approve	Strongly Approve
a. Smoke one or more packs of cigarettes every day	1	2	3	4	5
b. Chew smokeless tobacco every day	1	2	3	4	5
c. Take four or five drinks of an alcoholic beverage (beer, wine, liquor) every day	1	2	3	4	5
d. Use marijuana regularly	1	2	3	4	5
e. Use heroin regularly	1	2	3	4	5
f. Use cocaine regularly	1	2	3	4	5
g. Use other drugs (uppers, downers) regularly	1	2	3	4	5

III. Alcohol, Tobacco, Other Drugs Use
   3. How many times have you tried the following in the *past 30 days*?

	None	Once	Two to Three	Four to Five	More Times
a. Cigarettes	1	2	3	4	5
b. Smokeless tobacco	1	2	3	4	5
c. Beer	1	2	3	4	5
d. Wine	1	2	3	4	5
e. Wine cooler	1	2	3	4	5
f. Liquor	1	2	3	4	5
g. Marijuana	1	2	3	4	5
h. Inhalants	1	2	3	4	5
i. Heroin	1	2	3	4	5
j. Cocaine (coke or crack)	1	2	3	4	5
k. Uppers (amphetamines, crank, ice, speed)	1	2	3	4	5
l. Downers (barbiturates, valium, ludes)	1	2	3	4	5
m. LSD, PCP, acid, mushroom	1	2	3	4	5
n. Steroids	1	2	3	4	5

IV. Background Information
   4. How old are you?
      13 or Younger   14   15   16   17   18 and Older   (Please circle your age on the left.)

   5. What is your sex?
      a. Male
      b. Female

   6. With which ethnic group do you identify yourself?
      a. African American (Non-Hispanic origin)
      b. Asian/Pacific Islander
      c. Hispanic
      d. Native American/Alaskan native
      e. White (Non-Hispanic origin)
      f. Other (please specify) _____

   7. In what type of community are you currently living?
      a. Large city
      b. In a small city or town
      c. In a suburb of a city
      d. In the country, not on a farm
      e. On a reservation
      f. Can't say, mixed

Source: CSR, Incorporated, 1400 Eye St. NW, Washington, DC 20005.

Parental Involvement Survey

Please answer the following questions with respect to your son or daughter. If you have more than one child, answer the questions with respect to the child who is closest to 14 years of age.

1. How many PTA meetings have you attended in the last year? _____
2. How many parent-teacher conferences regarding your child have you attended in the last year? _____
3. List any youth organizations (e.g., Scouts, sports teams, music groups, church groups) you are involved in at least once per week.

    _____
    _____
    _____

4. How often do you know where your child is outside of school hours?
   never   1   2   3   4   5   always
5. How often do you know with whom your child is outside of school hours?
   never   1   2   3   4   5   always

The following questions should be answered with the following scale:

    1 = never   2 = once a year   3 = monthly   4 = weekly   5 = daily

6. How often do you spend time with your child in sports or athletics?
   1   2   3   4   5
7. How often do you and your child go to movies together?
   1   2   3   4   5
8. How often do you and your child go camping, fishing, hunting?
   1   2   3   4   5
9. How often do you and your child go on vacation together?
   1   2   3   4   5
10. How often do you and your child visit relatives?
    1   2   3   4   5
11. How often do you instruct your child in some skill/activity?
    1   2   3   4   5
12. How often do you and your child participate in purchased activities (e.g., concerts, sporting events, going out to dinner) together?
    1   2   3   4   5
13. How often do you and your child talk about day-to-day things?
    1   2   3   4   5
14. How often do you and your child eat together at home?
    1   2   3   4   5
15. How often do you and your child watch TV together or engage in some other spontaneous activities at home?
    1   2   3   4   5

Source: Southeast Regional Center for Drug-Free Schools and Communities, Atlanta, GA, 1989.

Parents' Attitudes About Teen Substance Use

Read each of these statements and indicate on a scale
of 1 to 5 how much you agree or disagree with each statement.

	Strongly Agree	Agree	Don't Agree or Disagree	Disagree	Strongly Disagree
1. It's okay for teens to smoke cigarettes if they have their parents' permission.	1	2	3	4	5
2. It's my job as a parent to keep my teen from picking up the smoking habit.	1	2	3	4	5
3. Whether or not a parent smokes cigarettes doesn't affect a teen's decision to smoke.	1	2	3	4	5
4. If my teenager began smoking, it would have a very serious negative effect on his/her health.	1	2	3	4	5
5. I would be really upset if I found out my teenager smoked cigarettes.	1	2	3	4	5
6. I would do everything possible to stop my son/daughter from smoking.	1	2	3	4	5
7. Most teenagers smoke cigarettes, so my son/daughter's smoking doesn't really bother me.	1	2	3	4	5
8. As a parent, there is little or nothing I can do to keep my teen from smoking cigarettes.	1	2	3	4	5
9. It should be illegal to sell cigarettes to teens.	1	2	3	4	5
10. It's all right for a teen to smoke cigarettes occasionally as long as they don't pick up the habit.	1	2	3	4	5
11. It is okay for teens to drink alcohol if they have their parents' permission.	1	2	3	4	5
12. It is my job as a parent to keep my teenager from using alcohol.	1	2	3	4	5
13. Whether or not a parent drinks alcohol doesn't influence a teenager's decision to use alcohol.	1	2	3	4	5
14. If my teenager began to use alcohol, it would have a serious negative effect on his/her health or adjustment.	1	2	3	4	5
15. I would be very upset if I found out that my teenager drank alcohol.	1	2	3	4	5
16. I would do everything possible to keep my son/daughter from using alcohol.	1	2	3	4	5
17. Most teenagers drink alcohol, so my son/daughter's drinking doesn't really worry me.	1	2	3	4	5
18. As a parent, there is little or nothing I can do to keep my teenager from drinking alcohol.	1	2	3	4	5
19. Adults who allow teens to drink at parties in their homes should be arrested.	1	2	3	4	5

	Strongly Agree	Agree	Don't Agree or Disagree	Disagree	Strongly Disagree
20. It is okay for teenagers to have one or two drinks as long as they don't get drunk.	1	2	3	4	5
21. It's okay for teens to smoke marijuana if they have their parents' permission.	1	2	3	4	5
22. It's my job as a parent to keep my teenager from using marijuana.	1	2	3	4	5
23. Whether or not a parent smokes marijuana doesn't affect a teen's decision to smoke.	1	2	3	4	5
24. If my teen began to use marijuana, it would have a very serious negative effect on him/her.	1	2	3	4	5
25. I would be very upset if I found out that my teenager used marijuana.	1	2	3	4	5
26. I would do everything possible to keep my son/daughter from using marijuana.	1	2	3	4	5

Scoring: The items form 6 subscales: (1) rejection of alcohol use, items 11(r), 12, 14, 15, 16, 17(r), 19, 20(r); (2) rejection of marijuana use, items 21(r), 22, 24, 25, 26, 27(r), 29, 30(r); (3) rejection of tobacco use, items 2, 4, 5, 6, 9, 8(r); (4) parental sense of helplessness, items 8, 18, 28; (5) parental modeling effects, items 3, 13, 23; (6) parental permission, items 1, 7, 10.

Items with an (r) should be weighted in the reverse of scoring (response of 5 should be added as a 1, response of 4 should be added as a 2, etc.).

Source: J. A. Linney, S. G. Forman, and M. C. Egan, *Assessment of Parental Attitudes Toward Substance Use*, Project SCOPE Technical Report 6, University of South Carolina, Columbia, SC 29208, 1990.

Parenting Skills Inventory

1. You expect different things from a child than from an adult.	True	False
2. Ignoring a behavior, say, a tantrum, will only make it worse next time.	True	False
3. The best way of gaining your child's attention when he is watching TV is to shout over it.	True	False
4. A 1-year-old child should be able to stop crying when the parent says to stop.	True	False
5. A behavior that is followed by praise or a smile is likely to occur more in the future.	True	False
6. One reason why your child may not do what you say is because there are other things going on at the same time as you are talking.	True	False
7. Children usually go through a stage where they try to show they are independent.	True	False
8. A good idea for parents is to leave well enough alone—that is, to attend more to the misbehaving child and less to the well-behaved child.	True	False
9. One of the first things to do when you want to get your child's attention is to make sure you have eye contact.	True	False
10. There is something wrong with a child who won't cooperate with what his/her parents tell him/her to do.	True	False
11. When a problem behavior continues even though it is punished, we should make the punishment last longer.	True	False
12. Children often tell parents what they are feeling by the way they sit or stand.	True	False

13. A 2-year-old child should be able to take care of him/herself (e.g., feeding, dressing).	True	False
14. To change a child's behavior, we first need to know why the child acts in a particular way.	True	False
15. Children have the same feelings as their parents, they just express them differently.	True	False
16. Babies like to put everything in their mouth because that is one way of learning about the world.	True	False
17. How frequently we reward a child should depend on his/her attention span.	True	False
18. Telling an angry child that you sense he's angry will only make it worse.	True	False
19. The only punishment that some children understand is spanking.	True	False
20. An adult's attention is one thing most children will work hard for.	True	False
21. The best parents never let their children know they are angry at them.	True	False
22. A 1-year-old child should be able to tell right from wrong.	True	False
23. Negative attention—scolding, warnings, being yelled at—are rewarding for a child if this is how they get attention.	True	False
24. It's not a good idea for parents to share their feelings with their children.	True	False
25. As children grow older, they think in different ways.	True	False
26. The best punishment is withholding reward.	True	False
27. Talking to a young child in "baby talk" is the best way to communicate with him/her.	True	False
28. Children who are toilet trained early will be smarter and better behaved when they get older.	True	False
29. Telling your child exactly what you expect from him is better than telling him to be "good."	True	False
30. Young children only listen to a loud voice.	True	False

Answer Key:

1—T	6—T	11—F	16—T	21—F	26—T
2—F	7—T	12—T	17—F	22—F	27—F
3—F	8—T	13—F	18—F	23—T	28—F
4—F	9—T	14—F	19—F	24—F	29—T
5—T	10—F	15—T	20—T	25—T	30—F

Source: C. F. Hereford, *Changing Parental Attitudes Through Group Discussion* (Austin, TX: University of Texas Press, 1963).

Parental Awareness Survey

Please answer the following questions with respect to the average response within your child's school. If you have more than one child, answer the questions with respect to the child who is closest to 14 years of age.

1. At what age do students who smoke cigarettes start smoking?
   a. Under 10
   b. 10–11
   c. 12–13
   d. 14–15
   e. 16–17
   f. 18–19
   g. Over 20

2. At what age do students who drink alcohol start drinking?
   a. Under 10
   b. 10–11
   c. 12–13
   d. 14–15
   e. 16–17
   f. 18–19
   g. Over 20

3. At what age do students smoke marijuana?
   a. Under 10
   b. 10–11
   c. 12–13
   d. 14–15
   e. 16–17
   f. 18–19
   g. Over 20
4. How often do students smoke marijuana?
   a. Once a year
   b. Six times a year
   c. Once a month
   d. Twice a month
   e. Once a week
   f. Three times a week
   g. Every day
5. How often do students use cocaine?
   a. Once a year
   b. Six times a year
   c. Once a month
   d. Twice a month
   e. Once a week
   f. Three times a week
   g. Every day
6. Where do students usually drink alcohol?
   a. Home
   b. School
   c. In a car
   d. Friend's home
   e. Other
7. Where do students usually smoke marijuana?
   a. Home
   b. School
   c. In a car
   d. Friend's home
   e. Other
8. Where do students usually use inhalants?
   a. Home
   b. School
   c. In a car
   d. Friend's home
   e. Other
9. When do students usually smoke cigarettes?
   a. Before school
   b. During school

c. After school
   d. Weeknights
   e. Weekends
10. When do students usually drink wine coolers?
   a. Before school
   b. During school
   c. After school
   d. Weeknights
   e. Weekends
11. Do students feel beer is harmful to their health?
   a. No
   b. Sometimes
   c. Very much
   d. Don't know
12. Do students feel marijuana is harmful to their health?
   a. No
   b. Sometimes
   c. Very much
   d. Don't know
13. Do students feel cocaine is harmful to their health?
   a. No
   b. Sometimes
   c. Very much
   d. Don't know
14. How easy is it for students to get marijuana?
   a. Cannot get
   b. Fairly difficult
   c. Fairly easy
   d. Very easy
   e. Don't know
15. How easy is it for students to get cocaine?
   a. Cannot get
   b. Fairly difficult
   c. Fairly easy
   d. Very easy
   e. Don't know

Responses on this inventory would be compared to incidence and prevalence rates from a local drug use survey. The closer the estimates from this inventory are to those of the drug use survey, the more accurately aware citizens and parents are of actual substance use.

Source: Southeast Regional Center for Drug-Free Schools and Communities, Atlanta, GA, 1989.

Evaluation Instrument for Drug and Alcohol Prevention Video Programs

Video Title: _____ Year of Copyright _____

Grade Level(s): _____ Total Program Length: _____ Price: Buy $ _____ Rent $ _____

Number of Segments: _____ Available for free-loan?   Yes   No

1. Quick Check for Minimum Requirements
   If you answer "no" to *any* quick-check item, do *not* recommend the video,
   and skip Part 2 of this evaluation.

Content Requirements

    a. The video clearly advocates no use of drugs and/or alcohol by students.   Yes   No

    b. The video includes current, accurate information about health,   Yes   No
         legal, and/or social consequences of drug and/or alcohol use.

Practical Requirements

    c. Video and audio quality meets your standards for classroom materials.   Yes   No

    d. The video—or its segments—is the right length for classroom use.   Yes   No

    e. The video's purchase or rental price is acceptable, or it can be free-loaned   Yes   No

    Meets all minimum requirements?   Yes   No
   If you answered Questions a–e "Yes," the video meets minimum requirements.

2. Quality Check
   If the video passed the Quick Check, rate it for the following on a 1–4 scale:
   1 = Poor   2 = Fair   3 = Good   4 = Excellent

Developmental and Cultural Appropriateness

    a. The video communicates in age-appropriate ways for the intended grades.   1   2   3   4

    b. The video's prevention messages are believable and relevant for your students.   1   2   3   4

    c. The video is culturally appropriate for your students.   1   2   3   4

    d. The video avoids negative racial, ethnic, religious, and gender stereotypes.   1   2   3   4

Potential for Affecting Students' Skills, Attitudes, and Behaviors

    e. The video avoids glamorizing drugs or being a primer on how to use drugs.   1   2   3   4

    f. The video models effective drug prevention skills such as peer resistance.   1   2   3   4

    g. The video models effective ways to seek appropriate peer or adult help.   1   2   3   4

    h. The video models positive, drug-free lifestyles for students.   1   2   3   4

    i. The video reinforces or supplements your current prevention curriculum.   1   2   3   4

    j. The video or printed guide includes effective teacher orientation materials and   1   2   3   4
         guidelines for beneficial follow-up activities.

Add scores for items a–j. If total is 30 or higher, the video is in the "good" to "excellent" range.

Other factors influencing decision to recommend or reject this video:

_____

_____

Evaluation Conclusions: _____ Video Is Recommended _____ or

Video Is Not Recommended _____

Evaluated by: _____ Date: _____

Attitude Scales

1. Drugs are basically an "unnatural" way to enjoy life.
   a. Strongly agree
   b. Agree
   c. Have no opinion
   d. Disagree
   e. Strongly disagree

2. I see nothing wrong with taking an LSD trip.
   a. Strongly agree
   b. Agree
   c. Have no opinion
   d. Disagree
   e. Strongly disagree

3. I'd have to be pretty sick before I'd take any drug, including aspirin.
   a. Strongly agree
   b. Agree
   c. Have no opinion
   d. Disagree
   e. Strongly disagree

4. Teachers ought to encourage their students to experiment with drugs.
   a. Strongly agree
   b. Agree
   c. Have no opinion
   d. Disagree
   e. Strongly disagree

5. Pep pills are a stupid way of keeping alert when there's important work to be done.
   a. Strongly agree
   b. Agree
   c. Have no opinion
   d. Disagree
   e. Strongly disagree

6. I wish I could get hold of some pills to calm me down whenever I get "uptight."
   a. Strongly agree
   b. Agree
   c. Have no opinion
   d. Disagree
   e. Strongly disagree

7. Students should be told about the harmful side effects of certain drugs.
   a. Strongly agree
   b. Agree
   c. Have no opinion
   d. Disagree
   e. Strongly disagree

8. All drugs should be made licit and freely available.
   a. Strongly agree
   b. Agree
   c. Have no opinion
   d. Disagree
   e. Strongly disagree

9. Even if my best friend gave me some hash, I probably wouldn't use it.
   a. Strongly agree
   b. Agree
   c. Have no opinion
   d. Disagree
   e. Strongly disagree

10. In spite of what the establishment says, the drug scene is really "where it's at."
    a. Strongly agree
    b. Agree
    c. Have no opinion
    d. Disagree
    e. Strongly disagree

11. As a general rule of thumb, most drugs are dangerous and should be used only with medical authorization.
    a. Strongly agree
    b. Agree
    c. Have no opinion
    d. Disagree
    e. Strongly disagree

12. I admire people who like to get stoned.
    a. Strongly agree
    b. Agree
    c. Have no opinion
    d. Disagree
    e. Strongly disagree
13. Taking any kind of dope is a pretty dumb idea.
    a. Strongly agree
    b. Agree
    c. Have no opinion
    d. Disagree
    e. Strongly disagree

14. I would welcome the opportunity to get high on drugs.
    a. Strongly agree
    b. Agree
    c. Have no opinion
    d. Disagree
    e. Strongly disagree

Attitude scale scoring: Odd numbered items are scored as follows: a = 5, b = 4, c = 3, d = 2, and e = 1. Even-numbered items are scored as follows: a = 1, b = 2, c = 3, d = 4, e = 5, and can range from 14 to 70. Higher scores represent antidrug, conservative attitudes; lower scores represent more liberal, pro-drug attitudes.

Source: *Accountability in Drug Education: A Model for Evaluation*, L. A. Abrams, E. F. Garfield, and J.D. Swisher, eds. (Washington, DC: Drug Abuse Council, Inc., 1973).

Self-Esteem

How would you describe yourself on the following characteristics? For each one, put a check in the column that fits you best.

	Very Much Like Me	Pretty Much Like Me	Not Much Like Me	Not Like Me
1. Confident				
2. Unreliable				
3. Happy				
4. Easy going				
5. Moody				
6. Friendly				
7. Easily angered				
8. Makes friends easily				
9. Gets along with teachers				
10. Responsible				
11. Intelligent				
12. Lazy				
13. Forgetful				
14. Attractive				
15. Punctual				
16. Generous				
17. Helpful				
18. Uncooperative				
19. Shy				
20. Open minded				
21. A leader				

Score this self-esteem measure by assigning a 4 to the most positive descriptive category, a 3 to the next most positive, a 2 to the next, and a 1 to the least positive. For example, on the characteristic "confident," if the student checked "Very Much Like Me," she would get a 4; if she checked "Not Much Like Me," she would get a 2. Add the scores for each item to get a total score for self-esteem.

Source: Adolescent Diversion Project, Department of Psychology, Michigan State University.

Alternative Activities Survey

1. How often are you bored outside of school?
   Never   Seldom   Sometimes   Often   Always

2. When you are with your friends, how often does it seem like there is nothing to do besides hang out?
   Never   Seldom   Sometimes   Often   Always

3. What activities are you aware of in your community for you to have fun, including those you do not participate in (e.g., sports clubs, music groups, church groups)? List them:

   _____

   _____

   _____

   _____

4. Put a check by any of the above activities that your have participated in within the past six months.

5. What activities would you like to have available that are not available?

   _____

   _____

   _____

6. What new activities have you started in the last year?

   _____

   _____

   _____

7. What makes an activity fun to you?

   _____

   _____

   _____

Source: Southeast Center for Drug-Free Schools and Communities, Atlanta, GA.

School Drug Policies

Examples of School Drug Policies

The following material is extracted from the school policy of a public school district. School policy deals with a wide array of issues, and not all rules and procedures that deal with ATOD use are found in the same place. Therefore, the narrative that follows is somewhat disjointed, as it has lost the integrity and flow of the original document. Nevertheless, it does exemplify language that may be included in a school's policy to address ATOD use and abuse.

Alcoholic Beverages and Controlled Substances Possession

It is the belief of the _____ County Schools that the use of illicit drugs and the unlawful possession and use of alcohol is wrong and harmful.

1. No pupil shall possess, use, sell, or transfer alcoholic beverages, narcotics, drugs, controlled substances, counterfeit controlled substances, look-alikes, and/or possess drug paraphernalia on or about school property or in school motor vehicles or in private motor vehicles located on or about school property or at any location of a school-sponsored activity or enroute to or from a school-sponsored activity. (This will include sporting events, dances, conferences, conventions, club-sponsored activities, bus trips, but not excluding any other school activity).
2. As used in this section
   a. Alcoholic beverage means distilled spirits, malt beverages, wine, and wine coolers.
   b. Controlled substance means any drug substance or immediate precursor that is listed in Schedules I through V which are contained in Chapter 318 of the State Revised Statutes and any other substance which the State Department

of Human Resources may add to said schedules by regulation pursuant to the authority granted in SRS 218A.020.

Simulated Controlled Substance Possession

1. No pupil shall sell, possess, or transfer any substance with the representation or upon the creation of an impression that the substance which is sold or transferred is a controlled substance. No pupil shall possess for sale or transfer any substance designed in any manner to simulate a controlled substance.

Tobacco and Smoking

1. No student shall possess or use (smoking, chewing, or dipping) cigarettes, cigars, pipes, or any tobacco products in any form in or about school buildings, school grounds, school buses, and premises of the district during school hours. In addition, no student shall possess matches or a cigarette lighter in or about school buildings, school grounds, school buses, and premises of the district during school hours.

Violations of the above policy shall result in the following actions by school administrators:

- First Offense: One day in the school's Alternate Learning Center (CAP program, ABC room, etc.).
- Second Offense: Three days in the school's Alternate Learning Center.
- Third Offense: Five days in the school's Alternate Learning Center.
- Any offense beyond the level described above will result in an immediate out-of-school suspension.

For Possession, Use, or Being Under the Influence

1. For possession, use, or being under the influence of alcoholic beverages, narcotics, drugs, controlled

substances, counterfeit controlled, or look-alikes and/or possession of drug paraphernalia the student will receive an immediate five-day suspension and the superintendent may recommend expulsion. A recommendation for expulsion may be waived if the student and his/her parent(s) or guardian(s) agree to the following:

a. To obtain, at their own expense, an evaluation of the student's alcohol/drug use from a qualified chemical dependency counselor acceptable to the school district.

b. To complete any and all counseling or other treatment recommended in the evaluation.

Failure to complete both the evaluation and treatment as recommended by the chemical dependency counselor shall result in the principal making a recommendation for an alternate school placement or requesting the superintendent to recommend expulsion depending upon the severity of the circumstances. Appropriate juvenile and police authorities will be immediately notified when violation of laws governing use, possession, sale or transfer of alcoholic beverages, narcotics, drugs, controlled substances, look-alikes, or counterfeit controlled substances has occurred. A second violation of the above policy at any time during the student's enrollment in any county school will result in an immediate suspension and a recommendation for expulsion will be made.

For Sale or Transmission

1. For sale or transmission of alcoholic beverages, narcotics, drugs, controlled substances, counterfeit controlled substances, or look-alikes, the student will immediately be suspended, and a recommendation for expulsion will be made.

Student Dress and Appearance—ATOD Related

Patches, emblems, and clothing depicting offensive messages, vulgarity, or advertising alcoholic beverages or illegal substances shall not be permitted.

Enforcement

Principals shall enforce the dress code in their schools.

Violations

This dress code is adopted in the interest of developing and maintaining a student body which is well groomed and neat and avoiding disruption of the education process. When violations of these policies occur the principal or his/her representative will inform the student of the violation and instruct him/her in the correction of the discrepancy. If the student then fails to follow the established policy, disciplinary action may result.

Policy Violation Student Due Process

1. Due Process—The following due process is to be followed in connection with the suspension or expulsion of a pupil from school.

   a. The pupil is to be given oral or written notice of the charges against him/her which constitute cause for suspension;

   b. The pupil is to be given an explanation of the evidence of the charge or charges;

   c. The pupil is to be given an opportunity to present his/her version of the facts relating to the charge or charges.

These due process procedures shall precede any suspension unless immediate suspension is essential to protect persons or property or to avoid disruption of the ongoing academic process. In such cases, the due process procedures outlined above shall follow the suspension as soon as practicable, but no later than three (3) school days after the suspension.

2. Student is to receive another copy of the drug and alcohol policy.

3. Student will receive a mandatory suspension for five (5) days and the superintendent may recommend expulsion to the Board of Education. A suspended student shall not be permitted to make up class activities, assignments, and examinations missed during the period of suspension. A suspended student shall not be permitted to participate in any school functions during the period of suspension.

4. Alternative to possible expulsion for first offense:

   a. Superintendent will not recommend expulsion if the student and parent(s) agree to seek, at their expense, an evaluation of the student's alcohol/drug use from a qualified chemical dependency counselor acceptable to the school district.

   b. The student completes any and all treatment and counseling as recommended in the evaluation.

   c. If no treatment as such is recommended in the evaluation, the school may also require that the student either agree to meet with a school counselor or member of the core team or the student assistance coordinator a designated number of times or complete a designated alcohol/drug educational program (for example: Insight Drug/Alcohol Support Group) in order to qualify for the waiver of the recommendation of expulsion. Failure to complete both the evaluation and treatment as recommended by the chemical dependency counselor may result in either an alternate placement or a recommendation by the superintendent to the Board of Education that the student be expelled.

5. If parents have been present during the due process conference, they should be given a copy of the "Notification of Suspension" form and the district's alcohol and other drug policy. If they have not been present, they should be notified of the suspension by phone and in writing. Include with the letter to parents a copy of the policy and notification requesting that the parent(s) meet with the school principal within five days.

6. In cases which involve students with disabilities, the procedures mandated by federal and state law shall be followed.

Criminal Violations

Students are accountable to their school in their role as students as well as to the law in their capacity as citizens. The criminal laws of the State and of the federal government apply to the conduct of all persons on school property. Violations shall be dealt with according to these laws and local school board policy. When criminal violations occur, persons committing these acts may be immediately turned over to the appropriate law enforcement officials.

Misconduct which constitutes a criminal act may result in the immediate removal of said person or student from the school and its environs, pending a hearing before the Board of Education.

Prior to the admission of a student to any school, if a student has been adjudicated guilty of the offenses of homicide, assault, or an offense relating to weapons, alcohol, or drugs, or has been expelled from school for homicide, assault, or an offense in violation of state law or school regulations relating to weapons, alcohol, or drugs, the parent, guardian or other person or agency responsible for the student shall provide to the school a sworn statement or affirmation that the student has been expelled from school attendance at a public or private school in the state or another state for the offenses set forth herein above.

When any student who has been expelled from a school in the state for homicide, assault, or an offense in violation of state law or school regulations relating to weapons, alcohol, or drugs requests a transfer of the student's records to a new school, the records shall not be transferred until the proceeding has been terminated and the records shall reflect the charges and any final disposition of the expulsion proceedings.

A person who is an administrator, teacher, or other employee of the school is required promptly to make a report to the local police department, sheriff, or State Police by telephone or otherwise if:

1. The person knows or has reasonable cause to believe that conduct has occurred which constitutes:
   a. a misdemeanor or violation offense under the laws of the State and relates to carrying, possession, or use of a deadly weapon or use, possession, or sale of controlled substances; or
   b. any felony offense under the laws of the State; and
   c. the conduct occurred on the school premises or within one thousand (1,000) feet of the school premises, on a school bus, or at a school sponsored or sanctioned event.

A person making the report in good faith shall be immune from any civil or criminal liability that might otherwise be incurred or imposed as a result of making the report and participating in any judicial proceeding that resulted from the report.

Search and Seizure

Lockers are property of the school and are subject to the Board's regulation and supervision. Locker inspection or searches are not carried out as a harassment technique, but as a duty when the health, safety, or welfare of students is involved.

In a search and seizure situation, the following procedures shall be followed:

1. A student's person will only be searched when there is reasonable suspicion that the student is in possession of evidence relating to an illegal act or violation of policies of the County Board of Education or the individual school.

2. Illegal items (drugs, firearms, etc.) or other possessions reasonably determined by the proper school authorities to be a threat to the student's safety, security, or others' safety and security may be seized by school officials.

3. Items which may be used to disrupt or interfere with the educational process may be temporarily removed from the student's possession by a staff member. These items may be returned to the student by that staff member or through the office.

4. A general inspection of school properties such as lockers, desks, etc., may be conducted on a regular basis. During these inspections, items which are school property may be collected. (Example: overdue library books.)

5. All items which have been seized will be turned over to proper authorities or returned to the true owner, depending on the situation.

6. The student will have the opportunity to be present when a search of personal possessions is to be conducted unless:
   a. the student is absent from school, or
   b. school authorities decide that the student's presence could endanger his or her health

Examples of Policy Violations and Action Taken

These are provided as general guidelines. Individual circumstances may require different actions.

Example #1   A student was caught in possession of a roach clip. It was obvious from the discoloration of the tip that it had been used to smoke marijuana. Student has a high absentee rate and is failing most subjects.

Action: Student was suspended from school for five days. Parent and student agreed to seek an evaluation and follow the recommendation.

Example #2   Two students admitted to being in possession of an alcoholic beverage on school property. Upon investigation by the school administration, several witnesses verified seeing the beverage in the locker. Apparently Student A brought the beverage to give to Student B. Student B then took the beverage home and drank it.

Action: No substance was ever found by the school administration. The only evidence provided was the admission of the students to being in possession of the substance. The two students were suspended for five days pending an evaluation. Students returned to school and were assigned to educational counseling with the school counselor on a regular basis.

Example #3   A student who was visibly ill went to the school principal and admitted to taking an unknown prescription pain medication from another student. Student A gave the medication to Student B for a headache.

Action: The school administration obtained some of the medication from Student A and contacted a pharmacist. Upon identification of the substance by the pharmacist, Student B's parents were contacted and asked to take Student B home. Both stu-

dents were sternly warned about taking another person's prescription medication.

Example #4   A student is caught in possession of a "non-alcoholic" malt beverage. The beverage looks and smells like beer. The beverage contains 1/2 of 1 percent alcohol. According to the State Beverage Control Board, this is a legal substance for minors.

Action: Student was suspended for violating County Board of Education's policy.

Guidelines for Intervention for Being in Possession of or Under the Influence of Alcohol or Other Drugs

Meeting With Parent(s) and Student When a Policy Violation Has Occurred

1. The purpose of meeting with student and parent(s) is to discuss possible evaluation, treatment, and counseling for alcohol/drug use (not to discuss guilt or innocence).
2. Explain specific violation. (For example: You were caught with _____ in your possession (or) you were caught under the influence of _____. This is a direct violation of school board policy.)
3. Student is given mandatory five (5) day suspension. This is immediately reported to the superintendent who may recommend expulsion of the student to the Board of Education.
4. Discussion of possible alternatives for first offense (orally explain all alternatives).
   a. Parents must agree to seek, at their expense, an evaluation of the student's alcohol/drug use from a qualified chemical dependency counselor acceptable to the school district. A list will be provided.
   b. Parents are responsible for student completing any and ALL treatment, at their expense, as recommended in the evaluation.
   c. If no treatment as such is recommended in the evaluation, the school may also require that the student either agree to meet with a school counselor, member of the core team, or the student assistance coordinator a designated number of times or complete a designated alcohol/drug educational program (for example: Insight Drug/Alcohol Support Group) in order to qualify for the waiver of the recommendation of expulsion. Failure to complete both the evaluation and treatment as recommended by the chemical dependency counselor may result in either an alternate placement or a

recommendation by the superintendent to the Board of Education that the student be expelled.

5. Parent(s) decide between evaluation and possible expulsion.

6. Parent(s) select a treatment/evaluation agency from the list provided by the principal.

7. Parent(s) sign a written agreement and consent for release of information form. They must initiate and make an appointment within two working days and notify the person with whom they had the conference.

8. Remind parent(s) that a second offense of policy will result in immediate suspension and that superintendent may recommend student for expulsion. Alternative of seeking evaluation from chemical dependency counselor will not be available.

9. Contact student assistance coordinator if he or she has not been involved in conference with parents and give details of the intervention.

Conducting a Student Intervention When a Policy Violation Has Not Occurred

The SAP counselor, in consultation with the members of the core team, will normally conclude that a formal intervention strategy is needed based on the following considerations:

1. There are general behavioral indicators of a problem (i.e., grades, attendance, conduct) from several sources (staff, parents, screening interviews, support group participation);

2. There is evidence of alcohol and/or other drug abuse;

3. It seems possible that chemical dependency or chronic drug abuse is at the root of a student's behavior problems or complicates attempts to correct them;

4. The student has been unwilling or unable to change his behavior utilizing other strategies and resources;

5. It is unlikely that the student and/or family will accept referral to professional help without the motivational power of a formal intervention;

6. It is unlikely that the student and/or family will follow through with professional recommendations (e.g., for chemical dependency treatment) without the motivational power of a formal intervention.

In arranging the intervention meeting the SAP counselor/coordinator should exercise care to select appropriate participants who are properly trained in intervention skills and who have been properly prepared

for this specific meeting. This Referral Team is typically composed of key members of the core team as well as others who have significant information about the student or who have an important relationship with him. In preparing for the referral or intervention meeting, the SAP counselor/coordinator should take into account a number of criteria for participants:

1. Who are the most meaningful and/or influential persons surrounding and familiar with the student? (e.g., The SAP counselor/coordinator, the building administrator, concerned teachers, a coach or advisor, other students, family members, community agency representatives, police, clergyman, etc.)

2. Does everyone have personal, firsthand experience of the student's behavior and/or alcohol/drug use?

3. Can everyone assemble in your office to prepare for the personal intervention meeting?

4. Do all the members of the Referral Team understand enough about the nature of alcohol and other drug abuse or dependency, and the student's history, to accept the need for personal intervention?

5. Do the participants understand the intervention process and their proper roles within it?

6. Are the participants emotionally adequate to the intervention? Can they participate with care and concern and without judgment or blame?

7. Who will be the moderator, or leader of the intervention session: The SAP counselor/coordinator, building administrator, agency ATOD counselor, etc.?

8. Is there a need for training or consultation from an ATOD agency counselor in preparing for and conducting the personal intervention?

The preparation process may take several days. When members of the Referral Team have been identified, the staff member(s) in charge of preparing for the personal intervention should assure that as individuals and as a team they are prepared for the intervention meeting:

1. Are all the participants generally prepared for the session? Do they understand the agenda, what will happen?

2. Are participants specifically prepared for the session? Do they have written lists or documentation of behavior, incidents, or patterns which legitimize their concern? Is there sufficient data to make the intervention successful?

3. Have various alternatives for referral been considered by the members of the intervention Referral Team? Will everyone agree to support the same referral goal?

4. Have the pertinent Referral Team members considered and decided upon appropriate consequences for the student's and/or family's failure to accept referral and improve in the areas of concern?
5. Have the Referral Team members anticipated the student's and/or family's defensive responses and discussed ways of responding to them appropriately?
6. Is there a moderator for the session? Is he or she aware of his or her role in:
   a. introducing the meeting; stating why everyone is here and how they got together;
   b. establishing ground rules;
   c. keeping the meeting on track;
   d. closing the meeting by summarizing the group's concern and offering the referral recommendations agreed upon by the Referral Team in advance?
7. Have members of the Referral Team decided upon an order of presentation of their information?
8. Does anyone need to be added to or eliminated from the Referral Team?

Code of Ethics for Prevention Professionals

The following code of ethics was developed by the Illinois Alcohol and Other Drug Abuse Professional Certification Association (IAODAPCA). Although it was specifically developed for drug abuse prevention specialists in that state, the principles are generic in nature and are applicable throughout the United States, Canada, and many other countries.

Section 1: Ethical Responsibilities to the Public and Profession

Principle 1.1
Certified ATODA [alcohol, tobacco, and other drug abuse] Preventionists shall strive at all times to maintain the highest of standards in the services they offer.

Responsibility 1.1.1
The maintenance of high standards of competency is a responsibility shared by all Certified ATODA Preventionists.

Responsibility 1.1.2
In circumstances where Certified ATODA Preventionists or Counselors violate ethical standards, it is the obligation of Certified ATODA Preventionists who have first hand knowledge of unethical activities to attempt to rectify the situation and report all ethical violations to IAODAPCA.

Principle 1.2
Certified ATODA Preventionists respect their professional status and standing.

Responsibility 1.2.1
Certified ATODA Preventionists will not misrepresent their professional qualifications and affiliations.

Responsibility 1.2.2
Certified ATODA Preventionists will not aid or abet a person not duly certified as an ATODA Preventionist or Counselor in representing himself/herself as a Certified ATODA Preventionist or Counselor or at a certification classification which is not true.

Principle 1.3
Certified ATODA Preventionists have an obligation to see that ATODA prevention services are provided by qualified, competent persons. Constructive efforts to ensure delivery of competent ATODA prevention services, such as preventionist certification, deserve support.

Responsibility 1.3.1
Certified ATODA Preventionists are required to submit accurate and honest information to IAODAPCA for the purpose of obtaining, maintaining, and recommending someone for certification.

Principle 1.4
In representing alcohol, tobacco, and other drug abuse prevention services, Certified ATODA Preventionists concern themselves with accuracy, fairness, and the dignity of the profession.

Responsibility 1.4.1
In promotional and marketing activities for ATODA prevention services, Certified ATODA Preventionists shall respect the dignity and confidentiality of the communities, organizations, groups, and individuals they serve.

Section 2: Ethical Responsibilities of Certified ATODA Preventionists in Personal Use of Alcohol, Tobacco, and Other Mind-Altering Chemicals

Principle 2.1
Certified ATODA Preventionists engaged in the delivery of alcohol and other drug abuse prevention services shall show respect and regard for the laws and norms of the communities in which they work. They recognize

that violations of legal standards will damage their own reputation and the ATODA prevention profession.

Responsibility 2.1.1
Certified ATODA Preventionists shall not abuse alcohol.

Responsibility 2.1.2
Certified ATODA Preventionists shall not abuse legal drugs.

Responsibility 2.1.3
In some circumstances, Certified ATODA Preventionists may use physician prescribed, mind-altering drugs for necessary and appropriate medical reasons. In such circumstances, Certified ATODA Preventionists should weigh their ability to perform in the delivery of ATODA prevention services.

Responsibility 2.1.4
Certified ATODA Preventionists shall not possess or use any illegal drugs under any circumstances.

Responsibility 2.1.5
Certified ATODA Preventionists shall not furnish communities, organizations, groups, and individuals to whom they provide ATODA prevention services with alcohol or other mind-altering chemicals.

Section 3: Ethical Responsibilities of Certified ATODA Preventionists in Professional Relationships

Principle 3.1
Certified ATODA Preventionists shall establish and maintain professional relationships characterized by respect and mutual support.

Responsibility 3.1.1
Certified ATODA Preventionists shall establish and maintain professional relationships for purposes of networking, mentoring, professional support, etc.

Responsibility 3.1.2
Certified ATODA Preventionists shall respect the confidences shared by other colleagues/professionals.

Responsibility 3.1.3
Certified ATODA Preventionists shall not knowingly solicit the clients of other colleagues/professionals.

Responsibility 3.1.4
Certified ATODA Preventionists shall not knowingly withhold information from colleagues/professionals that would enhance their professional effectiveness.

Responsibility 3.1.5
Certified ATODA Preventionists shall not knowingly accept for a client any communities, organizations, groups, and individuals who are receiving similar prevention services from another professional except by agreement with that professional or after the termination of services by that professional.

Responsibility 3.1.6
When working in a prevention team or with other professionals, Certified ATODA Preventionists will not abdicate their responsibility to protect and promote the welfare and best interests of those they serve.

Responsibility 3.1.7
When working in a prevention team, Certified ATODA Preventionists will work to support, not damage or subvert, the decisions made by the team.

Principle 3.2
When making recommendation for positions, advancements, certification, etc., Certified ATODA Preventionists shall consider the welfare of the public and the profession above the needs of the individual concerned.

Responsibility 3.2.1
Certified ATODA Preventionists shall not use another professional as a reference without first obtaining that person's permission.

Responsibility 3.2.2
Certified ATODA Preventionists shall not lead a person to believe that he/she will receive a favorable recommendation when, in fact, such a recommendation will not be given.

Section 4: Ethical Responsibilities of Certified ATODA Preventionists in Employer/Employee Relationships

Principle 4.1
Certified ATODA Preventionists shall establish and maintain an employer/employee relationship characterized by professionalism and respect for the agency's rules of operation.

Section 5: Ethical Responsibilities of Certified ATODA Preventionists to the Communities, Organizations, Groups, and Individuals They Serve

Principle 5.1
The welfare and dignity of those to whom prevention services are provided are to be protected and valued above all else.

Responsibility 5.1.1
Certified ATODA Preventionists shall not physically abuse those they serve.

Responsibility 5.1.2
Certified ATODA Preventionists shall not verbally abuse those they serve.

Responsibility 5.1.3
Certified ATODA Preventionists shall not sexually exploit those they serve. Certified ATODA Preventionists shall not engage in sexual relationships with those they serve.

Responsibility 5.1.4
Certified ATODA Preventionists shall not financially exploit those they serve.

Principle 5.2
In the delivery of alcohol, tobacco, and other drug abuse prevention services, Certified ATODA Preventionists shall establish and maintain relationships with those they serve characterized by professionalism, respect, and objectivity.

Responsibility 5.2.1
Certified ATODA Preventionists shall not discriminate against those they serve in any way (e.g., on the basis of ethnicity, race, religious belief, disability, sex, sexual orientation, etc.).

Responsibility 5.2.2
Certified ATODA Preventionists shall ensure that services are offered in a respectful manner in an appropriate environment.

Responsibility 5.2.3
Certified ATODA Preventionists shall not charge or collect a private fee or other form of payment for prevention services provided to a community, organization, group, or individual who is charged for those same services through the preventionist agency.

Responsibility 5.2.4
Certified ATODA Preventionists shall avoid continuing to provide prevention services for personal gain or satisfaction beyond the point where it is clear that the community, organization, group, or individual is not benefiting from the services.

Responsibility 5.2.5
Certified ATODA Preventionists shall not give or receive a commission, rebate, or any other form of payment for referral services.

Principle 5.3
The Certified ATODA Preventionist's most critical responsibility is to provide competent professional ATODA prevention services.

Responsibility 5.3.1
Certified ATODA Preventionists shall not offer prevention services outside the boundaries of the ATODA profession unless otherwise educated and trained, licensed or, certified.

Responsibility 5.3.2
Certified ATODA Preventionists shall not offer any services outside their range of competency.

Principle 5.4
Certified ATODA Preventionists shall preserve, protect, and respect the rights of those they serve to confidentiality.

Responsibility 5.4.1
Certified ATODA Preventionists shall comply with the federal and state laws, rules, and regulations pertaining to confidentiality.

Responsibility 5.4.2
Certified ATODA Preventionists shall guard professional confidences and shall reveal such confidences only in compliance with the law or only when there is a clear and imminent danger to an individual or society.

Principle 5.5
Certified ATODA Preventionists shall strive to obtain the best professional services to meet the needs of those they serve.

Responsibility 5.5.1
Certified ATODA Preventionists are responsible for obtaining adequate and appropriate professional services to meet the individual needs of the communities, organizations, groups, and individuals they serve.

Section 6: Ethical Responsibilities of Certified ATODA Preventionists to Family Members and Significant Others

Principle 6.1
Certified ATODA Preventionists accept and understand that alcohol and other drug abuse and dependency affect the family members and significant others of the person abusing or dependent upon alcohol and/or other drugs. Therefore, Certified ATODA Preventionists demonstrate concern and respect for the welfare of the families/significant others of the person abusing or dependent upon alcohol and/or other drugs.

Responsibility 6.1.1
Certified ATODA Preventionists shall at all times adhere to all applicable federal, state, and local laws, regulations, and rules pertaining to the reporting of child abuse and/or neglect, and will promptly notify the proper authorities when they suspect that child neglect or abuse has occurred.

Section 7: Ethical Responsibilities of Certified ATODA Preventionists Engaged in Research

Principle 7.1
In the conduct of research, Certified ATODA Preventionists should adhere to the highest standards and follow appropriate scientific procedures.

Section 8: Ethical Responsibilities of Certified ATODA Preventionists in Teaching

Principle 8.1
When Certified ATODA Preventionists accept the responsibility of teaching ATODA prevention or of supervising/mentoring ATODA preventionists, they should discharge these responsibilities with the same high regard for standards required of all other professional activities.

Principle 8.2
Certified ATODA Preventionists will always cite their sources when engaged in the presentation of information whether in teaching or in the delivery of prevention services.

Section 9: Ethical Responsibilities of Certified ATODA Preventionists as Authors/Editors

Principle 9.1
As authors or editors, Certified ATODA Preventionists shall adhere to high standards, abiding by the traditions established in the academic arena.

Responsibility 9.1.1
Certified ATODA Preventionists will always, through byline credit or other means, cite the actual author or source of any materials researched or used in their articles, books, or other writings.

Source: Illinois Alcohol and Other Drug Abuse Professional Certification Association, Inc.

Abstinence syndrome Synonymous with *withdrawal symptoms*.

Acupuncture A component of traditional Chinese medicine that has been exported to the West. Needles are inserted into specific body locations to induce anesthesia or healing. It is remarkably effective in the Orient, but has shown limited value in Western society.

Addiction Continual and repetitive use of a drug in spite of medical, psychological, or social harm. Addiction may be physical dependence, which includes tolerance and withdrawal, but may also be psychological dependence, which occurs when the drug's properties reinforce certain behaviors and emotions. The word is sometimes applied to other compulsive behavior, such as overeating or gambling.

Administrative agency A governmental body charged with administering and implementing particular legislation.

Affective learning Intellectual processes that involve emotions, feelings, attitudes, beliefs, and values.

Aftercare All of the activities, programs, and services that follow formal treatment. Its main purposes are to discourage relapse and reorient the user to unimpaired living and normal social behavior.

Agent A portion of the public health model that refers to the immediate source of damage. In a generic sense, the agent may be a germ, a weapon, or a hazardous chemical. Alcohol, tobacco, and other drugs are considered agents.

Alcoholism Addiction to alcohol, usually accompanied by excessive alcohol consumption, greatly increased tolerance, and significant medical, personal, and social problems.

Analgesic A drug that relieves pain, usually without diminishing consciousness. Prescription analgesics often are based on the opiate family of drugs (e.g., morphine). Many nonopiate over-the-counter analgesics (e.g., Tylenol) are also available.

Analysis of variance (ANOVA) A statistical tool used to determine the odds that the difference between two or more means is not due to chance. It also compares the intragroup variation with the intergroup variation.

Angina pectoris Chest pain caused by inadequate circulation through the blood vessels that course through the heart muscle. Angina may be mild or very severe and is a sign that heart attack is very likely in the future. For many people with angina, pain occurs with physical exertion or emotional stress.

Antecedent Something that promotes, stimulates, or cues consumption of alcohol, tobacco, or other drugs. For example, stress is often an antecedent of smoking.

Antihistamines Drugs that counteract the inflammation that is a natural response to infectious microorganisms or substances to which we are allergic. Inflammation causes pain, swelling, heat, and redness. In the nose, it may cause congestion or running of mucous secretions. Antihistamines may cause drowsiness.

Antihypertensives Drugs that lower elevated blood pressure, usually by eliminating excess fluid in the circulatory system or diminishing muscle tension in artery walls.

Assertiveness The free expression of one's desires, needs, values, and beliefs from a place of genuineness.

Assessment A formal interview in which a person's behavior, including drug consumption, is systematically explored. Also included are inquiries about family relationships and problems at school, work, and home. Assessment should be documented with a standardized form.

Atherosclerosis A principal underlying mechanism of coronary disease that leads to heart attacks. It is characterized by a narrowing and stiffening of the blood vessels, increasing blood pressure, and a predisposition to clot formation and blockage of blood flow.

Behavioral objective A statement of intermediate-term intention, in measurable terms, that targets actions, such as smoking or drunk driving.

Behavioral signs External indications of a drug problem. Examples include declining performance, unexplained absences, continuous episodes of illness, and frequent interpersonal conflict.

Best practices Science-based strategies, activities, or approaches that effectively delay or prevent ATOD use.

Biological equivalence Drugs made by different companies that have the same ingredients may still have different effects because of differing manufacturing processes or different quality standards. The FDA allows some deviation from the stated dosage; for example, a 250-mg tablet may have slightly more or slightly less than 250 milligrams. One company's version may be consistently over the target dosage, whereas another company's version may be consistently under it.

Bipolar depression An emotional disorder characterized by severe mood swings ranging from extreme energy and hyperactivity (mania) to extreme lethargy and hopelessness (depression). Once commonly called *manic depression*.

Blood alcohol level (BAL) The concentration of alcohol circulating in the bloodstream. It is measured by the number of milligrams of alcohol in 100 milligrams of blood. Alcohol effects begin to occur at around 0.04%, while death may occur at a level of 0.4%.

Brand name The commercial name given to a drug by the company that owns the patent and by which it is known to consumers and providers. A drug eventually can have several brand names but only one generic name.

Carbon monoxide A chemical by-product of combustion. It is found in high concentration in tobacco smoke. When it enters the blood, it becomes bonded to the hemoglobin molecule, blocking the ability of red blood cells to carry oxygen.

Central nervous system Refers primarily to the brain and spinal cord.

Character education A program that addresses the complex nature of the decision-making process, the weighing of values and beliefs to make value-laden decisions.

Chemical name The original name assigned by chemists to describe the molecular structure of a drug.

Chemotherapy Any medical treatment that uses drugs can be called chemotherapy. The word is associated most with cancer treatment, but all use of medications is chemotherapy.

Chi-square test A statistical tool used to determine the extent to which the observed frequencies of some variable or value are different from what is expected. It does not test significance but suggests associations and relationships between variables.

Classical conditioning Associates an unconditioned stimulus with a conditioned stimulus so that with enough experience, the conditioned stimulus by itself causes the same response as the unconditioned stimulus. Ivan Pavlov used classical conditioning to get dogs to salivate at the sound of a bell.

Codependency A loosely defined word that applies to individuals in an addict's life. When these individuals behave in ways that are emotionally or socially disabling to themselves, they may be codependent. The line between codependency and appropriate caring and concern for the problems of loved ones is poorly defined.

Coercive strategy A strategy to compel compliance or constrain obedience.

Cognitive learning Intellectual processes that involve knowledge, comprehension, application, analysis, synthesis, and evaluation.

Cohort effect When people who were born at about the same time, such as during a given year or a particular decade, share various characteristics as a group (e.g., conservatism, credit card purchasing, home ownership, cigarette smoking). For example, the per capita consumption of alcohol has declined, partly because the cohort of people over 50 years of age, who tend to drink less, has proportionately increased.

Collaboration Linking the efforts of several organizations or agencies to promote community health.

Community A geographic area or a collection of people (a population) who have a common cause or set of beliefs and values.

Community health promotion Efforts that target the educational, social, and environmental actions conducive to the health of a population.

Comprehensive health education A documented, planned, and sequential program of health instruction for students in grades preschool through 12.

Conflict resolution A process that is used to resolve conflict through discussion, problem solving, negotiation, and compromise, with the intention of avoiding anger and violence. It is taught in schools, but it also may be used in many other settings.

Congenital malformations Birth defects ranging from superficial and cosmetic abnormalities to disabling or life-threatening problems. Malformations may be due to genetic inheritance, chromosomal defects, or prenatal exposure to microorganisms or toxic substances.

Cooperative learning An interactive teaching method in which groups of three to five students accomplish a particular task.

Coordinated school health program The collaborative effort between schools and communities that includes health education, healthful school environment, physical education, nutrition services, counseling and psychological services, health promotion for faculty and staff, health services, and parent/community involvement.

Cross-tolerance Tolerance for one drug transferred to a similar drug. For example, having developed tolerance to heroin, a person will also have tolerance for methadone, even if the latter drug has never been used before.

Decriminalization Reducing or eliminating the criminal penalties for possession of small amounts of illegal drugs, thereby targeting the force of the criminal justice system on traffickers rather than users.

Denial A defense mechanism in which a user is not able to admit that he or she has an alcohol or other drug problem. Denial manifests itself in these ways: refusing to admit to abnormal behavior, blaming other people, rationalizing mistakes, or trying to prove to others that no problem exists. Significant others, such as family members and coworkers, are also vulnerable to denial, and may cover up or make excuses for the user's drug problem.

Designer drugs Synthetic derivatives of several types of illegal drugs, especially the opiate group (e.g., China White) and mescaline (e.g., Ecstasy), a hallucinogen.

Detoxification The process of eliminating drugs from the tissues and organs of the body. It may be done with the assistance of medical support or unaided by any treatment. Detoxification is usually accompanied by withdrawal symptoms.

Developmental assets Internal and external building blocks of healthy development.

Diuretic A property of many drugs that causes the body to increase urine output. Diuretics often are used to treat high blood pressure or congestive heart failure. However, many drugs will cause diuresis as a side effect.

Dose dependent The magnitude of a drug's effects are directly related to its concentration and dosage.

Drug Any substance that has mind-altering properties or in other ways interacts with and modifies the structure and function of the body.

Drug abuse Chronically consuming a drug in a way that will probably be harmful to health, psychological well-being, or social functioning. Drug abuse usually coincides with addiction, but not always.

Drug education Teaching and communicating to help people avoid harm caused by the abuse of various drugs.

Drug misuse Consuming a drug in a way that is likely to cause harm, but only as an isolated episode, not as a chronic pattern of behavior.

Drug use Consumption of a drug in a way that is beneficial or at least not harmful. Controversy is generated when this term is applied to illegal drugs or to youth and alcohol.

Dual diagnosis The coexistence of a drug addiction and some other diagnosed mental disorder in the same person at the same time.

Ecological model A model that focuses on the interaction of environmental and individual factors for ATOD abuse prevention.

Empirical concept Relying on experience and observation without benefit of scientific methods of study.

Empowerment A social action process that promotes participation of people, organizations, and communities in gaining control over their lives and their community and larger society. With this perspective, empowerment is not characterized as achieving power to dominate others, but rather as power to act with others to effect change.

Endemic The continuous or permanent existence of a health or social problem, as opposed to a sudden outbreak or isolated occurrence.

Endorphins A category of substances (including endorphins, enkephalins, and dynorphins) produced in the brain that mimic the effects of opiate drugs. More correctly, the opiates mimic the endorphins (endogenous morphine). Though not fully understood, endorphins are thought to have natural pain-relieving properties, play a role in the response to stress, and contribute to the effects of acupuncture.

Environment A portion of the public health model that refers to the physical and social surroundings of the individual. Examples are social attitudes and peer pressure concerning drugs, mass media appeals to use alcohol or tobacco, or family influences concerning marijuana use.

Epidemic A sudden and large outbreak of a health or social problem.

Epidemiological study A research method that relies on data gathered from population surveys, medical records, and other kinds of community data and demonstrates relationships between variables. The focus is on using communities as laboratories, looking for patterns of health or social problems as influenced by population variables.

Evaluation A comparison of program elements against some measure of quality or success. Evaluation may assess the way in which prevention activities were done and their impact. It may be done early in the course of prevention programs in order to make ongoing program adjustments, or it may be done at the completion of the program in order to assess the program's effectiveness.

Family therapy Treating a drug addiction in the context of family relationships. It may include resolving or at least recognizing dysfunctional behavior, trying to normalize relationships, encouraging participation of family members in support groups or therapy, and enlisting the cooperation of family members in the addict's rehabilitation.

Fibrocystic breast disease A disorder experienced by half of all women; characterized by breast pain, lumps, or cysts (an enclosed sac or cavity filled with gas, liquid, or solid material). Though sometimes it requires treatment, this disorder is benign and is not a precursor to breast cancer.

Gateway drug A drug that leads to use of another drug. Young people do not select equally from all drugs for their first drug experience, but are more likely to choose inhalants, alcohol, or tobacco. The significance is that preventing or postponing the use of gateway drugs may prevent the use of other drugs such as cocaine, heroin, or LSD.

Generic name The name given to a drug by its developer once the drug is thought to have useful applications and has been patented. This name is the one by which it is known in the scientific community.

Goal A statement of long-term intention, synonymous with *mission* or *purpose*, that is nonmeasurable.

Group dynamics Interactions among members of a small group that trigger communication and learning that might not occur with individuals alone. Although group dynamics can be desirable, relationships within groups and the attitudes and motives of group members can also create barriers to communication, learning, and productivity.

Group guidance A situation in which guidance counselors teach classes on various issues of emotional and social development. Examples of issues include puberty changes, parent-child relationships, dating and sexuality, and interpersonal conflict. These sessions may be designed by the guidance counselor or may be structured around a standardized curriculum.

Habituating A word that can mean the same thing as addiction or that implies frequent use without the objectionable aspects of addiction.

Halfway house A residential facility that provides a supportive transition between a formal in-patient treatment program and independent living. Such facilities usually serve small numbers of clients, require participation in 12-step programs, and expect outside employment or at least work within the halfway house. Clients usually stay only a few months or less.

Hallucination Distorted perceptions or experiences of sound, sight, smell, touch, or taste that are not real, though they seem real to the one hallucinating. Some people can recognize the hallucination as distorted reality; other people cannot.

Harm reduction An approach to alcohol and other drug use prevention that is based on lessening the damage done by drug consumption, not necessarily eliminating drug consumption per se. An example is making clean needles available to IV drug users rather than only trying to get them to quit.

Health A state of complete physical, mental, and social well-being and not merely the absence of disease.

Health Belief Model (HBM) Behavior change model that states that behaviors are chosen on the basis of individual readiness, environmental influences, and individual behaviors and skills.

Health education A continuum of learning that enables people, as individuals and as members of social structures, to voluntarily make decisions, modify behaviors, and change social conditions in ways that are health enhancing.

Health promotion The aggregate of all purposeful activities designed to improve personal and public health through a combination of strategies.

High risk Conditions identified as most likely to increase the probability of a problem (such as alcohol or drug abuse) occurring.

High-risk youth Young people with weak emotional adjustment and deficits in social and environmental supports who are more likely to experience alcohol and other drug problems.

Hormone A chemical messenger that circulates in the bloodstream, delivering instructions to various organs and tissues. Examples include insulin, adrenaline, thyroid, and estrogen.

Host A portion of the public health model that refers to the individual—both his or her biological makeup and his or her emotional and intellectual capacities and traits.

Hypnosis A state of mind, usually induced by a therapist (or hypnotist), in which the subject is abnormally susceptible to the will of the therapist. Hypnosis is used to get patients to mentally return to an earlier time in their life to understand significant events and recall buried memories. In this context, hypnosis is used to effect posthypnotic suggestions, in which suggestions (e.g., do not smoke) made during hypnosis are carried over into the waking state.

Imaging A process that requires a person to imagine a situation or consequence that is desired or, conversely, to be avoided. It instructs a person to focus in great detail to make the imagined experience as real as possible.

It is used in a wide variety of counseling situations. Also known as *guided imagery,* this process can be done by an individual alone or with the assistance of a therapist.

Impairment A loss of the ability to function normally and meet responsibilities. Impairment may occur in a single episode, such as driving under the influence, or may be a chronic problem, such as an inability to complete tasks on the job.

Incidence The new cases or instances of some health or social problem that occur during a designated time period, typically a year. For example, the number of students who drop out of school because of drug-related problems during a given year is a measure of how rapidly a problem is changing or growing.

Indicated prevention Strategies designed to address subpopulations who are already manifesting ATOD initiation or risk factors such as behavioral problems in school.

Information model A common approach to using education for behavior change, based on the assumption that behavior is contingent upon knowledge possessed; that is, when people know the facts about some health problem or harmful behavior, they will make changes and behave in a rational way to avoid harm. The information model has very limited effect.

Instructional objective A statement of immediate intention, in measurable terms, that targets learning outcomes, such as the ability to name, define, explain, describe, illustrate, categorize, or compare.

Interdiction Efforts to block, intercept, or confiscate illegal drugs before they enter the country. Interdiction is done primarily at land borders, at airports, in harbors, and along sea coasts.

Intervention The counterpart of the term *early diagnosis and treatment* that is used in medical care. It includes activities, programs, and systems to identify drug abuse problems at an early stage of development. The hoped-for outcomes are cessation of the drug abuse and minimization of the harmful consequences.

Intramuscular injection Injection directly into a muscle.

Intravenous injection Injection directly into a vein.

Local anesthetic A drug that has a short-term numbing effect on a limited area of tissue, such as gums or skin. Local anesthetics deaden nerves that are sensitive to pain without causing unconsciousness.

Long acting When the effects of a drug become apparent slowly and subside slowly over a period of hours.

Materialistic Relating to the surrounding world with the expectation that everything has an explainable cause

and is governed by consistent laws that are rational and logical.

Metabolite A chemical substance that is a by-product of the body's metabolism and internal physiological processes.

Migraine headache One of the most severe types of headache. Characterized by distorted vision, throbbing pain, and sometimes nausea and prostration.

Modeling An interactive method of learning that occurs through imitation.

Mutual help/self-help group A small gathering of people who have some problem or traumatic experience in common. Meeting and talking to others in a similar circumstance to provide support, encouragement, understanding, fellowship, and unconditional acceptance.

National Institute on Drug Abuse (NIDA) The lead federal agency for drug abuse research.

Nicotine A chemical that is a central nervous system stimulant and is the principal addictive substance in tobacco.

Noncoercive strategy A strategy used in schools and communities that focuses on education and skills building.

Nonregulatory agencies Federal and state agencies that are responsible for dispersing sums of money for programs that promote particular goals.

Nostrum A fraudulent or useless remedy.

Objective A precise, specific action designed to meet the expectations of a goal.

Oncologist A medical doctor who specializes in the treatment of cancer.

Open-ended question A question that cannot be answered with a simple response, such as yes or no, but requires subjective opinion and points of view.

Outcome An action or behavior that results from a lesson or program.

Paradigm A model or way of looking at the world.

Paradigm shift A change in models; in the context of ATOD abuse prevention, viewing and working with communities in a fundamentally different way. For example, instead of proceeding on the assumption that all prevention work must be done by experts, a paradigm shift would allow critical contributions to be made by grassroots coalitions.

Paranoid delusions A type of hallucination characterized by a morbid fear that others are trying to do harm or the belief that one is very important, perhaps historically renowned, but is being denied a rightful position in society (delusions of grandeur).

Patent medicines Liquids, pills, and ointments sold for every imaginable disease or health problem. Patent medicines were formulated with a basis in fancy or fraud rather than modern principles of pharmacology. Typically, ingredients were hidden from consumers, and the medicines were attributed with curative value for a wide variety of disorders, in contrast to the specificity of modern drugs.

Peer resource model A program that uses children and youth to work with or help other children and youth.

Planned Approach to Community Health (PATCH) model A model that uses a bottom-up rather than a top-down approach to community development, with community empowerment as a fundamental component.

Policy The general principles by which governing bodies or organizations are guided.

PRECEDE-PROCEED model Community health promotion planning model that consists of a diagnostic (needs assessment) component and a developmental component.

Premenstrual syndrome (PMS) A disorder that affects 90% of menstruating women. It includes many diverse symptoms, and there is disagreement on whether it is actually a distinct disease or many different problems experienced in conjunction with menstruation. The most common symptoms are nausea, mood swings, appetite loss, crying, fatigue, and irritability. Treatment varies depending on the particular symptoms of each woman.

Prevalence The total number of cases of some health or social problem that exist at a specific point in time. For example, the proportion of students who are regular users of smokeless tobacco at the time a survey is done is a measure of how large a problem is, not how rapidly it is changing.

Prevention A dynamic, assertive process of creating conditions or developing personal attributes and skills to promote the wellness of individuals, families, and communities.

Price sensitive The degree to which purchase and consumption of a consumer good are affected by price. Basic food commodities are less price sensitive than luxury items because people are more compelled to buy food than nonessential items. Both alcohol and tobacco are price sensitive, even for those who are addicted to them.

Primary prevention Efforts directed at a time before a disease or unwanted behavior begins.

Proactive Initiating change prior to the onset of a problem rather than reacting to a problem after it arises.

Prognosis The probable outcome of a disease or health problem. A disease with a poor prognosis is not expected to improve but to get worse.

Program objective A statement of long-term intention, in measurable details, that targets health (accident fatality, lung cancer) or social (employment, graduation) status.

Protective factors Activities, programs, and practices that can alter an individual's opportunities, risks, and expectations.

Psychosis A severe emotional disturbance characterized by hallucinations and delusions, severely disturbed thought and behavior patterns, and an inability to think rationally. Examples include schizophrenia and paranoia.

Psychosocial model A model that emphasizes life skills training and peer refusal techniques.

Psychotherapy Individual or group work with a psychologist or psychiatrist. It emphasizes feelings and emotions and understanding the roots of dysfunctional behavior. Colloquially known as *talk therapy*.

Public health model A model that addresses health or social problems in a comprehensive way. It considers human factors, characteristics of the source of harm, and the environment, identifying causes and suggesting possible ways to intervene.

Quitting skills Behavior techniques and strategies that help a person quit smoking. Examples include avoiding persons and places associated with smoking; getting rid of tobacco products, matches, lighters, and ashtrays; and posting signs around the house and office that remind the smoker to quit.

Rebound anxiety An anxiety reaction a user has after the effects of a depressant drug subside and before return to a normal mood.

Recidivism Repeating a problem behavior after steps have been taken to rectify it. The term may apply to repeat offenders who have been incarcerated for criminal behavior or to those who go through drug treatment programs, relapse, and enter treatment again.

Regulation A rule or order prescribed by an authority to direct actions under its control.

Regulatory agencies Federal and state agencies that have the authority to regulate the economic activities of individuals and businesses (e.g., the Interstate Commerce Commission).

Reinforcement value The power or appeal of an object or experience such that it is sought after or repeated.

The perceived benefit or pleasure of a reward. Addictive substances or behaviors have high reinforcement value.

Reliability The consistency with which respondents answer questions or get the same score on a survey or test instrument.

Resilience Positive attributes and conditions that protect a child from engaging in problem behavior. Circumstances and characteristics that allow some high-risk youth to counterbalance their risk characteristics, enabling them to be successful in school, employment, and social relationships. It is thought that some counterbalancing factors may be promoted to enhance resilience.

Resource objective A statement of intention to provide the resources necessary for learning and behavioral objectives to be achieved. Examples include making available smoking cessation materials, organizing a student support group, and planning a Project Prom event.

Role playing An interactive teaching method that gives students the opportunity to take a role not normally their own or, if it is their own, in a place where the event does not normally occur.

Search Probing or exploration for something that is concealed or hidden from the searcher.

Secondary prevention Efforts that occur at a stage where ATOD use is first manifested or has just begun.

Secondhand smoke Cigarette smoke that is inhaled by nonsmokers from smokers' cigarettes. Also called *environmental tobacco smoke.*

Sedatives Drugs designed to relieve anxiety. Although sleep is not a primary purpose of the drug, it may occur as users become more relaxed.

Seizure Forcible or secretive dispossession of something against the will of the possessor or owner.

Selective prevention Strategies designed to address target groups or subgroups of the population, such as children of alcoholics or underachievers.

Self-esteem Measured by the degree to which the real self (the "as is" self) and the ideal self (based on filtering images and cues) differ.

Short acting When the effects of a drug become apparent quickly and subside quickly, perhaps in only minutes.

Sobriety The ability to live unimpaired by alcohol or drug addictions. In Alcoholics Anonymous and Narcotics Anonymous, *sobriety* has the connotation of abstaining from alcohol or other drugs.

Social development model A model that focuses on reducing risk factors and increasing protective factors.

Social marketing campaign The systematic and planned use of mass communication to influence and change individual behavior. An example is the use of billboards, print ads, radio announcements, and TV spots to promote smoking cessation.

Statute A particular law enacted and established by the will of the legislative branch of government.

Subcutaneous injection Injection into tissues just underneath the skin.

Supply reduction A wide variety of efforts designed to reduce the availability of illegal drugs.

Support group An association of people who have a specific problem or experience in common. Support groups may involve informal discussion and fellowship, but may be more structured, with the use of the 12 steps of Alcoholics Anonymous and similar programs. These groups provide mutual understanding and a forum for honest sharing of feelings.

T lymphocyte A special type of white blood cell that moves about the body to fight infection or cancer cells.

t-test A statistical tool used to determine the odds that the difference between observed mean scores is due to chance. It may be used with two groups or twice with the same group.

Tar A group of substances contained in tobacco smoke that are carcinogenic, that is, tend to cause cancer.

Target group The community or set of people that is the focus of program efforts. Examples include students in a school system, residents in a community, or employees of a corporation.

Teacher-proof curriculum Curriculum designed in a cookbook fashion so that everyone who uses the product will have the same results.

Tertiary prevention Efforts that occur when ATOD use behaviors are already fixed.

Test-retest method A single test is administered twice to detect changes that occurred in the interim. Also used as a measure of an instrument's reliability.

Tolerance Adjustments the body makes over a period of time to the effects of drugs in order to maintain a steady state (homeostasis) of functioning. This results in diminishing effects with a continuous dosage; to achieve the desired drug effects, dosage must be increased.

Transcendence An experience, not hallucinatory, that provides insights beyond ordinary perception and perspective; a sense of ultimate reality.

Transtheoretical model Behavior change includes pre-contemplation, contemplation, preparation, action, and maintenance stages.

Treatment Services that are designed to eliminate an addiction to a drug. Treatment may be provided on an individual basis or within groups and in an inpatient or outpatient format; the amount of professional involvement needed varies.

12-step program Twelve steps of personal development that are designed to help a person eliminate certain thinking and behavior. These 12 steps are the foundation of Alcoholics Anonymous and have been adopted by many other support group organizations, such as Narcotics Anonymous, Gamblers Anonymous, Emotions Anonymous, and Overeaters Anonymous.

Universal prevention Strategies designed to address large populations, such as all students in a school or district.

Upper respiratory The top half of the respiratory system that includes the nose, throat, larynx, and trachea.

Validity The degree to which a questionnaire accurately measures what it is designed to measure. The question "Have you had five or more drinks in a row in the last two weeks?" is a more valid measure of potential alcohol abuse than "Have you ever in your life had any alcohol to drink?"

Values Those things that one holds in high regard, such as truth, fame, specific persons or groups, and equality. Values exert strong influences on attitudes and behavior, but individuals may be unaware of their values or the influence they have on their actions.

Values clarification Process of encouraging people to examine their values.

Valuing process Arriving at values by the intelligent process of choosing, prizing, and acting.

Volatile chemical A chemical that readily changes from a liquid to a gas, making it easy to inhale.

Wellness Achieving and maintaining balance among the various components of health.

Withdrawal symptoms A variety of physical and emotional symptoms that occur when an accustomed dose level of a drug is cut off. Withdrawal symptoms vary between individuals and drugs, sometimes being very mild and other times being quite severe. Withdrawal is not the same as a hangover, which is recuperation from acute intoxication.

Disease model, 250
Domestic violence, 104–105
Drug abuse
    See also Treatment
    defined, 6
    factors that protect against, 10
    historical, 15–16
    youth at high risk for, 10
Drug Abuse Resistance Education
    (DARE), 197
Drug Abuse Warning Network
    (DAWN), 12, 82, 92, 269
Drug and Alcohol Services
    Information System (DASIS),
    247, 269
Drug education
    challenges facing, 4–5
    defined, 4
    target group for, 9–11
    terminology, 6–7
Drug Enforcement Administration
    (DEA), 206
Drug-Free Schools and
    Communities Act (1986), 208,
    210–211
Drugs
    See also under name of
    caffeine, 66–68
    club, 93–94
    depressants, 84–87
    hallucinogens, 90–93
    inhalants, 70–71
    misuse, 6
    naming, 59–60
    narcotics, 80–84
    over-the-counter, 60–64
    prescription, 64–66
    steroids, 68–70
    stimulants, 75–80
    use of term, 6
Drug use
    historical, 15–16
    in the 19th century, 16–19
    in the 20th century, 19–20

surveys on, 11–12
Drug use, illegal
    See also under type of drug
    1920 to 1960, 20–21
    1960 to present, 21–22
Dual diagnosis, 249
Dunn, Halbert, 147
Dysfunctional family roles, 230

E

Early Warning, Timely Response:
    A Guide to Safe Schools, 116,
    117
Ecological model, 154, 156–157
Ecstasy, 90, 91, 93
Education Development Center,
    Inc., 195
Eighteenth Amendment, 20, 287
Elder abuse, 105
Elders, Jocelyn, 123, 291
Elementary and Secondary
    Education Act, Title IV of, 211
Empirical concepts, 17
Employee assistance programs
    (EAPs), 237–239
Empowerment, community, 152,
    167
Endemic, 19
Endorphins, 15
Enlightenment model, 251
Environment, 11
Epidemic, 19
Epidemiological study, 23
Ethics, code of, 327–330
Evaluation
    analyzing data, 279–281
    disseminating findings, 281–282
    forms and questions, 309–319
    impact, 277–278
    outcome, 278
    problems with, 265–266
    process, 276–277
Evaluators, role of, 282

F

Fairness Doctrine, 293
Family
    dysfunctional roles, 230
    intervention and relations with,
        227–228
Family-Based Approaches to
    Prevention, 133
Family resource and youth service
    centers (FRYSCs), 233,
    236–237
Family Support America, 237
FBI, 103, 206
Femeldine, 253
Fetal alcohol effects (FAE), 42
Fetal alcohol syndrome (FAS), 42
Fibrocystic breast disease, 67
First Amendment, 291–295
Flay, B. R., 157
Focus groups, 268
Food and Drug Administration
    (FDA),
    tobacco and, 53
Freedom from Union Violence Act
    (1997), 106
Freud, Sigmund, 19
Fry, Edward B., 183

G

Gateway drugs, 45
Gender differences
    binge drinking and, 35
    blood alcohol levels and, 38
    drug treatment and, 247
    smoking and, 46
Generic name of drugs, 59
Geographic differences
    alcohol consumption and, 36
    smoking and, 46
GHB (gamma hydroxybutyrate),
    93–94
Goals, 180–181

School Health Curriculum Project, 195

School Health Policies and Programs Study, 177, 178, 179

Schools, health in. *See* Coordinated school health programs (CSHPs)

Science-based curricula, 194–197

Science-Based Practices in Substance Abuse Prevention: A Guide, 128, 132–133

Search and seizure issues, 217–218

Seattle School Development Project, 196

Secondary prevention, 124–125

Secondhand smoke, 24, 50–51

Self-esteem, 158–159

Self-help, 248, 253–255

Sensible Advertising and Family Education Act (1992), 293, 295

Sexual assault, 105–106

Short-acting drugs, 87

Sinclair, Upton, 19

Smoking. *See* Tobacco

Social context model, 164

Social control theory, 154

Social development model, 153–154, 155–156

Social learning theory, 154

Social marketing campaign, 280

Social services, 178

Special-needs students, 182–183

Spousal abuse, 105

Stages of change model, 152–153

Statutes. *See* Laws

Steroids, 68–70

Stimulants, 75–80

Strategy of Preventive Medicine, The (Rose), 143

Student assistance programs (SAPs), 230–233, 234–236, 277

Students
referral procedures for, 217
suspension or expulsion of, 218–219

Subculture theory, 154

Subcutaneous injection, 81

Substance Abuse and Mental Health Services Administration (SAMHSA), 145, 146, 207, 247

Substance Abuse Information Database (SAID), 205

Surveys
administration of, 273
anonymity, 272
conducting, 269–273
household, 274
mailed questionnaires, 273
reliability, 271–272
sampling, 272
telephone, 274
validity, 271

Synanon, 252

Synar, Mike, 53

Synar Amendment (1994), 53

T

Tar, 47

Target groups
defined, 11
for drug education, 9–11

Taxation as a prevention policy, 295–297

Teacher-proof curricula, 137

Teacher training, 217

Teaching methods, traditional, 185, 186

Teenage Health Teaching Modules (THTM), 195

Temperance movement, 20, 127

Terrorism, 106–107, 108

Tertiary prevention, 125

THC (tetrahydrocannabinol), 88–89

Therapeutic communities, 252–253

Thinking, critical, 159–162

T lymphocytes, 90

Tobacco
advertising of, 51–52, 191–192, 292
challenges to the prevention smoking, 51–54
death from, 48, 49
economic costs, 48
effects on the body, 47–50
First Amendment issues, 291–295
gender differences, 46
geographic differences, 46
illnesses/diseases from, 49
19th century use of, 17
products, 45–46
secondhand smoke, 24, 50–51
smoking and chewing cessation, 259–261
statistics, 46
trends in consumption, 46–47
20th century use of, 22–24

Tolerance
cross-, 18
defined, 6

Training
parent, 217
teacher, 217

Transtheoretical model, 152–153

Treatment
defined, 7, 249–250
need for, 246–249
who provides, 250

Treatment methods
aversion therapy, 256, 257, 260
behavioral self-control training, 256–257
California social model, 256
conflicting views on, 258
medications for, 253, 260
methadone maintenance, 251–252
Minnesota Model, 255–256
self-help and mutual support groups, 248, 253–255
smoking and chewing cessation, 259–261

therapeutic communities,
252–253
Trigger films, 194
t-test, 280

U

Uniform Crime Reports (UCR),
103
U.S. Coast Guard (USCG), 207
U.S. Surgeon General, 116

V

Values, affective education model,
129–131
Valuing process, 130
Vehicle accidents, alcohol consumption and, 41
Violence
abortion, 106
domestic, 104–105
drug abuse and, 100–101
factors that promote, 113–115
labor disputes, 106
nature and extent of,
101–104
need to address, 111–113
by police/government officials,
107
prevention strategies,
115–117
resources on, 116
risk for, 102
sexual assault, 105–106
school, 109–111, 115, 117
sources of information on,
103–104
terrorism, 106–107, 108
trends and incidence of,
107–111
workplace, 106
Vitamin supplements, 61–63
Volatile chemicals, 70–71

W

Web of Influence model, 141–142
Weekly Reader, 30–31
Wellness, defined, 147
Wine coolers, 30–31
Withdrawal, defined, 6
Women's Christian Temperance
Union (WCTU), 127
Workplace violence, 106
World Health Organization
(WHO), 103, 147
Writing objectives, 274–276

Y

Youth Risk Behavior Survey
(YRBS), 12, 103, 109, 269

Z

Zyban, 260